vaccine WARS

KIM TOLLEY

vaccine
WARS

The Two-Hundred-Year Fight
for School Vaccinations

JOHNS HOPKINS UNIVERSITY PRESS | Baltimore

Johns Hopkins University Press
2715 North Charles Street
Baltimore, Maryland 21218
www.press.jhu.edu

Library of Congress Cataloging-in-Publication Data is available.

ISBN 978-1-4214-4761-2 (hardcover)
ISBN 978-1-4214-4762-9 (ebook)

A catalog record for this book is available from the British Library.

Chapter 2 includes several pages of text from Kim Tolley, "School Vaccination Wars: The Rise of Anti-science in the American Anti-vaccination Societies, 1879–1929," *History of Education Quarterly* 59, no. 2 (May 2019): 161–94. Copyright © History of Education Society 2019. Reprinted by permission.

Special discounts are available for bulk purchases of this book. For more information, please contact Special Sales at specialsales@jh.edu.

Contents

Contents

Tables, Figures, and Charts

Tables

Figures

Charts

Acknowledgments

This book would not have been written without the help of many individuals. Scholars from a wide range of fields have been generous in providing useful feedback on conference papers and early book drafts. My thanks go to Kenneth Ludmerer, Simone M. Caron, Sevan Terzian, Lucy Bailey, and Campbell Scribner. I am grateful for the support and constructive criticism I received over the years from the wonderful women in my writing group at Notre Dame de Namur University: Marianne Delaporte, Therese Madden, Pearl Chaozon Bauer, Jennifer Murphy, and Jennifer Kinder.

I am also grateful to the many librarians who helped me navigate special collections at a number of institutions, including the Historical Medical Library of the College of Physicians of Philadelphia; the Wilson Library at the University of North Carolina, Chapel Hill; Stanford University's Green, Lane, and Cubberley Education Libraries; and the San Francisco Public Library. Kathy Kearns and Kelly Roll deserve special thanks for their assistance with the historical textbooks and state and city school reports housed in the Cubberley Education Library.

Many organizations made this research possible. Notre Dame de Namur University sponsored my travel to the College of Physicians of Philadelphia in 2015 and also supported my research in the Stanford University libraries. I'm also indebted to the North Caroliniana Society at the University of North Carolina, which awarded me an Archie K. Davis Research Fellowship a number of years ago— this book draws on some of that earlier research. Because of protocols established in response to the COVID-19 pandemic, during the past two years, many libraries and archives have been shut to outside researchers. I am deeply thankful for the organizations that have made historical documents freely accessible by placing them online. The "Archival and Digitized Sources" section in this book lists the sites that provided me access to rare books, government reports, oral histories, diaries, letters, historical newspapers, and other artifacts dating from the late eighteenth century to the present.

I have been fortunate in having the help of wonderful editors on this project. I thank Greg Britton for his assistance in bringing this project to Johns Hopkins University Press. The comments of the anonymous external reviewers were incredibly helpful. Additionally, Juliana McCarthy adroitly managed the editing process from start to finish, and Beth Gianfagna's exceptional copyediting greatly enhanced the book.

My deepest thanks go to my family. I became interested in the history of school vaccination in 2015, when a campaign emerged in California to eliminate nonmedical exemptions from vaccination requirements. When I expressed some hesitation about writing on such a controversial topic, my husband encouraged me to proceed, and my sister Lesley Higgins and brother-in-law Pete King added their voices to his. Although the work was delayed by other priorities during the following years, I am most grateful for Bruce Tolley's support throughout the entire process. He read every chapter and never ceased to provide valuable feedback. He is—as always—my better half and best reader.

vaccine
WARS

Introduction

On March 11, 2020, the World Health Organization announced that the coronavirus known as COVID-19 had become a pandemic.[1] Two months later, news outlets reported that a five-year-old boy in New York had become the first child in the United States to die from the disease.[2] As more cases appeared in the news, some states passed laws designed to keep children safe from infection in K–12 schools.

Eventually, protests erupted over these mandates. When California's governor announced that students would soon be required to be vaccinated against the disease, some parents stormed school board meetings, holding signs stating, "Our children our choice" and "Our kids are not lab rats!"[3] When states began passing laws requiring school staff to be vaccinated, some teachers refused, leaving schools struggling to both keep classrooms staffed and create a safe environment for students.[4] Referring to the new COVID vaccines, a speaker at a Staten Island protest warned, "If they're going to push this on the kids . . . I can guarantee you one thing: Town halls and schools will be f——king burned to the ground." Hearing this, his audience burst into cheers and waved American flags.[5]

Angry protests over school vaccination requirements are nothing new in American history. Given the world's quest for effective vaccines to protect against serious epidemics, understanding the factors that historically have led people to accept or reject vaccination is critical. This book contributes to such an understanding by analyzing American attitudes toward vaccination in the context of conflicting interests and evolving views about school vaccination policies among doctors, education authorities, local public health departments, families, and anti-vaccination groups. The resulting story reveals the historical nature of the ongoing struggle to reach a national consensus about the importance of vaccination.

I focus here on three overarching questions: Throughout history, how have Americans understood the role of schools in the transmission and prevention of contagious disease? How have schools balanced their duty to educate with their responsibility to protect children from illness? Why does opposition to vaccination persist?

Others have tackled some of these questions as well. Twentieth-century historians generally portrayed the early anti-vaccinationists as cranks and charlatans and dismissed their arguments as baseless.[6] More recent studies have provided a more balanced view, interpreting twentieth-century anti-vaccination protest as a form of grassroots struggle against medical authority. These works have expanded our understanding of how anti-vaccination dissent has illuminated questions central to liberal democracies, including the proper reach of government power, the relationship of the citizen to the state, and the place of expert knowledge and science in society.[7] Most researchers, however, have focused on issues of public health policy and rarely have discussed issues relevant to education. With few exceptions, schools themselves have had only a marginal presence in this body of scholarship.[8]

Why focus on schools? Schools have always been important in the history of public health. As sites where students are in close contact for hours each day under the same roof, they inherently foster disease. Many of the deadliest diseases of earlier centuries, including smallpox, diphtheria, whooping cough, and measles, spread through airborne viruses and bacteria. A laugh, a touch, a sneeze—any one of these actions can transmit illness. Near the end of the nineteenth century, contagious diseases accounted for nearly half of the deaths of children below the age of fifteen.[9] Native American children, who had no immunity to the diseases Europeans brought to the continent, were particularly susceptible. Virtually every treaty the federal government signed with Native American tribes included educational provisions. Federally funded boarding schools, where children lived and studied together in overcrowded rooms, served as breeding grounds for diseases like tuberculosis, influenza, and measles. By 1902, there were more than 150 such schools. Most had their own graveyards.[10]

On the other hand, schools became critical in the prevention of contagious disease through their admission requirements. The first vaccine available protected against smallpox. The disease killed about 25 percent of its victims throughout most of the nineteenth century. Some states passed laws authorizing authorities to exclude unvaccinated students from school during outbreaks; others passed laws making vaccination a standing requirement for school attendance, as discussed in chapter 1. Such laws aimed to keep children safe in school. Acceptance of the germ theory in the nineteenth century led to a better understanding of the way in which one child from an infected family could bring a disease like smallpox to school, where it could spread to others who would then carry the infection back to their own homes. During the twentieth century, states added more vaccines to the list of those required for school attendance. By 1980, every state in the country had passed legislation making vaccination a requirement for school attendance whether disease was present in the community or not. As a result of state laws requiring students to be vaccinated before attending school, some of the deadliest childhood diseases were almost completely eliminated within two decades, as shown in chapter 6.

Some writers have portrayed the development of school vaccination policy as a top-down process driven by public health bureaucrats or state legislators, but throughout history, grassroots advocacy groups and court rulings have also shaped policy.[11] For instance, in 1855, Massachusetts passed the nation's first statewide school vaccination law in response to multiple petitions from citizen groups concerned about the spread of smallpox, as discussed in chapter 1. From the early 1940s to the late 1960s, the nationwide voluntary campaign to immunize children against polio would not have been possible without the active participation of large numbers of community volunteer groups, parents, and schools, and that widespread voluntarism encouraged legislators in many states to pass laws requiring additional vaccines to protect against other diseases. The 2015 campaign of the advocacy group Vaccinate California is another example of a highly influential political campaign initiated by parents concerned about their children's safety at school, as examined in chapter 8.

Of course, not everyone supported vaccination. At various times in history, parents opposed to vaccine mandates have disrupted school board meetings, pulled their children from classrooms, and hauled school districts into court. Nor have the schools themselves always supported vaccination. Although schools have historically served a pivotal role in keeping students safe from contagious disease, school leaders have not always consistently enforced state vaccination laws. Some school officials thought vaccination was simply not their business. Others felt that the laws interfered with their mission to educate by requiring the exclusion of unvaccinated students. Many feared the loss of enrollment funding that would occur if unvaccinated students remained out of school for long periods. As shown in chapter 4, some education leaders actively sought to overturn the laws, as happened twice in California during the Progressive Era (1890–1920).

This lack of support extended to the curriculum. Throughout most of the nineteenth century, the subject was largely absent in elementary and secondary schoolbooks. Only gradually did writers begin to include information about the germ theory of disease and immunization. Textbooks improved in the early twentieth century, when some authors began overtly countering anti-vaccination claims. Later, during the campaign against polio, publishers began adding content about the nature of the disease, the process of immunization, and the progress toward finding a vaccine. Nevertheless, once polio vanished from the scene, the subject of immunization once again became a low priority in American classrooms (chapters 4, 5, and 8).

Some of the most intense local battles over compulsory vaccination laws have involved schools. Overseen by elected school boards, public schools have long served as community hubs in their localities. Through school board meetings and local elections, parents opposed to any aspect of school policy can become involved in the democratic process and join together in political action. As a result, public schools have often been sites of participatory democracy and battlegrounds for social concerns. In the early nineteenth century, parents attended board meetings to weigh in on the question of prayer in schools, the proper education of girls, or temperance.

During the Progressive Era, some of the most heated conflicts were over vaccination against smallpox. During the twentieth century, protests erupted over sex education, school integration, school busing, and civil rights issues related to equity and access. As new concerns about vaccine safety developed in the 1990s, anti-vaccination protests and anti-vaccine rhetoric reappeared.

Some writers have tried to draw a direct line from the vaccine opponents of the Progressive Era to the anti-vaccine protesters of more recent periods, concluding that their arguments remain unchanged.[12] There are certainly similarities across eras—for example, vaccine opponents have always raised concerns about safety in the wake of very rare but serious vaccine-related injuries. As this book shows, activists in all eras have included some practitioners and supporters of alternative medicine who rejected vaccination because they subscribed to philosophies of healing at odds with the practices and theories of scientific medicine. And throughout US history, opponents have advanced constitutional arguments regarding liberty and freedom of choice in efforts to prevail in the courts.

Nevertheless, the differences are great. As this book demonstrates, public policies and American attitudes toward vaccination have shifted by era (table I.1). From the early 1800s to the 1920s, documentary sources reveal a shift from broad support for the smallpox vaccine to complacency, hesitancy, and eventually opposition. The voluntary campaign against polio, which relied on persuasion, ushered in a sea change in the way Americans viewed vaccines. During the polio campaign, the United States witnessed a new era of widespread support for vaccination, but inevitably the earlier pattern of support followed by complacency, hesitancy, and opposition was repeated in the context of expanding school vaccination mandates.

Some of the factors influencing opposition to vaccination have remained constant over time. Opposition to vaccines based on safety

Table I.1. Policy trends, timeline of selected vaccines, and public attitudes toward vaccination, 1800–2021

	1800s–1860s	1870s–1920s	1930s–1950s	1960s–1980s	1990s–2021
Public policy trends	Development, distribution, and policy formation	State regulation and control	Persuasion	Eradication	Expansion
Timeline of selected vaccines	Vaccine against smallpox (1796)	Vaccines against rabies (1885); pertussis (1914); tetanus antiserum (1890); diphtheria antitoxin (1895)	Vaccines against polio: Salk (1954); Sabin (1959)	Vaccines against measles (1961); rubella (1964); mumps (1967); hepatitis B (1986); chicken pox (1988)	Vaccine against HPV (2006)
Overall public attitudes	Support and complacency	Support, hesitancy, and opposition	Support and complacency	Support and hesitancy	Support, hesitancy, and opposition

concerns has always risen in the wake of reports of adverse effects. During eras when Americans believed there was no threat from disease, or thought their children's risk of infection was very low, or believed vaccines were ineffective, they have hesitated to accept vaccination. Social cues—the means by which people learn about a disease and methods of prevention, whether through news sources, social media, or other channels—have also influenced the way people evaluate the necessity for a given vaccine and regard its effectiveness.

Yet the social and cultural factors influencing opposition have not been constant—they have evolved in tandem with new developments in science and technology. For instance, opposition based on alternative health ideology emerged in the 1870s, a time when the germ theory of disease was still controversial. Controversies and disputes about new discoveries and theories are common among scientists. Often it can take decades for disagreements to be resolved. Resolution of disputes can occur through the accumulation of empirical evidence, repeated testing, and the confirmation of hypotheses, but when dissention persists, resolution can also occur through the creation of symbolic boundaries that are reflected in new norms of conduct, standards of interpretation, and certification and membership requirements that exclude dissenting parties.[13]

As shown in chapter 2, the first national anti-vaccination society came into being in large part as a result of this kind of boundary-work during disputes over the germ theory of disease, a time when allopathic, or so-called conventional doctors, aligned with empirical science and supported the germ theory and vaccination, while alternative physicians rejected both. Over time, as the germ theory came to be widely accepted among scientists and the American public in the twentieth century, many alternative doctors also came to accept the theory and endorse immunization.

Advances in vaccine development have sparked resistance from religious groups. None of the major religions formally opposed vaccination throughout the first half of the nineteenth century. Most of the lawsuits against school vaccination based on religious objections began to appear after the founding of the Church of Christ, Scientist in 1879, which advocated healing through prayer. As states added religious and philosophical exemptions to school vaccination laws, opposition from Christian Scientists and other groups practicing faith healing declined. During the mid-twentieth-century campaign against polio, all of the major religious groups encouraged their members to accept vaccination for the common good. Renewed opposition—this time from Catholic and conservative religious groups active in the anti-abortion movement—followed the use of fetal cell lines in vaccine research. Additionally, the development of new vaccines capable of preventing diseases transmitted through injection drug use and sexual activity sparked opposition from both liberal and conservative parents who found them inappropriate for school-age children, as discussed in chapter 7. By 2021, resistance to the COVID-19 vaccine was more widespread among evangelical

Christians than almost any other demographic group, as discussed in chapter 8.

Furthermore, advances in technology have greatly expanded the means by which people access information about vaccines—from newspapers, pamphlets, and books in the nineteenth century to radio, television, the Internet, and social media in subsequent centuries. Unfounded claims about vaccines have always had a long shelf life. Nineteenth-century anti-vaccinationists claimed that smallpox was not contagious, that a water bath could cure diphtheria, and that vaccines would permanently poison the blood. In the twenty-first century, the expansion of social media has allowed more people to read and share new kinds of false claims: that vaccines cause autism, that following the vaccine schedule recommended by the Centers for Disease Control and Prevention will overwhelm the child's immune system, that vaccines contain the cells of aborted fetuses, that COVID-19 vaccines cause infertility, or that the US government places microchips into COVID-19 vaccines to track people's movements.

Finally, as discussed in chapter 8, one of the greatest differences between earlier and later eras is the emergence of partisan politics in debates over vaccination. By the time COVID-19 was declared a pandemic in 2020, one's stance on vaccination had become a symbol of partisan identity, with more Republicans than Democrats opposed to vaccine mandates.

Organization and Scope of the Book

The chapters in this book are divided into two parts to reflect these changing trends in vaccine opposition. Those in part I analyze a long societal shift, from broad support of vaccination against smallpox in the early nineteenth century to organized opposition in the Progressive Era (1890–1920). These chapters are arranged thematically to introduce issues that have persisted throughout more recent history: safety concerns and controversies over vaccines, organized opposition to vaccination, lawsuits and court rulings, and the occasional noncompliance of schools with vaccination laws. With the polio era serving as the pivot point, the chapters in part II analyze a similar trajectory, tracing a shift from broad acceptance of immunization policy in the mid-twentieth century to increasing criticism of vaccines in the 1970s and 1980s, followed by a new era of organized opposition originating in the 1990s.

The book's conclusion analyzes points of continuity and discontinuity in the history of school vaccination and outlines some of the ways America's response to the campaign against COVID-19 has been shaped by this history.

Some aspects of public health in schools are beyond the defined scope of this study. Because my focus is primarily on efforts to achieve immunity in schools through vaccination, there is little discussion of other notable diseases for which vaccines did not exist at the time, including tuberculosis, typhoid fever, influenza, and others. Additionally, preschools and institutions of higher education appear rarely in the following pages, because until the late twentieth century, few states required vaccination for admission to schools at these levels. Throughout much of this book, the term *schools* refers to public or private primary, elementary, and high schools. Moreover, although international vaccination efforts and anti-vaccination protests abroad influenced attitudes and practices in the United States, discussion of international developments is limited. There now exists an excellent and growing body of scholarship on the history, sociology, and politics of vaccination abroad and in America, and readers will find some references to these works in the book's notes.

Definitions

A few definitions are in order, starting with the term *compulsory education*. The US Constitution does not provide the right to an education, nor does it mention public health or vaccination—instead, the states have authority over both. Education laws have always varied by state. Some state constitutions give children the right to attend public schools, some simply require the state to provide educational services, and others hardly mention education. By 1918, every state had passed compulsory education laws requiring children to attend school, but before 1960, only two states—North Carolina and Wyoming—defined education as a fundamental right. Maryland joined them in 1960. In 1976, the California Supreme Court ruled in *Serrano v. Priest* that education was a fundamental right under the state's constitution. Shortly after that, courts ruled similarly in Connecticut, Washington, and West Virginia, and soon other states began recognizing a fundamental right to education in their constitutions.[14]

Compulsory school vaccination laws have also varied. This book uses the term *standing law* to refer to a law that makes vaccination for admission to school compulsory, even when disease is not present. Not until 1980 did every state in the country have such laws—they were relatively rare before the mid-twentieth century. In contrast, the terms *contingent* and *discretionary* refer to non-standing laws. *Contingent* school vaccination laws gave public health or school authorities the authority to require vaccination for admission to school only during disease outbreaks or when disease threatened a community. *Discretionary* laws allowed a designated authority to require vaccination for school attendance whenever that authority deemed it necessary. In states with few episodes of disease, contingent and discretionary state laws were rarely imposed, with the result that

Americans' experience with compulsory school vaccination could vary enormously across the country.

The passage of standing vaccination laws in the late twentieth century was part of a national effort to achieve *herd immunity* against long-standing childhood diseases. Herd immunity—also known as *community immunity*—refers to the degree of protection against contagious disease in any herd or large group of people, whether from natural exposure or immunization. US livestock veterinarians first used the term during the 1920s, as they worked to prevent epidemics among cattle and sheep. Soon, scientists studying contagious disease among humans began using the term. During the campaign against polio in the 1950s and 1960s, and throughout the effort to eradicate childhood diseases during the 1970s, the term appeared frequently in the news media as scientists estimated the share of the population that would need to be vaccinated to eliminate disease outbreaks.[15]

The vaccination rate required to provide herd immunity varies by type of disease. For example, the herd immunity threshold is between 93 and 95 percent for a highly contagious disease like measles, between 92 and 94 percent for whooping cough (pertussis), and between 80 and 86 percent for polio.[16] Community immunity helps everyone, from newborns to the elderly and all those in between. Newborns cannot receive vaccines until after a certain period of time—two months for polio, whooping cough, and diphtheria, and a full year for measles. In addition to newborns, people with compromised immune systems benefit as well, including those who have had chemotherapy or a transplant, or those who have an inherited condition that makes vaccination impossible. Finally, community immunity protects all those who have been vaccinated but still may become ill. Vaccines have greatly reduced the threat of contagious disease around the world, but they never provide 100 percent protection—there is always a risk of breakthrough infections during any spate of disease. When everyone is vaccinated, herd immunity acts like a shield, making everyone's chance of infection far less likely. Of course, for this level of protection to exist, a large majority of the population must agree to support vaccination.

Misinformation has often been a significant force in anti-vaccination campaigns. *Misinformation* is defined here as any information claimed to be factual that is unsupported by available evidence. Historical context is important in evaluating whether any claim about vaccination constitutes misinformation. During periods of uncertainty and dispute over medical theories, some claims may be eventually supported by evidence, while others may be disproven through the scientific processes of experimentation, peer review, replication, and verification. The unsupported claim that vaccines cause autism is a case in point. When a claim like this circulates in public for long periods of time after it has been overturned, it becomes misinformation. Regardless of whether misinformation is circulated with intent to deceive, it contributes to public ignorance and harms the body politic.[17]

Vaccine Wars tells the history of efforts to achieve and maintain immunity in schools through vaccination. The story begins in 1800, with the introduction of the smallpox vaccine and an era of widespread public support for vaccination. It ends with the COVID-19 pandemic in 2021, a year that saw a dramatic decline in the routine childhood vaccinations required for school and a growing partisan divide over public health mandates to protect against the coronavirus. Along the way, the book underscores recurring themes that have roiled political debates over school vaccination time and again, including the proper reach of state power; the intersection of science, politics, and public policy; the nature of individual liberty in a democracy; and the responsibility each of us bears to protect—not only our own children—but also the children of others.

PART I

The Long Fight against Smallpox
From Support to Complacency and Opposition

1

The Rise of School Vaccination Laws

In the fall of 1887, an outbreak of smallpox began to spread across California, killing 12 percent of those infected. The first deaths were in San Francisco, where the number of cases quickly spiked.[1] Some blamed the increase on a lack of communication between San Francisco's health and police departments. When men in the city jail showed symptoms of smallpox, the jailer released them with directions to walk to the city hall and obtain a permit to enter the hospital. As a result, a procession of smallpox victims threaded through the crowded downtown streets, infecting scores of people.[2] By the end of January 1888, the city's board of health declared the outbreak had become an epidemic and appointed additional vaccinators, but it was too late to prevent the spread of disease.[3]

Some towns moved quickly to minimize contagion; others did not. When thirteen cases appeared in Sierra City, northwest of Lake Tahoe, the town's board of supervisors swiftly appointed a health committee, erected a "pest house" to sequester the sick, and adopted strict quarantine measures, proclaiming, "None can leave town under penalty of forty days in the County Jail or a fine."[4] Not every town followed Sierra City's model. After visiting the Sierra foothills to examine the spread of disease, Dr. Gerrard G. Tyrrell, secretary of the state board of health, found quarantine measures were few and far between. In the town center of Murphys, he "saw a man cutting meat with the smallpox pustules yet fresh on his face."[5] Even where local health officials imposed strict quarantine, smallpox was so contagious that the usual measures were not always effective. In the town of Redding, a child reportedly became infected after petting a dog belonging to a man quarantined a quarter of a mile away.[6]

Schools played a central role in the transmission of disease. More than a decade earlier, research conducted in England had demonstrated this connection. Infected children could bring contagious diseases to crowded schoolrooms and infect others, who would then carry illness to their own homes. In this way, smallpox radiated from each school to the surrounding districts and along travel routes to neighboring towns.[7]

The rapid spread of the disease prompted Tyrrell to urge schools everywhere to exclude all unvaccinated students: "No child should be permitted to enter any school until it is successfully vaccinated."[8] Like many other states at the time, California did not require students to be vaccinated to attend school. Tyrrell hoped his recommendation would stop the outbreak, but he was disappointed. In some areas, families hid sick children and adults to avoid quarantine and vaccination, and the epidemic spread.[9]

The widespread noncompliance with public health recommendations and the personal and financial costs of the 1887–88 epidemic led California to pass a compulsory school vaccination law the following year. By mandating vaccination of all the students in the public schools, state legislators hoped to keep everyone safe and ensure the protection of the "rising generation."[10] Although they never used phrases like *herd immunity* or *community protection* in their debates—terms that would become common in the second half of the twentieth century—the idea of providing immunity for an entire generation was very similar. Essentially, they aimed to protect everyone in the state.

Only eighteen states had passed some form of school vaccination law at the time, even though school and health officials knew that schoolrooms were prime sites for the transmission of contagious diseases. Of these, few states passed standing laws similar to those of the late twentieth century that required students to be vaccinated to attend school at all times—even when there was no threat of disease in their communities.[11]

Why the long delay, and what motivated state legislatures to act when they did? Although there was public support and acceptance of vaccination during the first decades of the nineteenth century, several trends contributed to the delay, including concerns about the safety of the vaccine and a growing complacency regarding vaccination in the absence of disease outbreaks. As happened in California, it took one or more significant triggering events to bring a state to the tipping point necessary to pass a compulsory school vaccination law, including recurring epidemics, high fatalities, substantial financial losses, and unemployment.

The Development and Deployment of the Smallpox Vaccine

For most of the nineteenth century, only one vaccine was available—the smallpox vaccine. Americans welcomed its arrival. There was no cure for smallpox, one of the deadliest diseases in human history.

According to one account, it killed a third of its victims during the colonial period. In seventeenth-century Massachusetts, more people died from the disease than from any other natural calamity.[12]

Smallpox was caused by the variola virus, which lived only in humans. Unlike cholera, the disease did not spread through sewage-tainted water, and unlike typhoid fever, it did not spread through contaminated food. Like diphtheria, scarlet fever, influenza, and COVID-19, smallpox spread exclusively through human contact. The miniscule particles, or virions, of the virus were invisible to the naked eye and could not be seen before the invention of the electron microscope—only in 1947 did Canadian and American scientists view them for the first time. Smallpox virions launched into the air when the infected victim sneezed, coughed, laughed, sighed, spoke, or simply breathed. When the virions gained access to another person's respiratory system, they began to replicate.[13]

An attack of smallpox either killed its victim or left the survivor with lifelong immunity. When the virus entered an isolated or self-contained community, it gradually infected almost everyone. Because it could not survive long outside human bodies, once the supply of susceptible humans disappeared, the virus was unable to replicate and died out. It took a steady stream of new susceptible arrivals for smallpox to become endemic in a community, whether through the birth of children or through migration.[14]

European immigrants brought smallpox to North America. As pioneers traveled across the continent into lands inhabited by indigenous peoples, they carried smallpox, diphtheria, whooping cough, measles, mumps, scarlet fever, chicken pox, and influenza with them. Because Native Americans had no immunity to these contagious diseases, outbreaks of smallpox often killed up to 50 percent or more of tribal members.[15] The disease followed transportation routes, periodically scouring the tribes of the Upper Missouri River. In 1837 a virulent form of smallpox appeared at Fort Clark, where close contact among tribal members and the fur trade post quickly spread the disease. The Mandan tribe suffered enormous losses. According to contemporary reports, there had been up to 2,000 Mandans living in the area when the epidemic broke out in the spring. By the fall, only 138 were left alive.[16]

Pioneer settlements along overland routes routinely experienced outbreaks. In 1857, Julia Louisa Lovejoy described a crush of new arrivals in Lawrence, Kansas: "Lawrence has been over-run by the thousands, that have swarmed the streets for weeks past—every house being literally full, and some densely packed. And, as usual, with such a rush, sickness has come too, and we are told, small-pox, measles, and scarlet fever, are now in Lawrence."[17] Smallpox became endemic the entire length of the Oregon Trail. In 1852, when Ohio resident John Hawkins Clark pulled up stakes to travel west on the Trail in hope of finding gold in California, he periodically passed graves containing smallpox victims. In one journal entry he wrote, "Met a young man with two small children returning to the states; said he had buried his wife and one child just beyond. We felt for the fellow as he every now and then turned his look toward the wilderness where lay his beloved ones."[18]

In a typical course of smallpox, the victim had a one-in-four chance of dying. However, there was a great deal of variation because of differences in viral strains and the differing susceptibilities of individuals and groups. In the most common cases, the smallpox blisters were "discrete"—normal skin was still visible between the pustules (figure 1.1). But in the severe, "confluent" cases, so many pustules erupted on the face and body that they fused together and lifted the skin from the underlying tissues. The fatality rate for cases of discrete smallpox could be as low as 10 percent, whereas for confluent cases, it could be 60 percent or more. In the worst cases, which

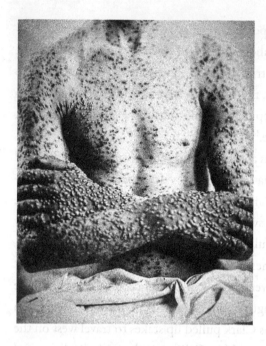

Figure 1.1. Variola virus, or smallpox. *Source*: George Henry Fox, *Photographic Illustrations of Skin Diseases*, 2nd ed. (New York: E. B. Treat, 1885), between pp. 20 and 21.

were almost always fatal, the victim's pustules could turn black or purple, making the body appear charred, and in a rare form, known as "hemorrhagic" or "black smallpox," the patient suffered explosive bleeding throughout the body.[19]

Before inoculation, the only weapon in the arsenal against smallpox was quarantine. Quarantine originated during the late Middle Ages as a strategy to isolate victims of the bubonic plague, the "Black Death."[20] It was a coercive strategy that prioritized protection of the community over the rights of individuals.

Quarantine was never popular—during the nineteenth century, some people argued that quarantine violated Americans' constitutional right to liberty. But the practice was universal during the colonial and early national eras. The American colonies gave local town leaders the authority to bar ships from ports, close roads, detain people with contagious diseases in their homes or hospitals, and punish those who refused to obey the quarantine laws. After the Revolution, every state enacted similar quarantine laws. For example, Rhode Island gave local town councils broad authority and police powers to take any compulsory measures necessary to prevent the spread of smallpox. Such measures included quarantining infected homes and boarding houses, relocating infected persons to isolated structures called pest houses, and sequestering the crew of any vessel infected with disease and seizing and disinfecting its "goods, wares and merchandizes," at a cost to be borne by the owners.[21]

In 1796, the US 4th Congress passed the first federal quarantine law, allowing the federal government to support state quarantines. In 1824, after a number of legal challenges, a case reached the US Supreme Court. In its ruling, the Court cited the Tenth Amendment to the Constitution in validating the authority of the states to impose isolation and quarantine to protect their citizens' health.[22] This ruling became a precursor to later Supreme Court rulings upholding the constitutional right of the states to pass and enforce school vaccination laws.

Quarantine remained an important weapon against smallpox throughout the nineteenth century. Since the disease traveled along transportation routes, some towns self-quarantined to stop its spread, closing all roads and tearing down their bridges. In the fall of 1868, a virulent outbreak of smallpox appeared in northern California. John W. Whitney, the local postmaster in San Juan Bautista, wrote to a Santa Cruz newspaper to report 23 deaths out of 122 cases in the town, a fatality rate of 19 percent.[23] When the town of Aptos received news that smallpox was "spreading badly" in nearby Santa Cruz, Aptos residents burned down the bridge between the two towns.[24] Similarly, during an outbreak near the lower Chattahoochee River in Alabama, residents in several counties tore up their bridges "to prevent the passage of persons and the spread of the disease." The newspaper that reported the story described the people in Alabama as "excited on account of the smallpox," but "excited" was probably not the best term to describe how they felt. It took time and money to build a bridge—no community would tear down its bridges unless it were terrified.[25]

Imposing quarantine reduced the spread of disease, but it often came with a cost: Quarantined persons lost much-needed income from work, and closed ports and roads resulted in lost trade and business revenue. For instance, during the outbreak in San Juan Bautista, townspeople who had been living on subsistence wages suffered greatly when work disappeared and had to rely on charitable assistance from residents in nearby Salinas and Santa Cruz.[26] But the only other option—to allow deadly diseases like smallpox to spread through communities unchecked—was far worse.

In the eighteenth century, American colonists had learned of another possible weapon against the disease. The first inoculation procedure against smallpox arrived in the colonies in 1721. Since antiquity, *variolation* had reportedly been practiced in China, India, and the Middle East, sometimes with successful results. Variolation involved taking pus from the pustules or scabs of a person infected with smallpox and inserting it in an incision the arm of a healthy person.

Variolation commonly induced a mild, survivable form of the disease and created immunity. By the eighteenth century, variolation had spread to Europe and England. During a smallpox outbreak in Boston in 1721, the Congregational minister and author Cotton Mather convinced a local physician, Zabdiel Boylston, to begin a campaign to inoculate residents using the procedure. Some residents protested, claiming Mather was acting against the will of God. After Boylston inoculated 287 people, some of them became ill, and six died. As a result, many Bostonians came to oppose variolation, including members of Mather's own church congregation and every physician in town except for Boylston.[27]

As was demonstrated in Boston, variolation carried serious risks. As many as one person in fifty died as a result, which could transfer blood-borne diseases to the recipient, including a more virulent form of smallpox itself.[28] Although the procedure saved lives, fear of its adverse effects led to protest. Opposition reached such a fever pitch that one night someone lobbed a bomb through a window into Mather's house, with this message attached: "Cotton Mather, you dog; damn you. I'll inoculate you with this, with a pox to you." Fortunately, the bomb's fuse burned out, so there was no explosion.[29]

In contrast to variolation, vaccination posed fewer risks. The procedure was similar to variolation, but it involved the use of cowpox, a disease that produced a mild illness in humans but still induced immunity against smallpox. In 1796, the English physician Edward Jenner (1749–1823) noticed that few dairy workers ever came down with smallpox. The workers themselves believed that exposure to cows infected with cowpox protected them from smallpox. To test this idea, Jenner lanced some pustules on the hand of a milkmaid to extract the cowpox material contained in the pus and inserted it beneath the surface of the skin on the arms of a young servant and several children. He then inoculated the servant and children with smallpox. In every case, the inoculated individuals appeared to have developed immunity against smallpox.[30]

After reading Jenner's 1798 publication on the use of cowpox in vaccination, Harvard medical professor Benjamin Waterhouse introduced vaccination to the United States in 1800.[31] Four of his children and two household servants were his first subjects, and after a successful result, he published a monograph: *A Prospect of Exterminating the Small-pox*. Excited about this news, Thomas Jefferson obtained some vaccine from Waterhouse to conduct an experiment of his own. He inoculated his entire family and as many of his neighbors who desired the vaccine—around two hundred people altogether. As for side effects, Jefferson reported, "Generally it gives no more of disease than a blister as large as a coffee-bean produced by burning would occasion."[32]

Success and Support

The first public trial occurred in 1802. Under the auspices of Boston's board of health, Waterhouse and six other physicians vaccinated nineteen boys and subsequently exposed them to the smallpox virus. The trial was a success, leading the board to announce that the "cowpox is a complete preventive against all the effects of the small-pox upon the human system."[33] After this, the practice of vaccination began to replace variolation in the United States.

In the context of deadly outbreaks of disease, most people sought the vaccine to protect themselves and their families. Although some may have hesitated to bare their arms for the vaccine, there was no overt or organized opposition to vaccination during this period. Although some Boston residents had opposed Cotton Mather's variolation campaign on religious grounds, religious groups did not oppose vaccination in the early nineteenth century.[34] Some of the earliest accounts of students receiving vaccination against smallpox are from North Carolina. Students at the University of North Carolina in Chapel Hill were vaccinated during an outbreak in 1802.[35] In 1812, when smallpox threatened the students at the Female Boarding School in Salem, the school published a notice in the newspapers assuring parents that students had been successfully vaccinated with the cowpox, or "kine-pox" vaccine.[36]

As reports of similar successes began to spread, demand for the cowpox vaccine increased, but supply was very limited. In some areas, one or more doctors with the skill and authority to transport and preserve vaccine matter from England established "vaccine institutes," but it was difficult to guarantee enough to meet the demand, and the vaccine did not always perform well after the long sea voyage to America.[37] To solve the problem, Baltimore physician James Smith obtained a sample of cowpox virus in 1802 from an American merchant and started producing his own vaccine. In 1809, Maryland appointed him to direct a vaccine institute in Baltimore, with the result that smallpox was eliminated in the state for a period.[38]

A decade later, the federal government became involved. Smith lobbied Congress and wrote to President James Madison suggesting a plan to distribute vaccines across the country with the goal of eliminating smallpox altogether. "[T]he very Existence of this Pestilence, within the limits of our Country, may be entirely destroyed," he wrote, "if the Confidence of the people can be preserved, and sufficient attention is paid, to keep up a *free*, and *general distribution* of the vaccine Matter among them."[39] After several years of deliberation, Congress agreed that the goal of eradicating smallpox was worthy of federal support. It passed "An Act to Encourage Vaccination" in 1813, which subsidized the distribution of vaccine matter through the US Post Office and authorized a federal vaccine agent to preserve and furnish vaccines to any US citizen who applied.[40] Madison commissioned Smith as the federal agent in charge of the program. Smith appointed agents in several states and directed them to vaccinate for free anyone seeking immunity against smallpox, regardless of age or social status. His agents began sending the cowpox vaccine via the US Postal Service to physicians and laypersons alike, along with detailed instructions for the procedure.[41] The program was met with enthusiasm, until disaster unfolded in North Carolina.

Controversy

The federal vaccination program lasted only nine years. In 1821, James Smith's vaccine institute accidentally sent North Carolina agent John F. Ward a sample of live smallpox virus. As a result, when Dr. Ward vaccinated fifteen people in the town of Tarborough, he infected them with smallpox.[42] On December 29, he wrote to inform Smith that twelve of the fifteen people had developed "the most alarming symptoms."[43] Soon a virulent outbreak of smallpox began to spread, sparking fear and outrage.[44]

The resulting epidemic in Edgecombe County killed ten people and impelled Congress to launch an investigation. Some congressmen argued that the federal government should never have given Smith monopoly over the distribution of vaccine. Others, fearful of any increased federal role in American society, argued against the 1813 Vaccination Act on the basis of laissez-faire politics. Ultimately, the tragedy in North Carolina not only led President James Monroe to revoke Smith's commission but also resulted in the repeal of the federal 1813 Vaccination Act.[45]

After the federal government withdrew its support of vaccination, states and local communities scrambled to obtain vaccine matter and the funding to pay for vaccines.

In the absence of federal subsidy, some communities taxed residents to support such programs. The practice was not without controversy. In Vermont, a conflict over local taxation for vaccination erupted in 1820. During an outbreak of smallpox in the town of North Hero, the selectmen hired a doctor to vaccinate the public, and when the bill came due, the town's inhabitants voted for a tax to raise money to pay for the expense. Not everyone agreed. When David Strong, the town's bill collector, asked resident Dan Hazen for his payment, Hazen refused. In response, Strong seized Hazen's cow and "sold her for the collection of such tax." Furious, Hazen sued. In 1830, the case of *Hazen v. Strong* ultimately reached the Vermont Supreme Court, where the judges ruled in favor of Strong, concluding that towns had the authority to vote to raise money through taxation, because under state law town selectmen had the broad authority *"to take the most effectual measures to prevent the spreading of the disease."* During later decades, a number of court rulings cited this case as evidence of support for the police powers of the community over the rights of the individual when smallpox threatened.[46]

Despite the existence of vaccine institutes in some cities, the vaccine remained in short supply in many areas. Early attempts to develop a vaccine in the United States failed, leaving vaccinators dependent on English suppliers.

Because vaccine matter was so scarce, once they had successfully vaccinated some patients with cowpox, American doctors often performed subsequent vaccinations using an arm-to-arm technique, which entailed taking pus from the cowpox pustule of one patient and inserting it in an incision in the arm of another. Physicians referred to this as "humanized virus" and used this technique extensively until around 1870, when private companies established the first American "vaccine farms" to manufacture cowpox vaccine directly from calves. Unfortunately, arm-to-arm vaccination was not entirely safe—if the donor had an asymptomatic disease like syphilis, the practice could transfer the disease to the recipient.[47]

Even when performed properly, the vaccination procedure came with risks. Before the federal government passed the Biologics Control Act in 1902, there was little oversight or control over vaccine production. At "vaccine farms" more focused on profit-making than quality control, vaccine matter sometimes became tainted with tetanus bacteria, which live in dust, soil, and manure. When doctors used tainted vaccine, vaccination could transmit tetanus to their patients.[48]

Additionally, even when carefully produced, the vaccine produced adverse effects in some people, ranging from mild to severe. More than a third of those vaccinated missed some days of work or school because of mild symptoms related to the vaccine. In the past, about one vaccinated person out of every thousand experienced serious adverse reactions, including corneal scarring and blindness, disfiguring skin conditions, brain damage or partial paralysis from encephalomyelitis, and for every one hundred thousand people vaccinated, up to five experienced life-threatening reactions. Those with weakened immune systems or certain skin conditions were at greater risk for adverse effects.[49]

Hesitancy and Complacency

Despite the risks, the practice of offering vaccination during outbreaks of smallpox became common in the states and territories during epidemics. As a result, despite hesitancy among some people to receive the vaccine, smallpox fatalities declined during the first three or four decades of the nineteenth century. Some areas that enforced compulsory vaccination during outbreaks saw dramatic declines. For instance, in 1809, Massachusetts law required towns to designate committees to oversee the vaccination of their residents. Compulsory vaccination was so successful in Boston that between 1811 and 1837, only thirty-seven people died from the disease, a rate of 2.7 deaths per 100,000 people. This was an enormous drop from the previous century, when rates ranged from 400 to 7,700 deaths per 100,000 people.[50]

Vaccination policies in Europe reduced the prevalence of smallpox even more dramatically. American newspapers in the mid-1820s pointed out that Denmark's government had completely eliminated smallpox, and in Prussia and Sweden, the disease had become almost nonexistent. In 1826, while a smallpox epidemic was spreading across Maine and other areas of New England, an editorial in a Baltimore newspaper pointed out that Denmark's success was due to stringent laws stipulating that no person could be admitted to a school, apprenticed to a trade, confirmed in a church, or married, without having been vaccinated or previously had smallpox. The author asked, "Does not the wide spread existence of this dangerous and loathsome disease admonish us that some legislative measures ought to be adopted in our country?"[51]

However, rather follow in European footsteps and pass more stringent laws, state and territorial governments grew more complacent after decades of declining fatalities.

As new generations of Americans grew up without ever having experienced a smallpox epidemic or the need for quarantine, they hesitated to seek vaccination. The *Polynesian*, a Hawaiian newspaper, cautioned readers about the phenomenon in the islands. For several years after a virulent smallpox epidemic in 1853, Hawaiians were very aware of the importance of vaccination, but after nearly a decade, "the slumber of a false security is creeping over the people . . . and we may have another eruption sweeping off a number of lives."[52] Massachusetts revoked its compulsory vaccination law in 1837 because many people believed it was no longer necessary. Unfortunately, over the next eighteen years, more than a thousand people died from smallpox outbreaks in the state.[53]

Given the adverse effects that came with the smallpox vaccine in that era, it took an epidemic for people to take vaccination seriously. As one health officer in Kansas put it, "The rule in regard to vaccination is hardly observed at all. . . . The people generally seem to think the regulations good, in a general way, but will not take the trouble to observe them until small-pox or cholera has secured a foothold in the county."[54]

Given the decline in vaccination and the growing numbers of potential victims without any sort of immunity, it was inevitable that the disease would begin to spread again near midcentury. In some states, new outbreaks spurred the passage of laws requiring that students be vaccinated to attend school.

The Rise of Laws Requiring School Vaccination

It fell to individual cities and towns to pass the earliest school vaccination laws. In 1827, Boston began requiring all students in town to show proof of vaccination before enrolling in the schools, becoming the first city in the Unites States to do so.[55] That year, Philadelphia's Infant School Society amended its constitution to require vaccination in its schools. By 1850, some other towns had passed similar mandates.[56]

Most state legislatures did not begin enacting school vaccination laws until the second half of the nineteenth century. In some areas, school vaccination laws followed closely on the heels of new laws requiring children to attend school. School education laws varied by state, but they all required children between certain ages to enroll in school for a minimum period of time or minimal level of formal educational attainment. From 1850 and 1914, tens of millions of culturally diverse migrants arrived in America. Concerned that they be educated and socialized in democratic values and alarmed about the relatively low number of students enrolled in school, states began passing laws compelling school attendance.[57] By 1918, every state had passed compulsory education laws requiring children to attend school at a certain age and for some period of time.[58]

Some historians have speculated that in light of concerns over the spread of disease in school, the enactment of compulsory school attendance laws naturally led states to pass school vaccination laws.[59] By the 1870s, American doctors were aware of research linking compulsory attendance laws to outbreaks of illness. The English physician William Squire published a study reporting that in London in 1870, "the first year of compulsory school-attendance under the School Board Act," there were more than six thousand deaths from scarlet fever outbreaks originating in schools.[60]

Yet despite increased awareness of the way smallpox could spread through the schools, only four states passed school vaccination laws within a few years of mandating school attendance: Connecticut, Massachusetts, Pennsylvania (the same year), and Wisconsin. Few other states followed this pattern. Many enacted school vaccination laws at least a decade before passing compulsory attendance laws (table 1.1).

Other scholars have mentioned the establishment of state health boards as a factor influencing school vaccination laws.[61] During the period from 1870 to 1890, as growing towns came to understand the importance of sanitary systems to reduce garbage, ensure clean water, and prevent the spread of contagious disease, the number of municipal health departments expanded across the country. In 1869, Massachusetts established the first state board of health, and the following year, California established the second. By 1910, virtually every state in the country had a state board of health with some degree of authority over local municipal health boards. In a few states, school vaccination

Table 1.1. Dates of school vaccination laws, compulsory school attendance laws, and creation of state boards of health, 1850–1919

State/territory (N = 25)	School vaccination laws	Compulsory school attendance laws	State boards of health
Massachusetts	1855	1852	1869
Maine	1856	1874	1885
New York	1860	1874	1880
New Hampshire	1861	1871	1881
Maryland	1864	1902	1874
Virginia	1870	1908	1872
Ohio	1872	1877	1886
Connecticut	1878	1872	1878
North Carolina	1879	1907	1877
Georgia	1881	1916	1875
Indiana	1881	1897	1881
Rhode Island	1881	1883	1878
Arkansas	1882	1909	1881
Illinois	1882	1883	1877
Wisconsin	1882	1879	1876
South Carolina	1883	1915	1879
New Jersey	1887	1875	1877
California	1889	1874	1870
Iowa	1889	1902	1880
Hawaii[a]	1892	1896	1850
Pennsylvania	1895	1895	1885
New Mexico	1901	1891	1919
Oregon	1901	1889	1903
West Virginia	1905	1897	1881
Montana	1907	1883	1901

Sources: Data compiled from August W. Steinhilber and Carl J. Sokolowski, *State Law on Compulsory Attendance* [Washington DC: GPO, 1966], 3; J. W. Kerr, *Vaccination: An Analysis of the Laws and Regulations Relating Thereto in Force in the United States,* Public Health Bulletin No. 52 [Washington, DC: GPO, 1912], 6; William Fowler, *Smallpox Vaccination Laws, Regulations, and Court Decisions* [Washington, DC: US Public Health Service, GPO, 1927], 3–5; US Department of Health, Education, and Welfare, *Historical Roster of State and Territorial Health Officers, 1850–1960* [Washington, DC: GPO, 1960].

[a] Although Hawaii was a territory during this period, it is included in the table because of its early experience with public health policy.

laws appeared soon after the establishment of state health boards, raising the possibility that the boards' reports and recommendations influenced the passage of state school vaccination laws.[62]

However, here too, states diverged. Some states enacted school vaccination laws years before they established a state board of health. For example, Maine and New Mexico passed school vaccination laws about two decades before they had state boards of health. Massachusetts passed the nation's first statewide school vaccination law in response to multiple petitions from citizen groups. New York enacted a law "authorizing school trustees to exclude from the schools all children who have not been vaccinated" in response to a petition from the New York Medical Society, whose members were concerned about a record number of smallpox outbreaks amid a growing neglect of vaccination throughout the state.[63] And advocacy for vaccination sometimes came from school boards, as occurred in Iowa in 1862.[64]

Whether a state passed a school vaccination law depended on its experience with smallpox outbreaks and the support of its voters. In the absence of any serious epidemics, few state legislators had the will to try to drum up backing for a law requiring vaccination for school attendance.[65]

Smallpox epidemics triggered the passage of school vaccination laws in many states.[66] This was the case in Massachusetts, which became the first state to pass a law requiring school vaccination in 1855. After decades with few outbreaks, smallpox fatalities rose in 1854, and the following year, a virulent outbreak produced a spike in deaths. More than half occurred in Boston, "largely among young children."[67] As popular momentum grew for legislation to protect the public from smallpox, citizen groups filed five separate petitions for vaccination bills. In response, the state passed a comprehensive law requiring the general vaccination of children and stipulating that officers of all state-supported institutions, including public schools, must "be vaccinated immediately upon their entrance thereto, unless they produce sufficient evidence of previous successful vaccination within five years."[68]

Smallpox outbreaks influenced legislation in other states as well. In Illinois, a financially devastating epidemic lasting from 1880 to 1882 with a fatality rate of "over 50 percent" among the unvaccinated led the state board of health to order all children to present evidence of "proper and successful" vaccination before enrolling in the public schools.[69] An outbreak in Iowa made national news when reporters learned the source was a medical student who had nicked himself after using a scalpel on a smallpox-infected cadaver. The resulting epidemic killed 12.6 percent of those who fell ill.[70] Worried about the spread of smallpox in schoolrooms, Davenport's school board petitioned the Iowa legislature for a law authorizing school boards to require pupils to be vaccinated. Davenport's petition failed, but after seven more years of outbreaks, a school vaccination law went into effect when Iowa's attorney general ruled that the state board of health had the legal authority to require the vaccination of students. Smallpox epidemics provided a strong rationale for legislation across the country.[71]

This is not to say that all epidemics led to school vaccination laws. For example, in 1883, a virulent form of smallpox erupted in Kentucky. Alarmed, the Kentucky state board of health proclaimed, "It is hoped that the next Legislature will make vaccination compulsory. . . . Health and school boards, everywhere, should co-operate in requiring vaccination as a condition of admission to all schools, public and private." Despite the recommendation, Kentucky's legislature did not pass such a law before the twentieth century.[72]

Each state responded differently to epidemics, depending on the virulence and duration of outbreaks, the financial cost of quarantine measures, and its residents' attitudes toward public health measures.

California's case is illustrative. The state had experienced virulent outbreaks in 1868 and 1873, but neither had led to calls for a school vaccination law. During these outbreaks, most residents complied with quarantine orders, because they understood the dangers posed by the disease. By 1887, however, as a national anti-vaccination movement was under way, popular attitudes toward vaccination and quarantine had changed. That year, smallpox appeared first in Los Angeles and then in San Francisco, with a fatality rate of around 12 percent. The personal and financial costs of that outbreak were enormous. City supervisors and health officials placed quarantine officers along land and water routes into California, ordering them to inspect every train and vessel, detain every person suspected of infection, and "vaccinate all passengers exposed." Business losses mounted as the quarantine orders disrupted the flow of goods and passengers coming from infected areas. Medical inspectors canvassing neighborhoods reported that many families were hiding sick children and adults to avoid quarantine. Dr. H. S. Orme, president of the state board of health, traced one case to a school "where children were in attendance from families in which were concealed cases of smallpox at the time."[73]

Orme reported that many citizens underestimated "the necessity for stringent measures, opposed and thwarted those who tried to prevent the spread of the disease. . . . Cases were actually kept carefully concealed by their friends, because they did not believe in vaccination, and did not wish to submit to the inconveniences of isolation, or the smallpox hospital. Thus, the contagion was allowed to spread to others."[74] The public's growing resistance to public health regulations raised the specter of unending, recurring smallpox epidemics. As the legislative report that year noted, "Smallpox in a community means the paralyzing of all trade and commerce. It means pecuniary loss, sickness, suffering, destitution, deformity, or death."[75]

The high degree of noncompliance with public health orders and the personal and the financial costs of the 1887–88 epidemic led

California legislators to pass a compulsory school vaccination law the following year. They believed that without intervention, epidemics would reoccur repeatedly: "In times of immunity from epidemics the practice of vaccination is neglected, hence in a few years there is accumulated in the State a vast array of unvaccinated persons who fall ready victims to the malady when it reappears from any cause." By passing the bill, the legislature hoped "to ensure the vaccination of the rising generation."[76]

In contrast to California, few other states faced the kind of statewide crisis that led to the passage of a standing law requiring vaccination for admission to school, even when there was no evidence of disease. By 1927, in response to advocacy from anti-vaccination groups, only twenty-eight of the forty-eight states had a compulsory vaccination law on the books (chart 1.1). Of these, only eleven had

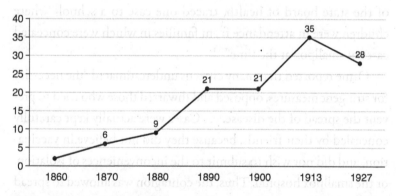

Chart 1.1. Number of states with compulsory school vaccination laws, 1860–1927. *Sources*: Data compiled from August W. Steinhilber and Carl J. Sokolowski, *State Law on Compulsory Attendance* (Washington, DC: GPO, 1966), 3; J. W. Kerr and A. A. Moll, *Communicable Diseases: An Analysis of the Laws and Regulations for the Control Thereof in Force in the United States*, Public Health Bulletin 62, July 1913 (Washington, DC: GPO, 1914), 132; William Fowler, *Smallpox Vaccination Laws, Regulations, and Court Decisions* (Washington, DC: GPO, 1927), 3, 4; William Fowler, "Principal Provisions of Smallpox Vaccination Laws and Regulations in the United States," *PHR* 56, no. 5 (Jan. 31, 1941): 169–70; HEW, *Historical Roster of State and Territorial Health Officers, 1850–1960* (Washington, DC: GPO, 1960).

laws similar to those of the twenty-first century, requiring students to show proof of vaccination for school attendance regardless of the presence or absence of smallpox.[77]

Most states had laws that were discretionary or contingent in nature. Six passed discretionary laws that empowered local school, town, or health authorities to require vaccination for school admission whenever they felt conditions merited the requirement.[78] Ten states passed contingent laws allowing schools to suspend unvaccinated students, but only when smallpox either existed in the community or was close enough to be a threat. West Virginia had both contingent and discretionary laws on the books.[79]

Discretionary and contingent statutes enabled communities to defeat epidemics, but they did little to prevent their recurrence. As the Medical Society of New York pointed out, "Whenever the pestilence prevails in any locality, the people of that locality, for the time being, seem to feel the importance of the preventive remedy, and vaccination is eagerly sought and obtained, to the complete arresting of the disease; and when this is accomplished, no further attention is paid to it until the public are again alarmed by the outbreak of the pestilence." As one group of law professors concluded, "That was like locking the door only when it looked as though the horse might be stolen."[80]

Conclusion

Americans welcomed the smallpox vaccine when it first became available. However, state and federal governments struggled to implement an effective vaccine distribution system, provide a constant supply of vaccine matter, and ensure safe inoculation procedures. As a result of poor policies, controversies, lax oversight, and the inevitable adverse effects resulting from unsafe vaccination methods, the public's attitude toward the vaccine shifted from broad support to hesitancy and complacency.

When Congress repealed the Vaccination Act in 1822, the states retained control over public health. Every state had the right to pass laws to protect its residents from contagious disease, as was expressed in early state quarantine and vaccination laws. Without a doubt, such laws infringed on individual liberty. Nevertheless, as explained in the Supreme Court's 1924 ruling on quarantine laws, the states had the authority to restrict individual liberty when necessary to protect the public from contagion. Of course, whether or not a state passed a compulsory school vaccination law depended on the will of its voters.

The early history of school vaccination in the United States is a story of increasing state legislation to gain control over a contagious disease, but it is also a story of the accommodation to public needs and demands that always occurs in a democratic society. To remain in power, elected legislators needed to be responsive to their constituents. In states where epidemics took the lives of children, destroyed economies, and threw people out of work, school vaccination laws passed easily. Passing such laws was far more difficult in states that remained relatively free of death and devastation from smallpox.

The absence of school vaccination laws in some areas of the country, and the patchwork nature of the laws in many states, ensured that the eradication of smallpox in the United States would take about 150 years. Whether a state passed a standing school vaccination law similar to the laws of the late twentieth century depended on its experience with smallpox outbreaks. Given the long history of problems with vaccine production and supply, most Americans preferred to accept vaccination only when smallpox threatened. As a result, most states passed discretionary or contingent laws that allowed school or health authorities to require vaccination whenever they felt it necessary, or when an epidemic threatened. On the one hand, such laws allowed families to avoid vaccinating their school-age children for long periods when disease was not present. But on the other hand, they also guaranteed that outbreaks would return.

It took one or more serious triggering events to motivate state legislatures to drum up backing for a standing law that required vaccination for school attendance, even in the absence of disease. A few states that had experienced recurring epidemics took this step, hoping to guarantee a more permanent protection for schoolchildren and their local communities. But from the 1880s onward, the political activism of organized anti-vaccination groups made it difficult to pass such legislation. Some of the strongest opposition came from national organizations committed to overturning school vaccination laws. As newspapers across the country publicized their arguments, health officials began talking about how to inoculate the public against a growing epidemic of anti-vaccination sentiment.

2

The National Anti-vaccination Societies and the Schools

In the early nineteenth century, the practice of arm-to-arm vaccination reduced the severity of smallpox outbreaks so dramatically that few people objected to the procedure, but it was never safe. Benjamin Waterhouse had warned against using the method in 1809, but when there was a shortage of vaccine, doctors often ignored his advice.[1]

Americans became more aware of the risk in the 1860s. During the Civil War, when smallpox spread through the Union and Confederate armies and vaccine was in short supply, panicked soldiers attempted arm-to-arm immunization to protect themselves. Because syphilis was prevalent among the troops, many became infected as a result.[2] After the war, as mortality rates from smallpox declined and the disease appeared far less threatening than vaccination itself, people opposed to the procedure began organizing societies to overturn school vaccination laws.

An era of opposition to vaccination arose, starting with the formation of the Anti-Vaccination League of America in 1879. There were three distinct phases in organized resistance to school vaccination: First, the period from 1879 to 1885, when physicians practicing alternative medicine organized the first national anti-vaccination society; second, the period from 1885 to 1906, when lay leaders came to predominate in the Anti-Vaccination Society of America and focused on overturning school vaccination laws; and third, the period from 1906 to the late 1920s, when anti-vaccinationists joined with business interests in the medical liberty movement. The rise of anti-vaccination discourse occurred within the context of broader social changes and scientific discoveries within each of these phases.

Some writers have tried to draw a direct line from the vaccine opponents of the late nineteenth century to the anti-vaccine protesters of more recent eras, claiming their arguments remain unchanged.[3] But while there are similarities, there are also substantial differences. Nineteenth- and early-twentieth-century opposition to vaccination was never solely about safety concerns—to a great extent, the first North American anti-vaccination movement was an effort to promote, protect, and preserve alternative forms of medicine.

The Rise of Alternative Medicine

Many of the arguments against vaccination were rooted in long-standing disputes over science and medical practice. Alternative approaches to traditional medicine flourished in the early nineteenth century, as many Americans became disillusioned with traditional treatments like bloodletting, purging, and the application of mustard plasters. Some of these treatments dated back hundreds of years. During the eighteenth century, doctors drew on medieval views of impurity as a cause of disease. They believed that to become healthy, a sick patient required bodily cleansing through purging and bloodletting to remove impurities from the body. As a result, they often prescribed emetics and laxatives to empty the stomach and colon, a practice that could induce severe dehydration.[4] The physicians attending President George Washington during his final days of illness in 1799 carried out an extreme version of this kind of treatment. When Washington developed an inflamed sore throat and a fever, the three doctors attending him recommended bloodletting, purging, blistering, and a tonic of molasses, vinegar, and butter. Through repetitive bloodletting, the doctors removed about 40 percent of the blood in his body, believing it necessary to constrict the blood vessels in his throat and reduce inflammation of his windpipe. Washington died after twelve hours of this treatment.[5]

Disenchanted with such methods, many Americans turned to alternative forms of medicine during this period. Samuel Thomson (1769–1843), a self-taught herbalist, attracted followers by arguing that doctors were completely unnecessary. His book *New Guide to Health, or Botanic Family Physician*, which appeared in multiple editions from 1822 to 1835, aimed to teach people to heal themselves using plants. "It is my opinion," he informed readers, "that you are better off with your own judgment and this book than with all the scientific ignorance, called knowledge, as taught in the schools."[6]

Wooster Beach, the founder of "eclectic" medicine, a precursor to naturopathy, established a medical practice in New York City in 1825 with a focus on plant-based medicines. He opened a medical school in New York in 1829, and his book, *The American Practice of Medicine*, became a national bestseller after it came out in 1833. His ideas and methods spread, and by 1874, there were nine eclectic medical colleges.[7]

Another influential form of alternative medicine was homeopathy. Developed in Germany by Samuel Hahnemann, homeopathy was based on the theory that disease could be treated with minute doses of drugs believed capable of producing in healthy people symptoms identical to those of the disease under treatment.[8] Homeopathy was among the most popular and influential alternative approaches to medicine during the nineteenth century. By 1911, there were thirteen homeopathic medical colleges in the United States.[9]

Although they rejected traditional medicine, the founders of homeopathy and eclectic medicine supported vaccination before the 1860s. In a letter written in 1831 to a colleague with a sick child, Samuel Hahnemann recommended arm-to-arm vaccination.[10] In 1836, Wooster Beach described smallpox as "no more to be dreaded than fire on the hearth. For this change we are indebted to inoculation."[11]

However, eclectic and homeopathic doctors began speaking out against vaccination as traditional doctors, also known as "allopathic," or "regular" doctors, embraced new forms of scientific medicine and the germ theory of disease. Louis Pasteur confirmed the germ theory in 1860, but the eclectics refused to accept the existence of bacteria and viruses capable of causing disease, and American homeopaths remained divided over the theory for decades.[12] By the end of the 1870s, allopathic doctors had embraced sanitary methods and given up older practices of bloodletting and purging, and they had come to view alternative doctors as hopelessly out-of-date and impeding the progress of scientific medicine.

Seeking to establish new professional boundaries to exclude the dissenting eclectic and homeopathic doctors, allopathic physicians began referring to alternative practitioners as "irregulars" and describing the fields of homeopathy and eclectic medicine as "medical sects." This was especially true of the doctors in the American Medical Association and those who worked in public health. As part of this kind of boundary-work, or professional exclusion, many public health departments refused to hire alternative practitioners as vaccinators and allowed only allopathic doctors to fill leadership positions. In an address before the Eclectic Medical Society of New York in 1869, Dr. Alexander Wilder described the barriers eclectic doctors faced: "At the present time the Eclectic practice is classified as 'irregular.' Its practitioners, however learned, skillful, or accomplished, are ostracized. They are eligible nowhere to honorable official appointments."[13] The chance to take a stand against an allopathic practice like vaccination galvanized alternative physicians who believed their treatments were entirely safe and beneficial.

The First Anti-Vaccination League of America, 1879–1885

On October 10, 1879, a small group of "earnest sympathisers" led by eclectic doctors Robert Gunn and Alexander Wilder met in the United States Medical College in New York to establish a national anti-vaccination society. Wilder was president of the Eclectic Medical Society of the State of New York, and two years earlier, Gunn had published a booklet denouncing the practice of arm-to-arm vaccination.[14]

By this time, New York's allopathic health officials had also condemned the practice of arm-to-arm vaccination. In 1870, Dr. Henry A. Martin of Boston introduced bovine vaccine to the United States. The following year, New York's board of health notified doctors to stop using the arm-to-arm technique and established a department to supply bovine virus material taken directly from calves, which did not spread syphilis or other diseases.[15]

But the fact that boards of health in New York and elsewhere were abandoning arm-to-arm vaccination did not stop Robert Gunn and others from organizing an anti-vaccination society. They opposed any form of vaccination, whether with humanized or bovine virus. To eclectic doctors, the injection of a nonbotanical substance like calf lymph into the human body was a form of blood poisoning. Like many of his colleagues, Gunn found it both harmful and inherently unnatural.[16]

Wilder chaired the meeting, introducing guest speaker William Tebb, cofounder of the London Society for the Abolition of Compulsory Vaccination. Tebb had come to speak about efforts to oppose vaccination in England.[17] Wilder said he wholeheartedly agreed with Tebb's goal of "creating an anti-vaccination sentiment that will find some legislative expression."[18]

Tebb riveted his listeners with accounts of the organizing strategies and tactics he and his colleagues were using in England to overturn the country's compulsory vaccination laws, including publication of *Vaccination Inquirer*, an anti-vaccination journal with impressively frightening illustrations on the cover (figure 2.1). He claimed that opposition to vaccination was growing in England, and he urged Americans to join the cause.[19]

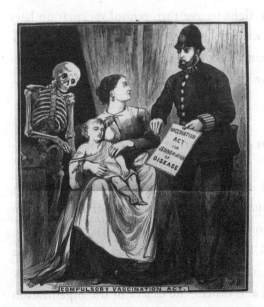

Figure 2.1. "Death the Vaccinator," published by the London Society for the Abolition of Compulsory Vaccination, late 1800s. *Source*: Courtesy of the Historical Medical Library of the College of Physicians of Philadelphia. Anti-vaccination Scrapbook Z8c 11, folder 60.

The audience was stirred to action by Tebb's remarks, and on Gunn's motion, voted to organize the Anti-Vaccination League of America to oppose vaccination and "all legislation for its enforcement." Wilder was elected president, and Gunn and Tebb were elected members of the executive committee. Five of the league's seven officers possessed a medical degree—four from the field of eclectic medicine and one from the field of homeopathy.[20] According to Tebb, who reported on this meeting after returning to England, the league's goal was "the emancipation of the American people from a medical despotism which... usurps parental rights and deprives the most thoughtful and intelligent parents who object to Vaccination of the use of the public schools for their children."[21]

Despite this stated goal, the league's leaders never actively engaged in any grassroots efforts to overturn legislation—instead, they concentrated on public communication. They published influential books and tracts, and as newspapers reported on the league's activities, popular knowledge about anti-vaccination spread across the United States. As the fight to overturn school vaccination laws continued, later anti-vaccination societies would reiterate league members' core arguments well into the twentieth century: that vaccination was ineffective, unnecessary, and dangerous.

Anti-vaccination Arguments in the News

News coverage of anti-vaccination activism increased dramatically after the league was founded. With the formation of a homegrown national anti-vaccination league, US newspapers were quick to publish the news (chart 2.1). Many printed just a brief notice: "The first Anti-Vaccination League of America has just been formed in New York by medical men and others, the object of the organization

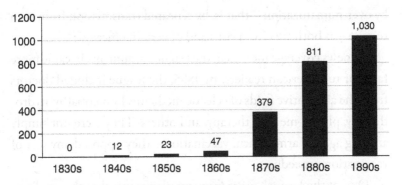

Chart 2.1. Number of US newspaper articles reporting opposition to vaccination, by decade, 1830s–1890s. *Source*: Data derived from a search conducted Jan. 10, 2021, of newspapers published between 1830 and 1900 on Newspapers.com using the phrase *opposed to vaccination*.

being 'to awaken the attention of the public to the evils of vaccination and to its inutility, to put an end to its practice and to prevent legislation for its enforcement.' "[22]

Some papers depicted the movement as a positive development, noting long-standing problems with the smallpox vaccine. The *Detroit Free Press* reported, "Mr. Tebb succeeded last week in organizing an anti-vaccination society in New York. If he can enforce more rigid regulations in regard to the purity of the virus, he will undoubtedly do good. If the vaccine were always taken from healthy young calves the unquestioned evils arising from the present too prevailing methods would be greatly reduced."[23]

Other papers derided the claims that smallpox vaccine was inherently ineffective and transmitted syphilis and other diseases. *Scientific American* pointed out that arm-to-arm vaccination was no longer recommended in the United States: "Our European friends, instead of trying to propagate their notions here, would do much better to study the methods employed in this country and try them at home. Vaccine virus, not contaminated and stripped of its virtue by over-humanization—that is, by repeated transmission from man to man—is both free from risks and of certain efficacy."[24]

As news coverage increased, the league's arguments became more familiar to American readers. By 1885, the league included doctors from the alternative fields of eclectic medicine, homeopathy, hydrotherapy, physio-medical therapy, and others. They were not simply arguing against arm-to-arm vaccination—they opposed any sort of vaccination procedure.

One of the league's more frequent claims was that the smallpox vaccine simply did not work. Wilder claimed, "Vaccination is useless, or, at least, perpetually uncertain as a preventive to smallpox."[25] Gunn wrote, "I believe the practice known as *vaccination* to be most absurd, and most pernicious. I do not believe that a single person has ever been protected from small-pox by it."[26]

To bolster their argument that vaccination was ineffective, Gunn and others pointed to evidence that previously vaccinated people had contracted smallpox. Gunn published a book explaining that he had come to distrust the efficacy of vaccination during a smallpox outbreak in New York City. Health authorities had claimed the city was "thoroughly protected by vaccination," and yet many people became ill and died during the epidemic. Other opponents of vaccination made similar arguments. In 1885 a major outbreak occurred in Montreal, Canada, resulting in over three thousand deaths. At the time, Dr. Alexander M. Ross collected statistics showing that nearly half of those who had died had scars on their arms, indicating they had been vaccinated previously. The argument that vaccination was ineffective persisted in anti-vaccination literature for decades. After the Philippine Insurrection (1898–1901), American anti-vaccinationists frequently cited the hundreds of smallpox deaths among vaccinated US soldiers in the Philippines to make the same point.[27]

However, in their speeches and writings, Gunn and Ross failed to acknowledge, or deliberately suppressed, what allopathic doctors had known for years—that the smallpox vaccine never provided life-long immunity. By the 1870s, allopathic medical journals commonly reported that immunity wore off five years after vaccination, and for this reason, public health officials commonly recommended periodic revaccination to ensure protection. Moreover, physicians knew that the vaccine was never 100 percent effective. In addition to production or storage problems that could render the vaccine material inert, for some people, vaccination simply "did not take," either because of blunders on the part of the vaccinator or because the individual's immune system did not respond to the vaccine.[28] As a result, breakthrough infections could occur in vaccinated people.

The intentional suppression of evidence like this is a well-known tactic in propaganda campaigns, but it is not possible to determine whether Gunn and Ross deliberately omitted information about breakthrough infections. The omission could have occurred through what historian Robert Proctor calls "passive ignorance"—the kind of ignorance that occurs when individuals limit themselves to the topics and sources of information they believe are most relevant to their own career interests and fields. The deepening divisions between "irregular" and "regular" physicians left each group in its own silo, with its own sources of information and expertise, disseminated through separate professional associations, conferences, and journals. In other words, Gunn and Ross may simply not have kept up with information about vaccine effectiveness that appeared regularly in allopathic journals.[29]

Although the anti-vaccinationists may have sincerely believed their statistics proved the smallpox vaccine was ineffective, it was impossible to draw any meaningful conclusions from their data, which never included the dates of previous vaccinations. During that era, investigators commonly looked for a smallpox scar on an arm as evidence of vaccination. When the anti-vaccinationists claimed to prove the vaccine did not work because vaccinated people had died from smallpox, they never acknowledged the possibility that such scars could be quite old. Immunity from smallpox vaccination never lasted forever.

Some English men of science joined the effort to repeal their country's unpopular compulsory vaccination laws, and American anti-vaccinationist leaders repeated their arguments that vaccination had no effect against smallpox. During the 1880s and '90s, Alfred Russel Wallace, celebrated for his codiscovery of natural selection, argued that the early-nineteenth-century experiments on vaccination were inconclusive. Wallace was a follower of spiritualism, the belief that the living can communicate with the dead. The spiritualist movement, which spread through the United States and Europe in the second half of the nineteenth century, emphasized the possibility of paranormal and supernatural influence in the world. Its followers, some of whom were doctors and scientists, pursued new methods of healing, including the use of electricity, magnetism, mesmerism, and crystal-gazing. Most spiritualists, including Wallace, opposed vaccination as an unnecessary and unsafe procedure. Wallace used evidence from mortality tables to support his claim that vaccination was not responsible for the decline in deaths from smallpox in England. For example, he cited statistics from Leicester, where deaths from smallpox had declined dramatically along with a decline in the vaccination of infants at birth.[30]

Wallace's evidence seemed compelling at the time—but the statistics he presented were incomplete. Recent research indicates that the elimination of smallpox in Leicester was due to a new method of controlling the illness that Leicester health officers implemented around the time that the number of smallpox cases began to fall. The method involved prompt notification of a case of smallpox to the health officer, isolation of all cases in the hospital, and quarantine for all the immediate contacts of the original cases. Leicester health officers also offered free vaccination to residents during smallpox outbreaks, and the number of people who chose vaccination during such times was not included in Wallace's statistics, which only displayed vaccinations at birth.[31]

A second argument league members made frequently was that vaccination was completely unnecessary, because existing sanitary practices could prevent smallpox. The notion that sanitary measures could defeat contagious diseases was common during this period. Before widespread acceptance of germ theory, many people explained the incidence and spread of illness without any awareness of the microorganisms that caused disease. In 1850, three main theories predominated: The *miasma theory* stated that disease was caused by poor climate or bad air or wind. The *filth theory* stated that unclean living quarters containing decaying matter or feces caused disease. The *germ theory* stated that miniscule organisms invaded the body and that a specific microorganism, or germ was responsible for a specific disease.[32]

By 1895, most American doctors had come to accept germ theory. This shift reflected the swift pace of discovery in medical science. In 1882, Robert Koch discovered the bacillus that caused tuberculosis and then isolated the cholera bacillus. Just two years later, Friedrich Loeffler isolated the diphtheria bacillus and Arthur Nicolaier discovered the toxins that caused tetanus; one year afterward, Pasteur successfully vaccinated a boy against rabies.[33]

Despite these breakthroughs, most of the doctors who rejected vaccination remained opposed to the germ theory of disease well into the twentieth century. Alexander Wilder sought to discredit the theory throughout his professional life, describing it as "purely a guess, without a solitary fact to sustain it."[34] Robert Gunn refused to believe that smallpox was contagious, describing it as "a filth disease that might arise from want of cleanliness, defective ventilation, bad physical conditions, etc., without the intervention of any contagion."[35] Alexander Ross argued that sanitary science alone could defeat smallpox, because epidemics only occurred "wherever the streets are narrow, the lanes and courts filthy."[36]

A third argument league members made against vaccination was that the calf lymph used in the smallpox vaccine poisoned the blood. In their opinion, abandoning the arm-to-arm technique would not eliminate the danger of vaccination, because the calf lymph itself was dangerous. "The act of vaccination," wrote Wilder, "is simply the contaminating of a patient's body with a blood-poison."[37] Newspapers across the country reprinted an article in which Wilder described the vaccine as "a disease working permanent corruption of the blood."[38]

The blood-poisoning argument persisted for decades. For example, in 1900, Dr. James M. Peebles published *Vaccination a Curse and a Menace to Personal Liberty*, a popular book that reiterated the arguments of those who had opposed vaccination in the 1870s and '80s. "The poisons concealed in calf-pus permanently affect the blood," he wrote. He believed that the calf lymph itself carried a range of diseases, including syphilis, cancer, and tuberculosis.[39] Although there was never any evidence that properly prepared calf lymph would poison the blood or transmit these diseases, throughout the 1920s, other authors published pamphlets and books reiterating these themes.[40]

As local anti-vaccination societies sprang up across the country, public debates over vaccination in newspaper opinion pages became common. Some editors rejected anti-vaccination claims. Referring to a city with a "flourishing anti-vaccination society," one Oregon newspaper editor noted, "These societies ought properly to be called 'societies for the spread of small-pox and the peopling of grave-yards.'"[41] According to the *Indianapolis Journal*, "Neither ignorance nor imbecility can justify any person in establishing himself as a distributing center of pestilence."[42] But others took league members' arguments and political goals more seriously. A California newspaper described the statistics presented at a league meeting in New York "concerning the alleged evils of vaccination" as "most appalling." More important, as discussed in chapter 3, over the next two decades, the individuals who filed some of the key lawsuits against school vaccination laws cited the league's arguments, often word-for-word.[43]

Despite the impressive reach of its messaging, the number of members in the league was small. In 1885, its secretary moved out of town, and regular meetings ground to a halt. As the league foundered, its remaining members made common cause with a new group in New York that was organizing a national organization under the name "The Anti-Vaccination Society of America" in 1885.[44]

The Campaign to Overturn
State Vaccination Laws

In contrast to the earlier league, the Anti-Vaccination Society of America (AVSA) was dedicated to overturning school vaccination laws. The group specifically targeted schools, sending anti-vaccination materials to principals and teachers and asking members to elect anti-vaccine candidates to local school boards.[45] "In every school district," urged Dr. Montague Leverson, secretary of the AVSA, "efforts should be made to secure the election of school trustees, pledged to refuse to carry out the laws of compulsory vaccination."[46]

The society incorporated in New York City on December 2, 1885. Dr. Peter M. Barclay was president, Dr. Montague R. Leverson was secretary, and Alexander Wilder, former president of the now defunct Anti-Vaccination League of America, served on the Executive Committee. Former league members took up familiar roles in the new organization: Robert Gunn became a vice president, and England's William Tebb became an "honorary vice president."[47] Members represented affiliated anti-vaccination societies in twenty-three states, England, and Canada.[48]

At first, doctors dominated the messaging and policies of the AVSA, but near the end of the century this changed as the proportion of physicians in the organization declined and nonmedical lay members became prominent in the society.[49] By 1900, the proportion of doctors among AVSA officers had fallen to 38 percent.[50]

Why did doctors leave the AVSA? Several reasons explain their exodus. For a start, theoretical disputes among researchers over the germ theory of disease were long over. In the face of new discoveries, it was not easy to maintain the belief that viruses and bacteria did not cause disease. Doctors now had access to the microscope, spirometer, electrocardiograph, and X-ray machine. Laboratory tests could detect the organisms responsible for tuberculosis, cholera, typhoid, pneumonia, diphtheria, gonorrhea, and syphilis, and new developments in microbiology facilitated the development of new vaccines against rabies, typhoid, cholera, and plague, along with antitoxins to fight diphtheria and tetanus.[51] Rapid advances in technology during the last two decades of the nineteenth century greatly improved medical knowledge about the ability of vaccines to prevent infectious diseases and methods to improve the safety of vaccination procedures. Decades earlier, statements that smallpox was not contagious or that sanitary methods could prevent all disease represented theoretical propositions, but by this point, with no evidence to support them, most doctors believed such claims represented misinformation.

Vaccines also became safer. In 1901, thirteen children died from tetanus after receiving tainted diphtheria antitoxin produced in St. Louis. Reportedly, the antitoxin had been taken from a horse that had developed tetanus, and the vaccine producers had no controls in place to detect the animal's infection. In response to pressure from the American Medical Association and other groups concerned about vaccine safety and anxious about anti-vaccine protests, the federal government passed the Biologics Control Act in 1902, also known as the Virus-Toxin Law. As a result, the government began regulating vaccine production, which increased the safety of the vaccination procedure.[52]

Additionally, by this time, many homeopathic and eclectic physicians no longer opposed the germ theory of disease. Although some homeopathic doctors continued to deny that germs caused disease and that vaccination could protect against contagion, in 1894 a writer in the *North American Journal of Homeopathy* expressed an opinion that many homeopaths had come to accept: "The consensus of opinion to-day undoubtedly is unanimous in adopting the theory of contagion. . . . Those who years ago stoutly denied the germ theory have had to amend their ideas under the light of scientific investigation."[53]

By 1903, much of the professional hostility between so-called allopathic or mainstream physicians and alternative physicians had subsided. That year, the American Medical Association revised its code of ethics. Although the AMA's code noted that physicians should not base their practice on "an exclusive dogma or sectarian system," the wording no longer included any mention of the sort of medicine doctors practiced. This ruling allowed homeopaths and eclectics to join the association.[54]

In contrast to doctors, who were members of professional associations and often voiced their opposition to vaccination by presenting conference papers and publishing books, lay members in the AVSA, some of whom were followers of spiritualism and believed strongly in alternative therapies and healing methods like hydrotherapy and magnetism, rolled up their sleeves and began organizing with the goal of overturning state vaccination laws. One of these was Frank D. Blue, a stenographer from Terre Haute, Indiana. He and his family had arrived there in 1888 from Pennsylvania, where he had worked as an office boy in Sunbury for the Philadelphia and Erie railway. By the summer of 1900 they had four children and worshipped in the local Catholic church.[55] Blue's opposition to vaccination was based on his health beliefs. He was a follower of T. V. Gifford, an Indiana hygeio-therapist and AVSA member who ran the Kokomo Invalid Sanitorium. Hygeio-therapy was "a system of curing the sick by and through natural methods only."[56] In 1893, when his son's school refused to admit the unvaccinated boy during an outbreak of smallpox, Blue had sued the school, and his case was now dragging through the circuit court. Another was Louis H. Piehn, president of the First National Bank of Iowa. Piehn's opposition to vaccination arose from tragedy—his daughter Alma Olivia had died after being vaccinated as a requirement to attend public school.[57]

In 1896, Blue and Piehn helped distribute AVSA literature in several states to bolster political advocacy against vaccination. A newspaper in St. Louis, Missouri, reported that Blue had arrived in town to establish an anti-vaccination society, armed with thousands of pamphlets.[58] A newspaper in Atlanta, Georgia, reported that Blue had sent a large package of anti-vaccination pamphlets to a judge, along with a letter castigating him "for his recent decisions in the cases against citizens who had refused to be vaccinated."[59]

In 1896, Piehn and Blue threw their support behind a Christian Scientist's refusal to comply with Wisconsin's school vaccination law. The resulting case, *State ex rel. Adams v. Burdge*, eventually reached the state's supreme court. Christian Scientists were natural allies in the fight against vaccines, because they viewed vaccination as a violation of their religious faith and freedom. Mary Baker Eddy had founded the Church of Christ, Scientist in Boston in 1879 based on the belief in the mind's power to prevent and cure disease through prayer, and the church grew rapidly, reaching forty thousand members by 1906. Near the turn of the century, wary of ongoing lawsuits involving the church's healing methods, Eddy issued a statement to her followers to follow the Bible's instructions and "Render Under Caesar the things that are Caesar's" by obeying vaccination laws, but despite her advice, individual Christian Scientists continued to avoid vaccination in later decades.[60] Piehn and Blue's propaganda efforts in support of the case gained them recognition and status in the AVSA. Montague Leverson announced to the membership that Wisconsin's supreme court had found the practice of requiring vaccination for school attendance "a violation of Constitutional Rights" in large part owing to their exertions.[61]

In 1897, Piehn became president of the AVSA, and Blue became secretary the following year. Under their leadership, a new slogan appeared on the back of the 1902 AVSA membership card: "Compulsory Education is an equal sharing of the national stock of acquired knowledge. Compulsory Vaccination is a distribution of the national stock of acquired diseases."[62]

Blue brought boundless energy and organizational skills to his role as AVSA secretary. A legal reporter and chief clerk in the office of the general counsel of the Vandalia Railroad, he was thirty-five years old when he purchased some typesetting equipment and began printing an anti-vaccination journal for the AVSA.[63] He started publishing *Vaccination: A Journal of Health, Justice, and Liberty* in Terre Haute, Indiana, in February 1898. Several months afterward, Leverson stepped down as AVSA secretary, and Blue succeeded him in the position.[64]

The first issue of *Vaccination* appeared in February 1898, reporting AVSA news and minutes along with snippets of information about the ineffectiveness and hazards of vaccination.[65] A recurring theme in the journal was the ability of natural and sanitary methods to defeat all disease. *Vaccination* called on AVSA members to oppose the "Germ faddists" and "keep intact the good health Mother Nature has given you" by compelling doctors to adopt "rational methods of treating the sick and sensible modes of Sanitation."[66] In some of his later articles, Blue went further and began recommending nature cures in line with the alternative forms of medicine he preferred. For example, he informed readers of a cure for smallpox "used by the Old Mammies in slavery days": the treatment involved drinking saffron tea and soaking in a barrel of hot bran mash for an hour or more. Describing one successful case, Blue reported, "Well about two doses cured him and in less than a week he was back at work. Now, I'd like to see some of your cultured, scientific, microbe hunters, beat that."[67]

The editorials and articles in *Vaccination* reiterated the anti-vaccination claims of former decades: that the smallpox vaccine did not work; that it poisoned the blood, and that germ theory was a delusion. Like their predecessors in the defunct Anti-Vaccination League of America, Blue and other AVSA leaders continued to discredit and denounce germ theory long after it had gained broad acceptance. *Vaccination* had rejected the idea from its very first issue in 1898: "Is Light Coming? The germ theory is getting some hard raps these days. . . . We always suspected there was more 'scare' than anything else in this theory."[68] Montague Leverson opposed germ theory for decades. In 1917, at the age of eighty-seven, when he was living in England, he sent a letter to the editor of *Health Culture* magazine explaining that he was working on a paper proving that Louis Pasteur was "a plagiarist and charlatan" and that the germ theory of disease was bunk.[69]

Rejecting germ theory meant dismissing the idea of contagion. Leverson and his colleagues refused to accept the idea that disease-carrying microorganisms could transmit disease from one healthy person to another. In their view, if a child became sick, it was because that child had become infected with filth, or was eating poorly, drinking impure water, breathing bad air, avoiding exercise, or had some inherited condition. Because Blue and Leverson did not believe in contagion, they could not accept the idea that students in crowded classrooms were in any danger of catching illnesses from others. The greatest risk, in their view, was the injection of any foreign matter into the blood through vaccination. As Blue put it many years afterward, "We believe health is contagious, not disease. Hundreds have died from vaccination."[70]

While this kind of rhetoric may have represented legitimate discourse during earlier decades, by 1900, Blue and Leverson were not publishing verifiable facts or plausible scientific theories—they were printing propaganda with the aim of gaining faithful followers to the anti-vaccination cause.

Blue used the journal to promote anti-vaccination activism in local school districts. The rhetoric about blood poisoning became politically useful in stirring parents to resist school vaccination, especially during the weeks before schools opened in the fall. "In our larger cities I note the annual vaccinating campaign is about to begin, to make a few cases of smallpox to serve as an excuse for poisoning all school children with vaccine virus," wrote Blue in August 1904.[71]

The National Anti-vaccination Societies and the Schools

He urged readers to "see that every member of your school board and all principals of schools receive a copy of *Vaccination* and a few of our tracts." Since few states had school vaccination laws on the books, "a knowledge of what vaccination is will always defeat them."[72]

Seeking to expand his readership among school officers and teachers, he asked former AVSA Secretary Leverson for help. As he explained, public health officers were meeting opposition from teachers in Pittsburgh who refused to exclude unvaccinated students from the schools. Blue wrote, "So the Death Board has announced that in the fall all unvaccinated will be rigidly excluded and if any teachers allow them to attend, they will prosecute the teachers. What I wish to do is to get some copies of *Vaccination* in the right hands in that city, especially in the hands of all the public school teachers." He asked Leverson if he knew "of a native of the place who could be depended upon to give or to get us lists of all public school teachers and officers."[73]

Despite the successful launch of *Vaccination* and Blue's unflagging activism, near the close of the century, the AVSA appeared to be foundering. Blue struggled to drum up subscribers to the new journal. As he described the situation to Leverson, "Anti Vaccination Leagues everywhere to be demoralized, Brooklyn is as bad as Chicago apparently. [The] T[erre] H[aute] League is also practically dead outside of three or four of us." In 1901, one almanac reported that the AVSA had two hundred members, but this figure may have been exaggerated. That year a reporter sent by the *New York Times* to cover a meeting of the local anti-vaccination league in Brooklyn found that "nine men, one boy, and seven reporters were present."[74]

The US Supreme Court's ruling on an anti-vaccination case in 1905 was the final nail in the AVSA's coffin. The case before the court involved Henning Jacobson, a minister living in Cambridge, Massachusetts. In 1902, he had refused to comply with an order to vaccinate members of his family during an outbreak of smallpox in the town. With assistance from the Massachusetts Anti-Compulsory Vaccination Association, Jacobson filed a lawsuit arguing that the Fourteenth Amendment to the Constitution gave him the right to refuse vaccination. To the dismay of those opposed to vaccination, the Supreme Court ruled that personal liberties could be suspended when the public's safety was at risk from disease, and it upheld the authority of the states to enforce compulsory vaccination laws through fines or imprisonment.[75]

In July 1905, Blue informed readers, "Now, I find in going over my list of subscribers, a great many have failed to renew their subscriptions." The journal's demise in 1906 was noted in the *Homeopathic Recorder*: "*Vaccination*, an anti-vaccination journal, edited by Frank D. Blue, has turned up its toes to the daisies."[76]

The Second Anti-Vaccination League of America, 1908–1930

Although the AVSA disappeared from view, anti-vaccination sentiment remained high in some areas. Soon Pennsylvania emerged as an important center for engagement. In March, the activist Lora Cornelia Little came to the state to lecture on the evils of vaccination. She was a steadfast opponent of the practice. Her only child, a seven-year-old boy, had died from diphtheria seven months after being vaccinated for smallpox, and she blamed the vaccination for his death. She published a Minnesota anti-vaccination magazine called the *Liberator*, which promoted freedom from medical science. She had also authored a little book titled *Crimes of the Cowpox*, which carried stories and photographs of children who had died or had experienced severe adverse effects after having been vaccinated.[77]

Pennsylvania's anti-vaccinationists embraced Little's method of publicizing vaccination's side effects. On May 16, 1906, John Pitcairn, a wealthy businessman and cofounder of the Pittsburgh Plate Glass Company, hosted a public meeting to discuss strategies to overturn the state's school vaccination law. A member of the Swedenborgian Church of North America and a follower of homeopathy, Pitcairn believed Pennsylvania's efforts to compel vaccination were unjust. Porter F. Cope, the son of a leading Philadelphia financier, spoke at the meeting and presented a grisly slide show depicting some of the rare but gruesome adverse effects of vaccination.[78]

The marshaling of evidence about the vaccine's adverse effects had a powerful impact, because many in the audience no longer viewed the disease as a death sentence. In 1906, there had been over fifteen thousand cases of smallpox in Pennsylvania, but only ninety were fatal. The decline in fatalities was a result of evolution in the smallpox virus. Although virulent outbreaks continued in many areas of the country well into the twentieth century, two new mild strains of the disease had appeared by the time of the meeting in Philadelphia. In contrast to the *variola major* strain, which generally killed about 25 percent of its victims, the new *variola minor* strains only killed between 0.01 and 2 percent.[79] Still, a fatality rate that killed one in a thousand victims was much higher than the fatality rate of the vaccine, which—despite improvements in production—now killed about one in a million people. Furthermore, smallpox survivors could suffer permanent side effects, including severe scarring and blindness in some cases. Nevertheless, to many of the men and women in the audience in Philadelphia, the adverse effects of the vaccine were far more menacing than smallpox itself.[80]

In September, Pitcairn, Cope, and others established the Anti-Vaccination League of Pennsylvania. The group was small, with only forty-eight dues-paying members that first year, ten of whom were women.[81] Members quickly began work on a campaign against compulsory school vaccination. They successfully lobbied for a bill in 1907, which passed in the House and the Senate. However, they lost the battle when Governor Edwin Sydney Stuart vetoed the bill. As was common among anti-vaccination societies—whose membership lists swelled during political campaigns and dwindled once the campaigns had ended—membership declined after the political defeat in 1907. By 1911 there were fewer than ten dues-paying members.[82]

Undeterred by their low membership numbers and desiring to advocate on a national stage, the leaders of the Pennsylvania league decided to reorganize as a new national organization called the Anti-Vaccination League of America (AVLA2) in 1908.[83] About fifty people attended its first conference at Griffith Hall in Philadelphia, including William Lloyd Garrison, the son of the famous antislavery leader; the ink manufacturer Charles M. Higgins of Brooklyn, New York; and Bernarr Macfadden, a well-known fitness buff from Battle Creek, Michigan, who was also the editor of *Physical Culture*, an alternative health magazine. John Pitcairn was elected president, Porter Cope became secretary, and Higgins became treasurer.[84]

The AVLA2 was significant in its emphasis on *medical faith*, defined as the constitutional right to freedom of faith in alternative forms of medicine. John Pitcairn proclaimed, "One of the foundation principles of our government is absolute freedom from interference in matters of religious faith. Shall we witness unmoved the establishment by that government of a practice that deprives us of freedom in matters of *medical* faith?"[85] This argument, which aligned freedom of belief in alternative medicine with freedom of religion, became common in later state-level and local efforts to win philosophical and religious exemptions from school vaccination laws.

In contrast to the earlier Anti-Vaccination Society of America, the AVLA2 abandoned the strategy of supporting lawsuits against school vaccination to focus on political campaigns aiming to abolish laws interfering with medical liberty. It threw its support behind the campaigns of the National League for Medical Freedom, a new organization opposed to any legislation designed to tighten the government's control over the practice of medicine. The National League aimed to protect people's right to select the practitioner of their choice and opposed any attempt "to put into power any one system of healing."[86] Like Pitcairn, the president of the National League, B. O. Flower, also talked about faith—specifically, the importance of respecting people's beliefs about medicine. This was a core tenet of the medical liberty movement. The nationwide league attracted a range of people opposed to greater federal oversight of health, including Christian Scientists, patent medicine manufacturers, and drugless healers like osteopaths, naturopaths, and chiropractors, along with their followers.[87]

In support of the National League's lobbying efforts, in 1910 the AVLA2 sent Porter Cope to testify before Congress against what came to be known as the "Owen Bill," legislation introduced by Senator Robert L. Owen (D-OK) during the 61st Congress to establish a federal Department of Public Health. Supporters of medical liberty opposed the bill on the grounds it would give the federal government and regular doctors too much centralized authority over state and local affairs. In the end, Flower and associates won their campaign, and the Owen bill went down to defeat.[88]

In later years, the AVLA2 continued to focus on advocacy for medical liberty rather than on the narrower question of school vaccination. For this reason, although its leaders had originally intended the organization to function as a national confederation of state and local anti-vaccination societies, the AVLA2 never attained the same level of prominence and reach of the earlier Anti-Vaccination Society of America, with its Terre Haute–based journal, *Vaccination*. Instead, local anti-vaccination societies arose sporadically here and there across the country in response to local issues without a national anti-vaccination society to direct or support their protests.[89]

Activism against school vaccination laws did not disappear, however. By 1918, a new national organization called the American Medical Liberty League had begun targeting school vaccination in its campaigns, headed by two activists well known in anti-vaccination circles.

The American Medical Liberty League, 1918–1930

The activist Lora Little was a cofounder of the new league. She had long felt that a national organization focused solely on mandatory school vaccination was no longer needed. In 1908 she had written to Pitcairn to recommend creation of a "National Health Defense League." "Otherwise," she said, "we win upon vaccination only to find ourselves bound hand and foot and subject to science."[90]

After moving to Portland, Oregon, in 1909, Little established a business offering nature cures, health coaching, and lessons in how to "be your own doctor."[91] From 1915 to 1917, she authored a regular health column in the *Mt. Scott Herald*. Some of her recommendations would be very welcome in the twenty-first century, including those about increasing whole grains and fresh fruits and vegetables in the diet. But as a follower of naturopathy, a term coined around 1985 denoting an alternative, nature-based approach to medicine, she also consistently discounted the danger of serious diseases and opposed all forms of drugs and vaccines.[92] In one column, Little urged her readers not to worry about the rising incidence of tetanus in Oregon associated with puncture wounds: "Eat right, live right, and all your injuries, of whatever kind, quickly disappear." She believed right living could cure everything, including cancer, because "it takes a cancerous constitution to produce a cancer."[93]

She was an indefatigable activist in the anti-vaccination campaign. In 1918, working as a field agent for a group called the North Dakota Freedom League, Little began distributing literature attacking the federal government's practice of requiring US troops to be vaccinated against smallpox and typhoid fever. Within a few weeks, a US marshal arrested her in Bismarck on March 29 on charges of sedition for violating the 1916 Espionage Act and claiming that the army was "in league with the 'medical trust.'" In her defense, Little argued that she fully supported the US military and only opposed the practice of vaccination. Ultimately, a federal grand jury refused to indict her on the charges, and the authorities set her free.[94] Little cofounded the American Medical Liberty League the same year. She served as its secretary, and by 1920, Frank D. Blue had joined her and was serving as the president of that organization.[95]

The economist Irving Fisher accused the medical liberty leagues of being funded by patent medicine interests, and the number of league officers involved in mail-order patent businesses supports Fisher's conclusion.[96] B. O. Flower, head of the National League for Medical Freedom, was president of R. C. Flower Medicine Company, a mail-order patent medicine business.[97] W. S. and D. W. Ensign, two of the founding members of the American Medical Liberty League, ran a mail-order patent medicine company and thus had a vested business interest in opposing any increased intervention and regulation by the government. In 1922, W. S. Ensign, president of the Ensign Remedies Company in Battle Creek, Michigan, was a director of the league, and D. W. Ensign was treasurer. The Ensigns published the *Truth-Teller*, a homeopathic anti-vaccination magazine devoted to alternative methods of medical treatment that all members of the American Medical Liberty League received as part of their membership subscription. Their patent medicine business sold small vials of granules advertised as "cell salts" and guaranteed to "cure all diseases by feeding the tissues." Their advertisements claimed that Ensign remedies would cure smallpox and virtually any other ailment, including abscess, acute appendicitis, asthma, bowlegs, bunions, cancer, cataracts, deafness, diphtheria, disappointed love, dullness and stupidity, eczema, epilepsy, gray hair, irritation, laziness, lack of ambition, lockjaw, paralysis, rheumatism, toothache, tuberculosis, warts, and wrinkles.[98]

An important factor in the persistence of anti-vaccinationism during this period is the very real threat posed by medical reformers to the livelihoods of the men and women practicing drugless forms of medicine, selling mail-order patent cures, or offering alternative health therapies. By March 1905, Frank D. Blue had taken a position as the new superintendent of alternative medical therapies in the Kokomo Sanitorium. He needed to fight for the survival of his new business in an increasingly hostile regulatory environment. That year, the AMA established a Propaganda Department to campaign against quackery and fraud in medicine, and the *Journal of the American Medical Association* began a regular column that investigated and exposed allegedly fraudulent practitioners, questionable medical schools, and medical organizations promoting unconventional therapies such as those Blue had recommended in *Vaccination*.[99]

In a related development in 1910, Abraham Flexner, with support of the Carnegie Foundation, investigated the state of medical education across the United States. After visiting 160 schools, he concluded that most of them should be closed because of the poor instruction they offered. He recommended stricter state laws, tighter standards for medical education, and examinations for certification to practice medicine. Soon after the so-called Flexner Report appeared, twelve medical schools closed or merged in response to its findings, as did another twenty-six in the two decades following. Many of the homeopathic colleges had received poor ratings from Flexner. Of twenty-two homeopathic colleges enrolling students in 1900, only two were still open in 1923.[100]

The physicians who practiced alternative medicine, the businesspeople who sold mail-order patent medicines and potions, and those who earned a living by writing and speaking publicly about health culture and alternative medicine had much to lose in an environment of increased regulation. For example, Dr. James Peebles, author of *Vaccination a Curse and a Menace to Personal Liberty*, founded the Peebles' Institute of Health in Battle Creek, Michigan, in 1902 and began selling mail-order epilepsy cures. In 1915, the *Journal of the American Medical Association* denounced his enterprise as quackery after having obtained samples of his potions and subjecting them to analysis in the lab—the Epilepsy Treatment was 8.44% alcohol and 15.18% bromide, with trace amounts of ammonia, potassium, and chloride. *JAMA* condemned Peebles's business as fraudulent.[101]

For some, sowing doubt and distrust in vaccination was a way to strike back at allopathic medicine. As the osteopath and occultist Reuben Swinburne Clymer put it, in a little book published by Frank D. Blue, "we are striking at the very root and foundation of so-called scientific or 'regular' medicine."[102] The American Medical Liberty League (AMLL) distributed pamphlets with attention-grabbing titles like "Toxin–Anti-toxin—How It Kills and Cripples Children," and "Medical Health Officers Syphilizing the Nation." At the league's annual meeting in Chicago in 1923, Blue gave a speech claiming that the antitoxin treatment for diphtheria was bunk and that hydrotherapy was "the only real antidote for disease."[103] The sad thing about this story is that diphtheria, which had taken the life of Lora Little's son two decades earlier, was a highly fatal disease that immunization could now prevent. It killed about 20 percent of its youngest victims, those below the age of five. After passage of the 1902 Control Act, which regulated the production of vaccines, the antitoxin employed to protect against diphtheria was very safe, and its use prevented thousands of unnecessary deaths among children.[104] There was never any scientific evidence that hydrotherapy—the popular practice of soaking in a pool of warm or cold water—had any effect on a contagious disease like diphtheria.

Much like the earlier AVSA, the AMLL threw its support behind the anti-vaccination lawsuits individuals filed against local school districts, including chiropractor William F. Rhea's successful suit against a public school in North Dakota in 1919.[105] Rhea rejected vaccination, characterizing it as an injection of animal poison that could never protect from smallpox or any other disease. When the Devils' Lake School District barred his two unvaccinated children from school, he sued.[106] After losing his case in the district court, he appealed to the state supreme court and won. One newspaper credited the "plucky woman, Mrs. Lora Little, secretary of the American Medical Liberty League" for propaganda helpful to the case.[107]

Scholars have depicted the anti-vaccination activism of this era as distinctively libertarian, but if so, it was a very narrow sort of libertarianism.[108] No anti-vaccinationist leader publicly opposed compulsory schooling—in fact, Frank Blue and other members of the AVSA had endorsed it openly on their membership cards. Nor did the medical liberty leagues oppose the compulsory payment of state and federal taxes or the compulsory draft that forced thousands of young men to risk their lives fighting in American wars. League members were libertarian only when it came to policies and practices at odds with their core beliefs about health and medicine.

These core beliefs formed an important part of the medical liberty leagues' collective identity and contributed to their social cohesion.[109] By itself, fear of the smallpox vaccine was rarely enough to sustain protest against the practice of vaccination. Parents who believed the vaccine was unsafe often joined anti-vaccination societies for a time to protest against school vaccination requirements, but once a specific campaign ended, most parents dropped out of the regular meetings and stopped paying the membership dues that kept the societies afloat. In contrast, opposition to vaccination based on shared health ideology allowed groups like the AVSA2 and the AMLL to survive over relatively long periods, even as their influence waned.

It is hard to know how many members attended league meetings during this period. Newspapers generally reported only the dates of annual conferences, the topics covered, and the names of officers. After its political victories in 1911 and 1912, the National League for Medical Freedom continued to publish a journal until it vanished from the national scene by 1916.[110] The AVLA2 dwindled during the 1920s and disappeared after Charles Higgins died in 1929, and the AMLL had disappeared from mention in newspapers by Lora Little's death in 1931.[111] The movement seems to have depended largely on the persistence of a dedicated few. Nevertheless, those few understood well the importance of maintaining a messaging campaign through public lectures and print media, and their pamphlets and tracts, which reiterated the arguments of the nineteenth-century anti-vaccinationists, were persuasive to many readers for many years.[112]

Conclusion

The era from 1879 to the late 1920s was a period of broad resistance and opposition to vaccination. The first Anti-Vaccination League of America arose in 1879 in response to concerns about the safety of arm-to-arm vaccination and the growing precarity of alternative medicine. Over the subsequent half century, the demographics, beliefs, and economic interests of the national anti-vaccination societies evolved. The nineteenth-century anti-vaccination societies had argued that Americans had a constitutional right to refuse vaccination for themselves and their children. The medical liberty leagues that arose in the early twentieth century appropriated and expanded this argument, claiming that Americans had a constitutional right to choose their own medical treatment and a right to freedom from medical interference, not only in the form of compulsory vaccination, but in all areas of social life.

On the one hand, the advocacy of the early anti-vaccination societies helped raise public awareness of the importance of sanitary methods and good health in reducing the spread of disease. Their warnings about the risks of vaccines also provided some of the impetus for reforms leading to greater vaccine safety. But on the other hand, they also did great harm in undermining the public's trust in vaccines and antitoxins capable of preventing some of the most dangerous diseases of that era.

By the second decade of the twentieth century, opposition to vaccination had become widespread and difficult to overcome. According to Detroit's health department, "The propaganda of the anti-vaccinationists is continually being circulated."[113] New York State's deputy commissioner of health claimed that newspapers "sympathetic to the anti-vaccinationists" contributed to vaccine resistance.[114] In places with severe outbreaks, children paid the penalty. In 1921, the secretary of California's state board of health reported that "as the number of unprotected children of school age increases through the opposition and influence of anti-vaccinationists . . . the number of smallpox cases among the young also increases."[115]

The leaders of the national anti-vaccination societies understood well the importance of maintaining a propaganda campaign through print media, and their arguments endured. Over the years, those who were convinced that the smallpox vaccine was dangerous and ineffective would test the strength of these arguments in the courts.

3

Taking Schools to Court
The Legal Battles

S hortly after California passed a compulsory school vaccination law in 1889, businessman D. K. Abeel sued the principal of the Santa Cruz High School for refusing to admit his unvaccinated son. At the time, a smallpox epidemic with a fatality rate of 12 percent was spreading through the state, but Abeel feared the vaccine more than the smallpox. Repeating a long-standing anti-vaccination claim, he told the press he believed the vaccine would infect his son with various diseases. Abeel had the financial resources to see his case through the courts. A cofounder of the *Kansas City Journal* in Missouri, he had sold his share of the paper and come to Santa Cruz in 1886 to build the Sea Beach Hotel.[1] When the district court ruled in favor of the high-school principal, he appealed, and *Abeel v. Clark* became the first school vaccination case in the nation to reach a state supreme court.[2]

California's supreme court ruled against him on May 31, 1890, finding the school vaccination law "a constitutional exercise of the police power of the legislature." In the court's ruling, Chief Justice Phil S. Gibson noted that smallpox remained both highly contagious and deadly, and that vaccination was the most effective known method to prevent it. The court found it reasonable and proper to require vaccination to protect both students and communities from the disease.[3]

The ruling in California did nothing to settle the question of school vaccination in other states. After *Abeel*, similar cases landed before state supreme courts, with varying results.[4] In 1905, a vaccination case known as *Jacobson v. Massachusetts* reached the US Supreme Court. Nevertheless, although the court's ruling clarified the extent and limits of the states' police powers in mandating vaccination, *Jacobson* did not consider the issue of school vaccination.

In the absence of legal clarity, school boards in many states were unsure of the extent and limits of their authority. How could a school refuse admission to an unvaccinated student when state laws guaranteed all children the right to a public education? Could a vaccination law trump a child's constitutional right to attend public school? These questions remained unresolved. As a result, lawsuits against school districts and state boards of education continued until 1922, when the US Supreme Court finally heard a case on this issue. Throughout this period, school districts across the country followed the outcomes of court cases to understand how to balance their duty to educate with their responsibility to keep students safe from contagious disease.

Motivations to Sue

Some historians have claimed that the appearance of a new mild form of smallpox after 1898 played an important role in ordinary Americans' opposition and litigation against school vaccination. From this perspective, as the disease became far less lethal, defiance of school vaccination requirements was understandable, particularly since the smallpox vaccine came with some significant side effects.[5]

There are two problems with this argument: First, serious smallpox outbreaks did not disappear, and second, few of the people who filed the most important lawsuits over vaccination could be considered ordinary. The fatality rate of a disease is a common measure of its seriousness. The most deadly pandemic in recent history was the "Spanish" influenza pandemic of 1918–19, which killed more than 50 million people worldwide, and for which there was no vaccine. That influenza strain had a case fatality rate of 2.5 percent.[6] In contrast, US newspapers and public health records reported a much higher fatality rate for many smallpox outbreaks of the late nineteenth and early twentieth centuries. Some of the most important lawsuits against school vaccination were filed during serious outbreaks of disease with fatality rates ranging from 2.5 to around 12 percent.

Moreover, few of the plaintiffs in these cases could be considered ordinary or representative of the population at large. In *Jacobson v. Massachusetts*, Chief Justice John Marshall Harlan cited six previous cases involving school vaccination as part of the legal precedent underlying the court's seven-to-two majority decision (table 3.1).[7] Most of these were initiated with the leadership or encouragement of alternative physicians, and the Anti-Vaccination Society of America (AVSA) had a hand in some of them. In none of these cases is there any evidence that plaintiffs claimed the smallpox vaccine was no longer necessary because the disease was no longer dangerous.

Why did people sue their local schools over vaccination? Newspaper accounts and court records show that parents sued the schools because they had come to believe the propaganda of the national anti-vaccination societies. Some claimed that the vaccine would cause syphilis, cancer, tuberculosis, and a host of other diseases. Others

Table 3.1. School vaccination cases cited in *Jacobson v. Massachusetts*, US Supreme Court (1905), by year of final decision

Case	State	Year of final court decision	Year of lawsuit	Anti-vaccination society involvement
Abeel v. Clark	CA	1890, state supreme court	1889	Unknown
Bissell v. Davidson	CT	1894, state supreme court	1894	New Britain Anti-Vaccination Society
Duffield v. Williamsport	PA	1894, state supreme court	1894	Philadelphia Anti-Vaccination League
State ex rel. Adams v. Burdge	WI	1897, state supreme court	1896	Beloit Anti-Vaccination Society; Anti-Vaccination Society of America
Blue v. Beach	IN	1900, state supreme court	1893	Indiana Anti-Vaccination Society; Anti-Vaccination Society of America
Viemeister v. White	NY	1904, New York appellate court	1904	Unknown

Source: Table compiled from school vaccination cases cited in "*Jacobson v. Massachusetts*, 197 U.S. 11," *American and English Annotated Cases*, ed. William M. McKinney, David S. Garland, and H. Noyes Greene (Northport, NY: Edward Thompson Co., 1906), 3:765–73.

rejected the idea that diseases were contagious or proclaimed that sanitary methods alone could cure smallpox. In other words, resistance to vaccination was rarely based on a rational assessment of the risks versus the benefits of the smallpox vaccine. It was often based on alternative health ideologies, a religious commitment to faith healing, misinformation, or fear.

The story of Frank D. Blue's lawsuit illustrates the importance of alternative health beliefs and the involvement of anti-vaccination societies in litigation. Blue, who later became secretary of the AVSA and editor of *Vaccination*, filed one of the earliest school vaccination lawsuits to reach a state supreme court. In 1893, when a serious smallpox epidemic broke out in Indiana, the Terre Haute school board followed the recommendation of the state board of health and prohibited unvaccinated children from attending the public schools.

Even though the fatality rate was very high, reaching 15 percent in the town of Muncie, Blue refused to have his son Kleo vaccinated. His stance was informed by his alternative health beliefs, which included the conviction that smallpox was not contagious. When school authorities suspended his son from school, he sued the teacher and the school principal. He was not alone in opposing the school board's action. Terre Haute schools refused admission to about a hundred children whose parents refused to comply with the vaccination requirement.[8]

Blue joined with a group of alternative physicians in Muncie to create Indiana's first statewide anti-vaccination society. Muncie's alternative physicians refused to vaccinate during the epidemic, and they became infuriated when Indiana's state board of health decided to quarantine the town for a two-month period in the fall.[9] In December, Muncie doctors Andrew R. Mock and Lewis Payton decided to hold a public town meeting with some of Indiana's notable anti-vaccination activists. Mock practiced the "clairvoyant diagnosis of diseases and magnetic and massage treatment," and Payton was a physio-medical practitioner. On December 12, they invited the homeopathic physician W. B. Clarke of Indianapolis, Frank Blue of Terre Haute, and the well-known hygeio-therapist T. V. Gifford to speak.[10] At the meeting, Gifford spoke about the importance of organizing against the school vaccination rules. Roused to enthusiasm, the audience resolved to form the Indiana Anti-Vaccination League and elected Gifford president and Blue secretary.[11]

The support of the newly formed group became very important to Frank Blue's case against his son's school in Terre Haute. Indiana anti-vaccinationists banded together to bear the costs, because they viewed it as an important test case.[12] On December 23, the first circuit court ruled in Blue's favor, but the ruling was later appealed, and the case dragged through the circuit court for nearly three years before the next judge ruled against him. Ultimately, Blue appealed to the Indiana Supreme Court in June 1896.[13]

While Blue's case was pending, an anti-vaccination society in New Britain, Connecticut, supported another important lawsuit: *Bissell v. Davidson*. This case arose in response to new school vaccination rules in the context of smallpox outbreaks in 1893. To control the spread of disease, Connecticut's state board of health urged all residents to be vaccinated and advised school boards "to enforce the statute relating to the vaccination of the pupils in the public schools."[14] Quick to comply, the school board in New Britain required all students to be vaccinated. According to a news report, school enrollments in the town dropped by one-third, not only because some children had not yet been vaccinated, but also "on account of the severe vaccination rules, which many parents do not favor."[15]

As had occurred in Indiana, alternative physicians were an important part of New Britain's anti-vaccination movement, recommending their own forms of treatment instead of vaccination. During this period, some homeopathic doctors had begun to administer tiny oral doses of the cowpox virus, based on the belief that this method would be safer and more effective than injection. Known as "internal vaccination" or *variolinum*, the approach was unproven to protect against smallpox and controversial among homeopaths, but the anti-vaccinationist doctors in New Britain endorsed it.

Concerned that some of the town's doctors were informing parents that vaccination by injection was unnecessary, New Britain's superintendent of schools wrote to William H. Brewer, president of the state board of health, to explain the situation and ask whether the method of swallowing a homeopathic remedy was as effective as traditional vaccination. Brewer wrote back to say that "any person claiming that such a practice is 'vaccination' is either a fool or a fraud."[16] His response reflected the allopathic view that had become uniform in state boards of health across the country. However, many New Britain residents, worried about possibility of adverse effects from the smallpox vaccine, remained convinced by their homeopathic doctors' arguments against traditional vaccination.

By April 1894, New Britain residents had organized an anti-vaccination society and begun holding meetings "at which prominent physicians made speeches and condemned the wholesale vaccination." Among the members was Henry Bissell, a congregant of the local Universalist Church. He decided to sue Edward H. Davison, the principal of the local high school, after he refused to admit Bissell's unvaccinated son. The New Britain Anti-vaccination Society supported his lawsuit as a test case.[17] Like almost every other denomination, the Universalist Church did not oppose vaccination, and court records show that Bissell did not sue Davidson on religious grounds. He sued because he believed the school had no right to exclude the children of any parent who "believes that vaccination is not proper treatment for the child or children under his control."[18]

There is no surviving evidence regarding the motivations of the other parents who banded together to support Bissell's case, but given the public's concerns about the adverse effects of the smallpox vaccine during this period, it is likely that whether they had always been followers of homeopathic medicine or not, many parents welcomed the homeopathic doctors' offer of an alternative method and were outraged when the school authorities refused to allow it. And they found the anti-vaccine arguments of the alternative physicians attending their meetings very persuasive.

It is not surprising that some people believed the arguments of the anti-vaccinationists during this era. Schools were among the most universal places of association for Americans below the age of fourteen, and yet few students had ever encountered adequate information about the prevention of contagious disease in their schools. School-books published before 1900 generally avoided the subjects of vaccination and the germ theory of disease. Only 17 percent mentioned vaccination, and only 33 percent mentioned germ theory (chart 3.1). Those that considered these subjects usually included just a sentence or two. Near the end of the nineteenth century, as the attention of educators and textbook authors shifted to temperance, with the goal of encouraging Americans to pledge to abstain from alcohol, discussion of the germ theory and vaccination remained minimal in most texts.[19]

Schoolbooks focused almost exclusively on the human body and sanitation, an emphasis that aligned well with the ideologies of alternative medicine. Books published near the mid-nineteenth century identified three causes to explain the spread of diseases like smallpox, cholera, and diphtheria: filth, bad air, and impure blood. These themes wove through nearly every nineteenth-century text, persisting for decades after confirmation of germ theory.[20] Why did

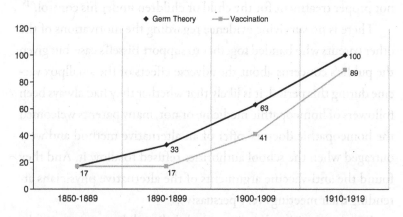

Chart 3.1. Elementary and secondary physiology, hygiene, and health textbooks mentioning germ theory or vaccination, 1850–1919 (in percentages). *Sources*: Chart created from analysis of sixty-seven textbooks housed in Cubberley Education Library, Stanford University.

this happen? In some cases, it is possible that authors' alternative beliefs about health and healing may have been an influence. However, research indicates the primary cause was what scholars call "curriculum inertia," a term denoting the slow pace of curricular change in the face of rapid social or technological developments.[21] The underlying cause of this lag was economic. Updating health textbooks involved extra costs for publishers and school districts. In some cases, authors or publishers did not bother to revise textbooks that sold well; in other cases, possibly because of the expenses associated with adopting new books, educational authorities continued to recommend older textbooks long after their content had gone out of date.[22]

The problem eventually came to the attention of the allopathic American Academy of Medicine, which in 1905 formed a committee to investigate the teaching of physiology and hygiene in elementary and secondary schools. After analyzing seventy-three textbooks published between 1883 and 1904, the committee concluded, "Distinctly scientific blunders are made. . . . Indeed it is safe to say that no book is free from a few such mishaps." Most of these "mishaps" involved outdated information about the transmission of contagious diseases. Many books taught that people could catch smallpox from filth, diphtheria from damp cellars, and malaria and typhoid fever from bad air.[23] Unfortunately, as anti-vaccination societies circulated claims based on this kind of outdated information, some Americans still found them plausible.

In Pennsylvania, anti-vaccination societies banded together to support a test case originating in Williamsport, where smallpox had broken out "and was epidemic in nearby towns."[24] Medical inspectors identified the first case of smallpox in Reading on January 24, 1893, and by the end of the epidemic there, on July 25, 1894, a total of 713 cases had been reported, with a fatality rate of 2.5 percent. The state board of health announced a general vaccination order two months after the first case appeared in Reading, which was located 106 miles southeast of Williamsport. Eleven months later, in December 1893, inspectors discovered a more serious outbreak with a fatality rate of 5.4 percent in the town of Danville, just thirty-four miles southeast of Williamsport. At the time, no one knew whether this epidemic would continue to inch closer or whether an even more virulent form of the disease would take root.[25]

Concerned, the state's Department of Public Instruction gave Pennsylvania school authorities the authority to require vaccination before admitting students. Once local newspapers announced that school boards could now enforce the vaccination requirement whenever they felt it necessary, outraged residents in Williamsport called for a meeting and quickly formed an anti-vaccination society. By the summer, anti-vaccination leagues had cropped up in other areas. In Philadelphia, a newly organized league held an open-air meeting that reportedly drew an audience of about three hundred men and women opposed to school vaccination. After the Williamsport school board refused admission to A. J. Duffield's unvaccinated child, Duffield decided to sue the board, and the Pennsylvania anti-vaccination societies rallied to his cause.[26]

Sometimes members of religious groups filed lawsuits, even when their churches did not oppose vaccination, and here too, alternative health beliefs, especially those associated with the home countries of immigrant groups, could have a role in the decision to litigate. For example, during an epidemic in 1894, when Lutheran minister John Schlerf's son was refused admission because he was unvaccinated, angry Milwaukee residents formed an anti-vaccination society to support Schlerf's lawsuit. Although the Lutheran Church did not formally oppose vaccination, Lutherans in the city began distributing anti-vaccination literature and encouraging parents to refuse to have their children vaccinated. At the time, Milwaukee was home to a large number of alternative physicians, with homeopaths comprising the largest group. According to historian Judith Leavitt, about one-third of Milwaukee's physicians agreed with the city's anti-vaccinationists and objected to the procedure, with homeopathic physicians divided over the issue. Many Lutheran immigrants had ties to Germany, where homeopathy originated, and they preferred homeopathic treatments for their illnesses and trusted the anti-vaccine messages of their own physicians. Opposition among Lutherans soon spread to other Wisconsin cities. The *Green Bay Weekly Gazette* reported, "The Lutherans of this city are going to fight the vaccination order of the State Board of Health."[27] However, the Lutherans lost their case when the judge decided the school board was within its rights to make and enforce the vaccination rule.[28]

The official beliefs of some religious organizations also motivated lawsuits against vaccination policies. The largest and most important was the Church of Christ, Scientist. A key tenet of Christian Science was that the mind had the power to prevent and cure disease through prayer. In 1896, a group of Christian Scientists in Beloit, Wisconsin, opposed on principle to any form of medical intervention, organized an anti-vaccination society to support a lawsuit against the state board.[29] The Anti-Vaccination Society of America threw its support behind this case, known as *Adams v. Burdge*, and this time the lawsuit succeeded.[30]

School Board Anxieties over Successful Lawsuits

News of successful lawsuits alarmed school authorities across the country. During the 1890s, the *American School Board Journal* (*ASBJ*) began regular reporting on school vaccination lawsuits and describing the steps school boards across the country were taking to enforce vaccination. Illinois boards breathed a sigh of relief in January 1894, when the state attorney general announced that school boards and officers who enforced the Illinois Board of Health rule requiring students to be vaccinated were "not liable for damages for suspending from attendance at school, children who refuse to submit [to] vaccination."[31] However, their relief was short-lived. Three months afterward, the *ASBJ* reported that school directors from Mount Erie, Wayne County, Illinois, had been "arrested and fined for enforcing the board's vaccination order." The Mount Erie school board appealed the case to county court in the hope that eventually the Illinois Supreme Court would "clearly define the powers of the state board and thus settle a puzzling and vexatious question."[32]

To avoid the risk of lawsuits, some school boards simply refused to comply with vaccination orders. Other boards were more assertive—in Sedalia, Missouri, after the city board of health revived the school vaccination requirement, the Sedalia school board asked the mayor and the board of health to repeal the "obnoxious ordinance."[33]

School boards everywhere followed the outcomes of lawsuits around the country with anxiety and pondered the implications for their own schools, should angry parents decide to sue. Over the years, it became clear that while some arguments were destined to fail in the courts, others had a good probability of success.

Legal Arguments and Rulings

The legal arguments against school vaccination evolved over time as plaintiffs refined their strategies to build on the successes or failures of previous cases. Some of the earliest arguments expressed the beliefs common in alternative medicine: that vaccination was ineffective, that improved sanitation and alternative health methods were far better treatments, and that smallpox vaccine poisoned the blood. As the *Indianapolis Journal* put it, after recounting the meetings of the newly formed society in Muncie, "The Anti-vaccination League just formed believe that a man is better able to make a fight against the smallpox with what pure blood he has in his system than to take into the blood cowpox, poisoning the blood and making a weaker man."[34]

However, arguments based on such beliefs were not persuasive to the courts. Although judges acknowledged the inherent risks of vaccination, they generally ruled in favor of vaccination requirements, pointing to the greater danger smallpox outbreaks posed to communities. As Chief Justice C. Gibson explained in the *Abeel v. Clark* decision:

> [California's school vaccination act] is designed to prevent the dissemination of what, notwithstanding all that medical science has done to reduce its severity, still remains a highly contagious and much dreaded disease. While vaccination may not be the best and safest preventive possible, experience and observation, the test of the value of such discoveries, dating from the year 1796, when Jenner disclosed it to the world, has proved it to be the best method known to medical science to lessen the liability to infection with the disease.[35]

Gibson's words echoed through the courts in subsequent years. On February 2, 1900, when the Indiana Supreme Court ruled against Frank Blue's case, Chief Justice James Henry Jordan quoted this passage from *Abeel* in his ruling, and in 1905 when the US Supreme Court ruled to uphold vaccination in *Jacobson v. Massachusetts*, Chief Justice John Marshall Harlan also repeated the passage, word for word. Harlan acknowledged that some laypersons and doctors did not believe in the effectiveness of vaccination. However, he emphasized the importance of the prevailing scientific evidence, "accepted by the mass of the people as well as by most members of the medical profession," that vaccination prevented the disease and was worth the risk. Citing *Abeel v. Clark*, *Bissell v. Davidson*, *Blue v. Beach*, and *Duffield v. Williamsport*, he noted that "statutes requiring children to be vaccinated in order to attend the public schools have generally been sustained by the courts."[36]

In contrast to arguments about the dangers of the smallpox vaccine, constitutional arguments found far greater traction in the courts. Judges carefully examined three aspects of plaintiff's lawsuits: first, whether a state had the constitutional right to require vaccination; second, whether existing state law authorized the school or health board in question to impose and enforce school vaccination requirements; and third, whether the imposition of the school vaccination requirements was "reasonable" in the context of current law.

The question of whether a state had constitutional "police powers"—the authority to make and enforce any laws necessary to preserve public health, safety, and general welfare—was generally settled by the late nineteenth century. The notion of police powers had deep roots in US history, originating from the English common law system used in the American colonies. A few months before the *Abeel* decision, a New York court of appeals defined the extent and limits of a state's police power to include everything necessary to maintain public health, safety, and morals. This earlier case, *Lawton v. Steele*, drew on scores of court decisions over questions of police power that stretched back to the early republican period.[37] California's supreme court decision in *Abeel* cited language from *Lawton*, concluding that the state's police power allowed it to order the compulsory vaccination of children. The court ruled the California school vaccination law was constitutional, because the state's constitution gave the legislature the power to pass laws for the public good. As Chief Justice Gibson wrote, "[I]t seems highly proper that the spread of small-pox through the public schools should be prevented or lessened by vaccination, thus affording protection both to the scholars and the community."[38]

Whether a state could enforce vaccination requirements for admission to school depended on its existing laws. Although the courts accepted that states had the authority to pass and enforce school vaccination laws to protect public health, not every state had such laws on the books, and that made a difference in case outcomes. The Christian Scientists in Beloit, Wisconsin, won their case in *Adams v. Burdge* for this reason. Unlike California, Wisconsin had never passed such a general school vaccination law. The 1876 law that established the state's board of health gave the board the authority to collect statistics, distribute information regarding matters of public health, and impose quarantine when they deemed it necessary.[39] The Wisconsin Supreme Court interpreted this language to mean that the health board could only impose compulsory vaccination when disease threatened the community. However, evidence presented during the case indicated that when the Beloit school board, following the state board of health's directions, refused admission to the plaintiff's two children, there had been no threat of smallpox in the town. As a result, Wisconsin's supreme court concluded that the state health board's power must be limited "to some particular condition or emergency in respect to the public health," and that in the absence of a smallpox outbreak or risk of contagion, "the powers of the state board of health, though quite general in terms, must be held to be limited."[40] After the Wisconsin decision, state supreme court judges in *Potts v. Breen*, an Illinois case, also ruled that without specific authority from the state legislature, it was unreasonable for a state board of health to require children be vaccinated for admission to school when smallpox did not exist in the community and was unlikely to appear.[41]

In their rulings, judges carefully considered whether the state in question had passed a law authorizing school or health boards to impose and enforce school vaccination requirements. The anti-vaccinationists lost their case in *Bissell v. Davison* because the Connecticut Supreme Court upheld a state law that gave school boards the authority to require vaccination as a condition of school attendance. In its ruling, the Connecticut court found the law both constitutional and reasonable: "It may operate to exclude [Henry Bissell's] son from school, but if so, it will be because of his failure to comply with what the legislature regards, wisely or unwisely, as a reasonable requirement, enacted in good faith to promote the public welfare."[42]

In some states, judges also considered whether municipal laws authorized school vaccination. Some state constitutions authorized cities to establish municipal charters, and in such cases, if a city's charter mandated school vaccination, the courts upheld that requirement as legally binding on the city's residents. A municipal charter defined the powers, functions, and organizations of the city government. In 1894, the anti-vaccinationists lost their case in *Duffield v. Williamsport School District* because Pennsylvania state law gave cities the authority to pass and enforce municipal ordinances, and the Williamsport city council had passed an ordinance requiring the vaccination of all students in the city's schools. As a result, the Pennsylvania Supreme Court found the school board's action to be proper in barring A. J. Duffield's unvaccinated son from school in response to a notification from the state board of health that smallpox had broken out in neighboring towns.

As explained in the court's decision, there had been no attempt to compel vaccination: "The school board do not claim that they can compel the plaintiff to vaccinate his son. They claim only the right to exclude from the schools those who do not comply with such regulations of the city and the board of directors as have been thought necessary to preserve the public health." In the court's opinion, the school board had the authority to "exclude such children as decline to comply with the requirements looking to prevention of the spread of contagion, provided these requirements are not positively unreasonable in their character."[43]

A year later, the St. Louis Court of Appeals also upheld the constitutional authority of a Missouri municipal charter in a case known as *Re Rebenack* in April 1895. In that case, the St. Louis school board had excluded lawyer August Rebenack's children from public school because he refused to have them vaccinated. Rebenack filed a mandamus to compel their readmission. However, because the municipal charter of St. Louis had authorized the school board to make all rules necessary for the government and management of its schools, the St. Louis court upheld the school board's authority to require the children be vaccinated as a condition of school attendance.[44]

By 1900, it was clear that if existing state or municipal charter law authorized the actions of health boards or school authorities in excluding unvaccinated students, the plaintiff's anti-vaccination lawsuit was very likely to fail and in the case of success, certain to fail on appeal. This is what happened with Frank Blue's lawsuit against Indiana teacher Fannie Beach and principal Orville Connor.

When Frank Blue's appeal finally reached the Indiana Supreme Court in 1900, his case rested on four main arguments: (1) vaccination poisoned the blood, frequently killed people, and did not prevent smallpox; (2) the state and local health boards did not have the legislative authority to make and enforce the school vaccination requirement; (3) although there was smallpox in Muncie, about 140 miles to the east, there were no cases of smallpox in Terre Haute when the school authorities barred his unvaccinated son from attending school; and (4) because the state constitution gave his son Kleo the right to attend public school without specifying the condition of vaccination, school authorities had no right to refuse his son admission.[45]

Indiana's supreme court set aside Blue's argument about the dangers and ineffectiveness of the smallpox vaccine, explaining that such matters were beyond the purview of the judicial courts and the responsibility of state legislatures and boards of health to determine. Instead, the court focused on what it considered the real question in the case: whether, in the absence of a state law expressly requiring vaccination as a condition of school attendance, the suspension of Kleo Blue from school could be justified.[46]

As for whether Indiana's state and local health boards had the authority to enforce the school vaccination requirement, the court decided they did, citing the 1891 statute that gave Indiana's state board of health the power to adopt regulations to prevent outbreaks of disease. This statute required all county boards of health to implement and enforce all of the state board's directives, and as the court pointed out, Terre Haute's city council had the power to create a board of health and invest it with the authority to make and enforce any rules it believed necessary to prevent the spread of smallpox. Moreover, the court cited a long list of previous cases establishing the authority of boards of health to create and enforce rules in pursuit of public health and safety.[47]

Next, the court turned to the question of whether the health board's actions were reasonable in requiring vaccination when there were no smallpox cases in town. Earlier, state supreme courts in

Wisconsin and Illinois had ruled against school vaccination laws, finding them unreasonable in the absence of any smallpox outbreaks. Judges used the concept of reasonableness to weigh whether the danger or urgency of the measure in question warranted interference with the liberty of the individual. As the supreme court of Georgia stated in 1898, "The natural right to life, liberty, and the pursuit of happiness is not an absolute right. It must yield whenever the concession is demanded by the welfare, health, or prosperity of the State. The individual must sacrifice his particular interest or desires, if the sacrifice is a necessary one, in order that organized society as a whole shall be benefited."[48]

Differences in court rulings from state to state generally hinged on the question of reasonableness. On the one hand, where the state legislature or municipal charter mandated school vaccination, the courts upheld the practice as a proper exercise of the state's police power for the protection of public health. On the other hand, where state and local boards of health had been granted general authority to protect the public from contagious disease, the validity of their policies and orders hinged on whether or not they were reasonable, leaving the question of reasonableness for the courts to determine.

Was the expulsion of Frank Blue's son necessary and therefore reasonable? Indiana's court noted that laws and regulations could not violate personal and private property rights unless they had "some relation to the end in view."[49] In this case, the court found the expulsion reasonable, pointing out that the Terre Haute health board had the authority to determine that smallpox, then threatening several areas of Indiana, might spread to the town's local schools, especially since some members of the community had been exposed to the disease. The court ruled that having made that determination, it became "the duty of the board to require that the pupils of such schools be vaccinated as a sanitary condition imposed upon their privilege of attending the schools during the period of the threatened epidemic of smallpox." The court found the health board's order entirely reasonable, since it was "intended and calculated to protect, in a time of danger, all school children, and the families of which they form a part, from smallpox."[50]

Finally, the court addressed the question of a child's right to a public education in Indiana. Did Kleo Blue's right to a public-school education mean that if he refused vaccination, school authorities were legally bound to admit him? The justices acknowledged that the privilege of children to attend public school without paying tuition was guaranteed by Indiana's constitution. Nevertheless, they pointed out that school authorities frequently denied this privilege to children who refused to submit to school rules. The court reasoned that if an expulsion could result from the violation of a rule intended to promote a safe and orderly school, then an expulsion intended to protect the health of the entire student body ought to be sustained.[51] As Chief Justice James Jordan explained, the Terre Haute health board did not force vaccination on Kleo Blue or strip him of his right to an education; instead, it simply gave him the choice of being vaccinated or staying out of school until the risk of contracting the disease had disappeared.[52] The court's decision upheld the state's police power to require vaccination in the face of threats to the public's welfare and confirmed the authority of schools to exclude unvaccinated students from school when smallpox threatened.

The decision in *Blue v. Beach*, however, did little to answer questions about school vaccination policies across the country. The differences in outcomes from state to state varied, creating a level of uncertainty that left many school districts in the dark regarding their proper position. Just prior to the ruling in *Blue v. Beach*, E. E. Collins, superintendent of public instruction in Pierre, South Dakota, wrote to his state attorney general to find out whether South Dakota's state board of health had the right to order district school boards to exclude unvaccinated students from school. As was true in some other states, South Dakota's board had the authority to create and enforce any rules necessary to prevent the spread of any contagious disease. Attorney General John L. Pyle wrote back describing the contrasting outcomes in important cases, including *Abeel*, *Duffield*, *Bissell*, *Adams v. Burdge*, and *Potts v. Breen*. Pyle was of the opinion that unless smallpox was prevalent, the health board's order could not be enforced. But he also allowed, "I have been besieged by letters from all parts of the State upon this subject," and he suggested interested health boards might "wish to look up the question for themselves."[53]

Four years later, when a vaccination case finally reached the US Supreme Court, the question remained unresolved. The case involved Henning Jacobson, a Lutheran minister living in Cambridge, Massachusetts. Jacobson opposed vaccination, not on religious grounds, but because he had experienced adverse effects when he had been vaccinated at six years of age in Sweden. In late 1901, Boston's board of health ordered everyone living in the greater Boston area to be vaccinated after a virulent strain of smallpox broke out with a fatality rate of 17 percent. Jacobson refused to comply. With help from the Massachusetts Anti-Compulsory Vaccination Association, he filed a lawsuit arguing that Section 1 of the Fourteenth Amendment to the Constitution, which proclaimed, "No state shall make or enforce any law which shall abridge the privileges or immunities of citizens of the United States; nor shall any state deprive any person of life, liberty, or property, without due process of law," gave him the right to refuse vaccination.[54]

Jacobson's case led the US Supreme Court to consider the extent of constitutional liberty in the context of vaccination. The case involved testimony from those in favor of vaccination and those opposed. When Chief Justice John Marshall Harlan issued the final ruling in 1905, he described the current state of the anti-vaccinationist movement: "It must be conceded that some laymen, both learned and unlearned, and some physicians of great skill and repute, do not believe that vaccination is a preventive of smallpox. The common belief, however, is that it has a decided tendency to prevent the spread of this fearful disease, and to render it less dangerous to those who contract it. While not accepted by all, it is accepted by the mass of the people, as well as by most members of the medical profession."[55]

Legal scholars have noted that *Jacobson v. Massachusetts* was significant on several levels. The court's ruling both upheld and placed limits on state powers. When Harlan delivered the majority decision, he noted that personal liberties could be suspended when the general public's safety was at risk, whether from military invasion or disease. As he explained, "[The] liberty secured by the Constitution of the United States to every person within its jurisdiction does not import an absolute right in each person to be, at all times and in all circumstances, wholly freed from restraint.... Real liberty for all could not exist under the operation of a principle which recognizes the right of each individual person to use his own, whether in respect of his person or his property, regardless of the injury that may be done to others."[56]

He also placed some limitation on the state's police powers, concluding that while the state could impose fines or imprison individuals who refused vaccination, authorities could not forcibly vaccinate them, as was then the practice in Massachusetts. Additionally, citing testimony from doctors opposed to vaccination, Harlan acknowledged that for some individuals who might suffer adverse reactions, requiring vaccination was an overreach of government power. This part of the ruling created a medical exemption from vaccination requirements under the Massachusetts health law, an exemption that some states had already adopted by the time of the Supreme Court ruling, and that every state in the nation adopted subsequently.[57]

Nevertheless, *Jacobson* was not a school vaccination case. Some state constitutions contained articles providing for the establishment of public schools and giving the state's children the right of attendance. The Indiana Supreme Court in *Blue v. Beach* had upheld the right of the schools to expel unvaccinated students during smallpox outbreaks, but neither the Indiana court nor the US Supreme Court addressed the question of whether a compulsory school vaccination law, one operative whether smallpox was present or not, could trump a child's constitutional right to attend public school.

In the absence of a state law specifically requiring school vaccination, if school authorities followed health board orders and expelled unvaccinated students, would they be violating the children's constitutional rights to education? School boards in many states across the country remained unsure. Not until 1922 would the US Supreme court hear a case on this issue.

Litigation against School Vaccination Laws from 1905 to 1922

Inevitably, although the number of lawsuits against school vaccination laws fell the year after *Jacobson*, newspapers soon began reporting more frequently on efforts to circumvent school vaccination requirements (chart 3.2). Some stories during this period focused on efforts among homeopathic groups to impel school authorities to accept their method of internal vaccination. Other articles reported ongoing efforts to overturn school vaccination laws.

After *Jacobsen*, some alternative physicians opposed to vaccination by injection tried a new line of attack, seeking to legalize the homeopathic alternative called *variolinum*, which involved ingesting by mouth a minute dose of cowpox virus. In 1904, the Iowa

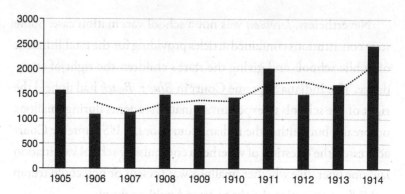

Chart 3.2. Number of US newspaper articles reporting opposition to vaccination, 1905–1914. *Source*: Data derived from a search conducted July 8, 2021, of newspapers published from 1905 through 1914 on Newspapers.com using the phrase *opposed to vaccination*.

Homeopathic Medical Society adopted a resolution defining vaccination "as the introduction of a cowpox virus into the system, either by the mouth or through the circulation by scarification of the skin." Soon homeopathic doctors in other states were advertising and recommending the oral method in letters and articles for local newspapers. Dr. William L. Morgan of Baltimore explained that patients could use the internal method without experiencing sore arms, scars, or the risk of infection from other diseases. Out in California, Bakersfield doctor S. C. Long proclaimed that hosts of physicians across the country were using the method.[58]

H. Evans, a parent in Des Moines, Iowa, filed the first successful lawsuit to force schools to accept variolinum as proof of vaccination. On February 17, 1902, he accompanied his daughter Doty to school to present a certificate of internal vaccination signed by Dr. Charles Woodhull Eaton, a homeopathic physician. After the teacher and principal refused to accept the certificate as proof of vaccination, Evans filed a petition for injunction in the district court, accusing the school board members, district superintendent, principal, and teacher of unlawfully excluding his daughter from school. His lawyers argued that because the state recognized homeopathy as an established school of medicine, boards of health could not prohibit any homeopathic method of healing or vaccination.[59] The court found this argument persuasive and granted the injunction. The growing custom of accepting internal vaccination in lieu of traditional inoculation underwent several legal tests in Iowa during the next few years, until a district court ruling in 1905 cemented the practice. On October 19 of that year, Judge N. W. Macy, of the fifteenth judicial district of Iowa, ruled that boards of health in Iowa had no authority to exclude any particular method of vaccination accepted and practiced by any school of medicine authorized by the state.[60]

Similar lawsuits over the homeopathic method called variolinum emerged in Pennsylvania and Missouri, but neither state followed in Iowa's footsteps. In 1908, the public school district in Edgewood, Pennsylvania, refused to accept an altered certificate of vaccination presented by eight-year-old Dorothy M. Lee. Dr. W. R. Stephens, a homeopathic physician who served on the Wilkinsburg board of health, had given Dorothy an oral dose of vaccine matter. Pennsylvania's official vaccination certificates required doctors to inoculate patients on an arm and confirm that they had observed "a resulting sore" on that arm several days after the procedure. The sore, which eventually turned into a small scar, indicated the vaccination had been effective. But oral doses produced no external sores or other visible signs on the body. Seeking to circumvent the requirement, when he signed Dorothy's certificate, Stephens crossed out the words "I find a resultant sore" so the certificate simply stated, "I find a result, which in my opinion means a successful vaccination." However, school authorities refused to accept the altered certificate, and when they excluded Dorothy from school, her father sued.[61] Henry E. Lee's lawyer argued that homeopathic vaccination should be accepted, because homeopathic doctors were recognized professionally under Pennsylvania law. The lawyer for the defense argued that the state board of health, which created the vaccination certificate, had the authority to make rules requiring its use to protect public health. When the court ruled for the defense, Lee appealed to the state supreme court.[62] Three years later, Pennsylvania's supreme court upheld the lower court's ruling, dealing a blow to the anti-vaccinationists and supporters of variolinum.[63]

In 1910, homeopathic physician L. M. Ottofy of St. Louis began a three-year legal battle to force the local school board to accept his two children's internal vaccination certificates as valid. Ottofy had been signing alternative vaccination certificates in St. Louis for years, and newspapers described his lawsuit as "representing homeopathists opposed to vaccination."[64] Unfortunately for Ottofy and his supporters, a district court in St. Louis ruled that the city's school board had the authority to compel the external vaccination of students, whether a smallpox epidemic was raging or not. Undeterred, Ottofy was determined to appeal, but his war against the school district unexpectedly ground to a halt after Mrs. Ottofy, on a day when her husband was out of town, "called in the assistant health commissioner and had her children vaccinated."[65]

After Ottofy's case fell apart, newspaper coverage of disputes over internal vaccination declined, most likely because few homeopaths supported the practice, and it gradually fell out of favor. The *Pittsburgh Daily Post* reported that "leading homeopaths say that there is not one of their school in a thousand who uses the internal method of inoculating against smallpox as opposed to the scarification or vaccination method." Still, the *Post* acknowledged that large numbers of homeopathic doctors in Pennsylvania believed the school vaccination law should be changed on the grounds that it interfered with medical liberty and individual rights.[66]

Some of the lawsuits that parents brought against school districts and health boards succeeded. Successful lawsuits generally hinged on the question of potential conflict between school admission requirements and existing state laws, municipal codes, and health board regulations. These cases fell into two categories: One type included situations in which smallpox threatened or was actually epidemic. If no state or municipal statutes existed to give schools the authority to require vaccination in such instances, anti-vaccination lawsuits of this sort sometimes succeeded. However, if such laws did exist, the lawsuits failed, because judges upheld laws giving school authorities the power to protect the public health. The other category included cases in which there was no danger from the disease. Louise Jenkins's suit against Chicago's city school board fell into the latter category. Chicago's board refused admission to the unvaccinated girl in response to a directive from the commissioner of health. Unfortunately for the board, the Illinois Supreme Court ruled in favor of Jenkins in 1908. According to Chicago's municipal code, the commissioner of health could impose any regulations deemed necessary, but only during an epidemic, and he had to submit such regulations first to the city council. The court found that not only had there been no epidemic at the time, but the commissioner had also failed to notify the city council.[67] Similarly, with help from the American Medical Liberty League in 1919, chiropractor William F. Rhea won a lawsuit against a public school in North Dakota because smallpox was neither epidemic nor threatening at the time, and the state had never passed a school vaccination law.[68]

Unsuccessful lawsuits included those in which plaintiffs argued that school vaccination laws violated their constitutional right to freedom of religion. In 1879, the US Supreme Court had ruled on the limits of religious liberty in *Reynolds v. United States*, a case involving a law banning polygamy. In that case, the Supreme Court unanimously ruled that the law did not infringe on the individual's right to the free exercise of religion, because Congress retained the authority to regulate actions that violated social duties or subverted the common good. Subsequently, numerous cases on the question of religious liberty cited this ruling.[69] In the absence of any state law allowing religious exemption from vaccination, this earlier ruling made it impossible to win an anti-vaccination lawsuit on the basis of religion, as illustrated by a case in Texas. When the city of New Braunfels required students to be vaccinated during a smallpox outbreak, Christian Scientist Fritz Waldschmidt sued on behalf of his children, arguing that the procedure violated their religious beliefs. In 1918, the Texas Supreme Court ruled against them, citing *Reynolds*. In its ruling, the court pointed out that just as the US Congress had the right to regulate actions for the common good, so too the Bill of Rights in the Texas Constitution did not "relieve one from obedience to reasonable health regulations."[70]

One of the most persistent issues in anti-vaccination lawsuits after 1905 was the possible conflict between compulsory education laws and school vaccination requirements. The issue remained unresolved, leaving educators in many areas struggling to know how to respond to public health board vaccination orders.

In Pennsylvania, the State Convention of School Directors reported, "The conflict between the compulsory attendance and vaccination laws is such that in many communities the authorities do not know how to act."[71] A lawsuit brought the issue to a head. When J. H. Reber, superintendent of the public schools in Waynesboro, expelled fourteen-year-old Grace Stull for refusing vaccination, her father sued, arguing that the state's school attendance laws meant she was legally entitled to attend the school. Newspapers reported that members of the local anti-vaccination society crowded the district courtroom in support of Edward C. Stull's lawsuit, but their presence made no difference in the outcome. The court ruled in favor of the school superintendent, concluding that compulsory attendance could not be enforced when it conflicted with the vaccination law.[72] Stull and his lawyers appealed the case to the state's highest court.

The Pennsylvania Supreme Court's ruling in *Stull v. Reber* established an important precedent in Pennsylvania for questions about the possibility of conflict between school admission policies and health board regulations. Chief Justice C. J. Mitchell noted that the main question in the case was whether the state's school vaccination law contravened the state constitution or was a valid use of the state's police power. Ultimately, the court ruled that the state's interest in preserving public health trumped the privilege of students to attend the schools: "the police power of the commonwealth in the preservation of the public health must, if necessity arises, sacrifice the less to the greater interest."[73] As the *ASBJ* noted in its regular column on school laws, this was the third time Pennsylvania's supreme court had upheld the law as constitutional.[74]

Over the next five years, more court rulings in Pennsylvania made it clear that if parents decided to keep their children out of school because they refused to vaccinate them, they could be found guilty of violating the state's compulsory education law. The first decision on this point was made in a case in 1916 involving James H. Aiken, who refused to have his eight-year-old daughter vaccinated. Following state law, the school principal sent her home. Aiken sued but lost his case. When it became clear after several months that Aiken, to avoid vaccinating his daughter, had not enrolled her in any school, Justice James W. Watson fined him two dollars for violating the compulsory education law. The local Anti-Compulsory Vaccination Society in Pittsburgh supported Aiken's lawsuit, but the superior court ruled against him. Similar cases had the same outcome.[75]

Although the issue appeared to be resolved in Pennsylvania, educators in other states still feared lawsuits from parents claiming that school vaccination requirements violated the compulsory education laws and their children's constitutional rights. Given the lack of uncertainty across the country, it was inevitable that a case would come before the highest court in the nation.

The US Supreme Court weighed in on school vaccination in 1922. Three years earlier, school authorities in San Antonio, Texas, had expelled dentist A. D. Zucht's children from school for refusing to be vaccinated. They did this because the city council had passed an ordinance requiring the compulsory vaccination of all students enrolled in San Antonio schools. The Zucht family argued that because there was no smallpox in town at the time, the vaccination requirement was unreasonable, and the children had been deprived of liberty without due process of law. Naming his eldest child as plaintiff, Zucht filed a lawsuit against the city's health board and school authorities, seeking damages of $10,000 for each of his three children: Rosalyn, aged fifteen years; Arthur, aged thirteen years; and Francis, aged ten years. The suit named Dr. W. A. King, the city health officer, the trustees of the school board, and the principal of the school his children attended.[76] After losing in district court, Zucht appealed to the Texas Supreme Court, which upheld the lower court's verdict. In response, Rosalyn Zucht appealed to the US Supreme Court, which agreed to take the case.[77]

Zucht's lawyers claimed that the city of San Antonio did not have the authority to require unvaccinated students to be expelled from school. They also argued that because San Antonio's health department required only students to be vaccinated and did not require vaccination of the entire populace, the vaccination order represented a form of class discrimination and thus violated the Fourteenth

Amendment of the US Constitution.[78] There had been no cases of smallpox in San Antonio when the city health director ordered school authorities to expel Rosalyn Zucht. For this reason, anti-vaccinationists across the country watched the case with interest, hoping the court would find the order unreasonable.

In a blow to the anti-vaccination movement, on November 13, 2022, the court upheld the validity of state laws and city ordinances that required the vaccination of children as a school admission requirement. The opinion in *Zucht v. King*, penned by Justice Louis Brandeis, cemented and extended the earlier Supreme Court decision in *Jacobson v. Massachusetts*. As Brandeis noted, drawing from previous case rulings, states had the power to pass and enforce compulsory vaccination laws to protect the public from harm. States could delegate this power to municipal governments. Moreover, states and municipalities could allow local authorities such as health and school boards "broad discretion required for the protection of health."

In other words, unless a state's laws had explicit wording limiting school vaccination to periods of disease outbreaks, the broad discretion allowed to state and municipal health boards included the authority to decide when to require vaccination as a condition of admission to school. Because the San Antonio vaccination ordinance was valid, as was the authority of the officials that carried it out in expelling her from school, the court found that Rosalyn Zucht had not presented a substantial constitutional question by simply asserting that San Antonio authorities had violated her Fourteenth Amendment right to due process.[79]

After *Zucht v. King*, the number of lawsuits against school vaccination fell, a development reflected in the declining coverage of opposition to vaccination in US newspapers. The decline in lawsuits reflected the greater clarity that state and federal supreme court rulings had brought to the issue of school vaccination requirements over the previous decades.

Conclusion

Many of the plaintiffs who sued their local school districts over school vaccination during the Progressive Era cited the rhetoric of the national anti-vaccination societies: that the smallpox vaccine caused a host of other diseases, that sanitation alone would protect against smallpox, and that injecting vaccine serum into the body was inherently dangerous. The surviving court records are a testimony to the long endurance of these arguments, even as they failed to gain traction in the courts. The legal arguments against school vaccination evolved as plaintiffs refined their strategies to focus on constitutional arguments more likely to succeed. Judges weighed three aspects of plaintiff's lawsuits: first, whether state law required vaccination; second, whether existing law gave school or health authorities the power to enforce school vaccination requirements, and third, whether the application of the law in the case was reasonable.

To the great relief of school districts everywhere, the U.S. Supreme Court ruling in *Zucht v. King*, which upheld the validity of laws that required the vaccination of children as a school admission requirement, finally resolved the apparent contradiction between compulsory education and compulsory school vaccination laws. In later years, court rulings would make it clear that there existed no conflict between a state's compulsory education laws and its compulsory vaccination laws. A child's right to education was not an absolute right—it could be suspended if the child or the child's guardians refused to follow school regulations, including regulations requiring vaccination. Requiring vaccination as a prerequisite to school attendance thus neither violated the child's right to a free public education, nor did it violate the state's compulsory education laws. Multiple rulings on this issue established the precept that safe schools were a precondition to education, and that it was well within the state's interest to require vaccination as a condition of attendance to ensure the safety of all students from contagious disease.

While the number of lawsuits waned after 1922, opposition to vaccination did not vanish—vaccine opponents simply shifted tactics. In some areas, local groups affiliated with the American Medical Liberty League began organizing to support state legislation allowing religious or philosophical exemptions from school vaccination requirements. California became one of the first states to pass a law allowing nonmedical exemption from its school vaccination requirements. And as the following chapter shows, that legislation had the full support of the state's school superintendents.

4

Schools against Vaccination Mandates
A Case Study

News reports of opposition to vaccination mandates often focused on anti-vaccination societies and parents' lawsuits, but school authorities also sometimes opposed the mandates. One of the most dramatic disputes occurred in Seattle, where in May 1895, the local health board identified scarlet fever in the city's south end. There was no vaccine to protect against the disease. Knowing that only quarantine could stop its spread, the health board ordered two schools in the affected area—Ranier School and South School—to close for the rest of the academic year. However, the school board opposed the order, claiming that only school officials had the power to deny admission to any member of an infected family.[1]

Determined to shut down the schools, the health board enlisted the help of local police. On May 16, when the principal, teachers, and students arrived at Rainier School, they found the doors locked and a health official and police officer standing guard outside. Undeterred, the principal walked to the back of the building and snuck into the basement through a window. The teachers followed him, and once the students saw their teachers were inside, they rushed the school, seeking entrance through windows and doors any way they could. Chaos erupted. The conflict in Seattle between the health and school boards was resolved only when the city council, concerned about recurring outbreaks of scarlet fever, passed an ordinance giving the health board the power to close the schools for as long as it thought necessary to control disease.[2]

In most cases across the country, educators' resistance to public health mandates was much more covert. For example, in a survey conducted in Kansas in 1885, county health officers reported that in many areas, school boards were not complying with vaccination rules. They were not actively opposing the rules—they were simply ignoring them.[3] This sort of recalcitrance was an endless source of frustration for public health officers across the country. As one New York health official complained, referring to the unwillingness of school officials to exclude unvaccinated children from the schools, "Unless WE make the arrangements very little is done."[4]

Arguably the most extensive and long-lasting conflict between educators and health officials took place in California, where for about three decades, from 1889 to 1921, school boards and superintendents across the state refused to enforce the school vaccination law. Some historians have portrayed such conflicts as power struggles between the professional medical elites appointed to the health boards and the amateur citizens elected to the school boards.[5] However, in California, apart from San Francisco and a few other cities, most health boards were composed of elected amateur citizens, just as were the school boards. Moreover, California was not that exceptional. Across the United States, mayors and town councils often appointed health board members, but in some areas, citizens elected them. This happened in at least ten other states besides California, including Alabama, Connecticut, Florida, Iowa, Massachusetts, Michigan, Nebraska, New York, Tennessee, and Texas. In California, no doctors served on the elected health boards of Los Angeles, Stockton, Santa Rosa, Chico, and other towns, and in some cities only one doctor could serve on the board, with no stipulation that the doctor practice allopathic, rather than alternative, medicine. And in these communities, the authority to refuse admission to unvaccinated students lay with school authorities, not the local health board.[6]

The growing tension between health and school boards in California was due to a perceived conflict in their respective roles and responsibilities. Educators believed their primary duty was to teach children, and effective teaching required that students regularly attend school. From the educators' perspective, the state's new vaccination law interfered with their core mission. Educators were not immune to the anti-vaccination rhetoric circulating throughout the state, but even those who supported vaccination on principle viewed it as tangential to their work in public schools. School leaders had long understood the importance of teaching children to improve and protect their health, but they did not always equate health with vaccination. In the opinion of many education leaders, enforcing vaccination was simply not their responsibility.

California's school superintendents took this position to an extreme, seeking for several decades to revise or overturn the school vaccination laws. Eventually their efforts succeeded, ushering in a new era of voluntary vaccination programs based on a policy of persuasion. Only then did the state's education leaders come to better understand the value of vaccination in providing immunity from contagious disease in the schools.

Opposition to the Law

Anti-vaccination activism became a widespread social phenomenon in California after the state passed a compulsory school vaccination law in 1889 in response to a serious smallpox epidemic. Opposition came from three sources: concerned parents, anti-vaccination groups, and school officials.

The first significant opposition arose when D. K. Abeel filed a lawsuit after his unvaccinated son was excluded from Santa Cruz High School. Abeel's case effectively suspended implementation of the law until the California Supreme Court ruled in its favor.[7] After the court's ruling, the state board of health secretary, Dr. G. G. Tyrrell, was confident there would be smooth sailing ahead: "The decision of the Supreme Court having now definitely settled the constitutionality of the law, we expect that no trouble will be experienced in having it enforced."[8] He could not have been more wrong. California's compulsory vaccination law sparked contentious debates in many communities, as illustrated by the growing number of newspaper reports on opposition to school vaccination between 1890 and 1909 (chart 4.1).

From the beginning, the law placed a financial and administrative burden on the public schools. It stipulated that school board trustees were to exclude from the schools "any child or any person who has not been vaccinated." For those unable to pay, the cost of inoculation would be taken from each district's school fund, and if any district had insufficient funds, the county superintendent would have to raise the money through a tax levied on the public.[9]

At first, San Francisco Bay Area school boards' resistance to the new law was covert. Some boards simply dragged their feet. In the fall of 1894, the *San Francisco Call* reported a persistent rumor that "Oakland, Berkeley and San Jose school directors had ignored the

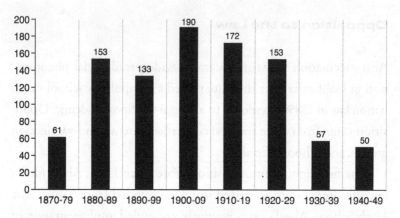

Chart 4.1. Number of California newspaper articles on opposition to school vaccination, by decade, 1870–1949. *Source*: Data derived from a search conducted June 12, 2022, of newspapers published from 1870 through 1949 in the California Digital Newspaper Collection (https://cdnc.ucr.edu) using the term *opposed to vaccination*.

law, and everything was running as smoothly with them as in other cities where vaccination was compulsory."[10]

The Anti-Vaccination Society of America's national campaign to elect anti-vaccinationists to school boards may have strengthened opposition in the region. Five well-known Bay Area anti-vaccinationists were AVSA members during this period, including Malinda Elliott Cramer, founder of the Church of Divine Science and an advocate of faith healing; two physicians from the fields of homeopathy and eclectic medicine; and two Oakland residents, one of whom was Wilbur Walker, secretary of the Merchants' Exchange of Oakland. One of Walker's children had died after having been vaccinated, and he came to exert an important influence in efforts to overturn the state's vaccination law in the district. However, it is difficult to assess the degree to which the AVSA influenced any school board elections, given the absence of any direct evidence.[11]

Berkeley's board was among the first to openly resist the law. During an outbreak of smallpox in 1896, the board protested the order that all unvaccinated pupils in the Berkeley schools be inoculated as a condition of school attendance. The following year the board decided to allow nonmedical exemptions, stating that parents must vaccinate their children unless they "absolutely refuse to comply with the law because they do not believe in its efficacy." Appalled, local allopathic physicians wrote an open letter to the *San Francisco Call* pointing out that this action did not conform to state law.[12]

The Berkeley board's provision that students be exempt from vaccination on the basis of belief came to be termed "conscientious exemption" in California. However, at the time, this notion failed to gain widespread acceptance. Protesters in other cities and towns did not agitate for conscientious exemption—they simply wanted the law repealed.

School boards everywhere had to respond to the concerns of anxious and angry parents who packed their meetings. Parent protests in Los Angeles prompted the city's school board to recommend repealing the law. By 1899, nine years after the California Supreme Court upheld the compulsory school vaccination law, the board still had not begun to comply. At a meeting in January of that year, the local health board pointed out that less than 40 percent of the city's schoolchildren had been vaccinated against smallpox. After some discussion, the school board agreed to require vaccination, but only if the board of health provided the lymph and hired physicians to vaccinate children whose parents were unable to pay.[13] Parents soon convened an "anti-compulsory vaccination meeting" at the music hall, and at the next meeting of the school board, angry protestors filled the room. In response, the board delayed implementation of the requirement by several weeks, telling the crowd that "the proper recourse lay in having the law changed by the legislature or by testing its constitutionality in the courts."[14]

In Los Angeles, over ten thousand citizens signed a petition asking their state representatives to overturn the law. In San Diego, more than eight hundred signed a similar petition. Aware that the state legislature would not meet again until 1901, those who wanted speedy action adopted a different tactic. Santa Barbara's *Morning Press* reported that the anti-vaccinationists threatened a lawsuit: "If the board of education requires all school children to be vaccinated or forfeit their right to attend school, a suit will be brought in the courts to test the law."[15]

Despite this flurry of grassroots activism, by 1903 the state's vaccination law was still on the books. The attempt to repeal the law had come too late to secure a hearing, and to the relief of school boards everywhere, a legislative attempt to allow plaintiffs to sue school districts and recover damages for adverse effects after vaccination failed to pass.[16]

The attempt to overturn the law gained traction in 1904 with the support of the state's school superintendents. The entry of county superintendents into the battle pitted education elites against the medical elites on some health boards. Whereas the authority of local health boards was rooted in the freeholder charters of cities and towns, the authority of school superintendents was embedded in California's constitution.[17] The conflicts between the professionals on the health boards and the professional superintendents in charge of city and county school districts were clashes between two different types of administrative authority and jurisdiction. School superintendents participated in professional organizations such as the National Association of School Superintendents, founded in 1865. Most elected to the position had risen up through the ranks of their profession, from teacher to principal to superintendent. They were accustomed to wielding power and authority—county superintendents supervised the work of local districts; in some cities, district superintendents served as the executive officers of their respective school boards.[18]

More important, the dispute between health and education officials arose from an unintended consequence of city charter and case law, whereby a local health board's decision to bar unvaccinated students from the public schools dealt a financial blow to the schools. State funds were tied to school enrollments. When schools barred unvaccinated students, they lost revenue for each day that students were absent from their classrooms.

Tired of dealing with angry citizens over the state requirements, fearful of the possibility of lawsuits in the case of any injury following the procedure, and unhappy with the financial burden of enforcing the law, superintendents proposed to relinquish all responsibility and oversight of school vaccinations. At the biennial convention of California school superintendents in Santa Barbara in May 1904, members unanimously adopted the following resolution: "Resolved. That it is the sense of the superintendents that the educational department of the state should not be burdened with the responsibility of carrying out the intent of the statute requiring vaccination; that the law should be so changed that the responsibility should fall upon the health department for enforcement independent of the school organization."[19]

Emboldened by the superintendents' resolution, more local school boards began to express opposition to the school vaccination requirements. In August, three hundred people met in Berkeley to form a new Anti-Compulsory Vaccination League to fight the state law. Dr. W. W. Allen, the president of Berkeley's school board, was elected league president, Eugenia C. Campbell secretary, and J. Stitt Wilson, a Methodist minister and Christian socialist, treasurer. Allen and Wilson claimed that vaccination did not prevent smallpox and was fatal. The organizers gave rousing speeches and read aloud letters of support from the Anti-Vaccination Society of America and from the Canadian anti-vaccinationist Dr. Alexander Ross. The *San Francisco Call* reported that the new league planned to establish affiliated groups "all over the state, organized specifically to fight for the repeal of the law."[20]

Two weeks after this meeting, Myrtle Conklin, a seven-year-old girl, died of tetanus, and Dr. Allen declared that her recent vaccination had caused her death. Outraged, members of the Anti-Compulsory Vaccination League proposed to sue those responsible, including the local board of education and the board of health "to test the constitutionality of the compulsory vaccination law."[21] Within a few days, local anti-vaccination groups sprang into action in other California cities.[22]

The movement gained supporters in the state legislature, and on February 21, 1905, legislators passed a bill banning compulsory vaccination from the schools. However, to the dismay of its supporters, Governor George C. Pardee vetoed the bill on March 8. Pardee was an allopathic doctor. He had obtained his medical degree from the Cooper Medical College after graduating from the University of California and had also spent time studying medicine in Germany.[23]

His remarks explaining his veto were widely reported in the press. He acknowledged that serious adverse effects, "and even death" could follow vaccination, but he pointed out that such cases were extremely rare. He also explained that by itself, the smallpox vaccine did not cause tetanus, or lockjaw, but that tetanus could occur when slight wounds became infected with the tetanus bacillus. "When vaccination is compulsory and the law is well administered," he said, "those protected by vaccination soon lose their fear of the dread disease. And turning their attention to the lesser evils of the vaccine virus, many of us conjure a fear not warranted by facts against the very thing that saves us from a much worse fate. And this I think, is what has called into being the bill which I now return to you unsigned." Pardee was convinced that if the bill were to become law, "vaccination would soon fall into practical disuse. And thus would be prepared among our children (not mine, for they shall always be protected) a field for smallpox to fairly revel in."[24]

The Senate found Pardee's candid explanation of the relative risks and benefits of vaccination compelling. By a vote of twenty-three to three, the senators refused to pass the bill over his veto.[25]

Undeterred, over the next few years, county superintendents continued to lobby to rescind the law. Even those who supported vaccination threw their support behind the cause. For example, at the 1906 Biennial Convention of California School Superintendents, San Francisco's superintendent argued for keeping the vaccination law, stating that public safety in San Francisco depended on it. However, he wanted it revised to apply to private schools as well. Dr. Charlotte Johnson Baker of San Diego also spoke at the meeting. Baker, an obstetrician and the first female doctor to practice in San Diego, was active in the fight to win suffrage for women in California and supported vaccination. She informed the audience that vaccination had proven its value in epidemics, but like many others at the meeting, she believed the state, rather than the schools, should have charge of vaccinating schoolchildren.

Baker favored a contingent vaccination law that would go into effect only when smallpox threatened the community. She explained that this was common practice in other states. When someone asked, "How do they enforce vaccination in most of these states?" she answered, "By a very simple method. They give people the choice between quarantine during the entire epidemic and vaccination. It usually doesn't take them long to decide." The audience erupted in laughter. At the end of the discussion, regardless of differences of opinion regarding vaccination, the superintendents unanimously adopted a resolution "that the public schools be relieved of the enforcement of the vaccination law."[26]

Over the next few years, county superintendents advanced two arguments to support their case: First, that excluding unvaccinated children from the public schools violated the state's 1905 compulsory education law, which required all students to attend school; and second, that enforcement of the law hurt student enrollments. At their 1907 convention, the superintendents unanimously voted to request the repeal of the law. As they explained in their motion, "The present law works against the public school and in favor of private institutions, many parents insisting on taking their children out of the public schools rather than submit to vaccination."[27]

During this period, as new outbreaks of smallpox began to emerge, few schools excluded unvaccinated students. Dr. Newel Kelly Foster, secretary of the state board of health in 1904, blamed both local health officers and school boards. Health officers had the legal authority to impose quarantine, but in some areas with smallpox, they were doing nothing. According to Foster, lax health officials had allowed infected people to roam the streets and travel by train and other public conveyances, allowing the disease to spread. He was also appalled that so few public schools obeyed the compulsory vaccination law in excluding unvaccinated students. "Such a stand taken by school trustees is more than a statutory crime; it is morally outrageous."[28]

For their part, educators highlighted the issue of enrollment loss repeatedly. In 1907, Berkeley's school board reported that by following the vaccination law, "several hundred pupils have been forced from the schools and the department has lost the state funds which would be due the town" had the children remained enrolled. To make matters worse, parents had begun enrolling their children in an independent school in Berkeley free of any vaccination requirements.

The board asked the district attorney to provide an opinion as to whether the vaccination law and the school truancy law were in conflict.[29] That year, an assemblyman from Berkeley introduced a bill to repeal the vaccination law, a measure the *Los Angeles Herald* reported as having the support of educators across the state: "The school superintendents of the state and other educational authorities have been the prime movers in having the law repealed, claiming that thousands of children were being denied an education on account of it." However, as happened with earlier bills, this one failed to pass.[30]

Two years later, at the state school superintendents' convention in Yosemite, the superintendents of San Diego and Los Angeles vowed to refuse to vaccinate. Boards in other cities reportedly continued to ignore the law. Some city health officers threw in the towel. As the health officer in Santa Cruz stated, "I know there is a very strong sentiment in this city against vaccinating children, and I know if we tried to enforce this law it would make lots of trouble."[31]

During this period, census reports showed the proportion of vaccinated students in the state's public schools plunged from just below 80 percent in 1906 to around 50 percent in 1910.[32] To put this in context, today scientists believe that to achieve the threshold percentage of immune individuals that would lead to a decline in outbreaks of smallpox, between 80 and 100 percent of the population would need to be vaccinated.[33] Public health officials were very concerned that the resistance against school vaccination would lead to more dangerous outbreaks of disease.

The battle between health and school officials reached a high point over a case in Watsonville, a town in the Monterey Bay Area. When Watsonville's school board, with backing from the county school superintendent, refused to bar unvaccinated students from the schools, the state board of health successfully petitioned state Superior

Court Judge Lucas F. Smith to exclude the unvaccinated children from the town's schools. The fight did not end there, however. The resulting case, *State Board of Health v. Board of Trustees of Watsonville*, went all the way to the state court of appeals.[34]

Watsonville's board argued that California's 1905 compulsory education law superseded and invalidated the older compulsory vaccination law. This argument was destined to fail, given earlier court rulings that found no conflict between compulsory education and compulsory vaccination laws, including the earlier Supreme Court ruling in *Abeel v. Clarke*. Not surprisingly, the court upheld the vaccination law as constitutional. As Judge Smith wrote, "The vaccination act of 1889 is not repealed or affected by the compulsory education act of 1905. . . . While parents must send their children to school under the latter act, if they desire to send them to the common schools, they must comply with the former act, which continues to apply to all common or public schools, and is not in any way modified or superseded by the latter act."[35]

However, this legal victory did nothing to slow opposition to the law—newspapers reported that anti-vaccination societies were still forming across the state.[36] The societies organizing across California included homeopathic and eclectic physicians still reluctant to accept the germ theory of disease, individuals who believed in faith healing or other forms of alternative medicine, medical libertarians opposed on principle to any form of compulsory medical intervention during outbreaks of disease, and individuals who feared adverse effects from the smallpox vaccine.[37] Now more than ever, these groups found common cause in the effort to overturn the state's compulsory vaccination law.

Some parents joined them and became active in political activism; others simply voted with their feet and left the public schools. In Long Beach, a city the *Morning Press* described as "one of the hotbeds of opposition to compulsory vaccination," so many parents had withdrawn their children from the public schools to enroll them in private schools free of any vaccination requirements, that there was "a conspicuous absence of many children" in public school classrooms.[38]

Worried about low vaccination rates, Secretary William Freeman Snow of the state board of health decided to survey Californians to discover their specific objections to vaccinating their children. His informal survey involved conversations and correspondence with members of the Berkeley-based Anti-Vaccination League, school superintendents, district school boards, and members of local communities.[39] As he wrote to one member of Santa Barbara's school board opposed to the state law, "This board is sincere in its determination to make a thorough study of all sides of this question.... [W]hile I personally believe in the principles of vaccination and its efficacy as a preventive measure when fully enforced, I desire to acquaint myself with every argument of those who do not so believe."[40]

The board of health published a narrative summary of the results, reporting that community members opposed to vaccination commonly held one or more of the following three beliefs: (1) that smallpox was not spread by germs, but by filth, and therefore sanitation, rather than vaccination or quarantine, would eliminate smallpox; (2) that injecting vaccine serum, a foreign matter, into humans was unnatural and therefore dangerous; and (3) that the smallpox vaccine would cause tuberculosis, tetanus, acne, and a host of other unrelated ailments.[41]

To address the claim that vaccination could spread a host of unrelated diseases, William Snow published a report pointing out that the scientific community accepted the germ theory of disease, the concept of contagion, and the effectiveness of vaccination. He explained that it was impossible for the smallpox vaccine to cause tuberculosis and that cases of tetanus at the vaccination site could only occur if the arm became infected after the injection through lack of proper care. As for the many other ailments opponents claimed resulted from vaccination, he argued that many people who had developed acne or the measles after receiving the smallpox vaccination might have developed those conditions even if they had not been vaccinated. He also sought to alleviate the concerns of the teachers, school boards, and superintendents who bore the brunt of anti-vaccination anger and outrage. He recommended, "Any differences of opinion among citizens over the details of this law should be referred to the State Board of Health for interpretation, rather than to the teacher or the local school trustees."[42]

Excerpts from the board of health's reports appeared in newspapers across the state, but they seem to have had little impact. By the fall of 1910, without mentioning any names, news media reported that anti-vaccination activists were once again circulating a petition throughout the state to repeal the compulsory vaccination law so that "school children shall not be compelled to be vaccinated in those cases where their parents object to such vaccination."[43]

Santa Barbara's *Morning Press* reported that opposition to vaccination was causing many parents across the city to consider moving their children to private schools that did not require vaccination. One parent had floated the idea of a segregated public school system, recommending the creation of a separate school in which teachers who opposed vaccination could instruct unvaccinated children.[44] In a panic, F. M. Fultz, Santa Barbara's school superintendent, informed the community that withdrawing children from the public schools would deplete the district's funding. He urged parents to go ahead and send their unvaccinated children to school, promising that things could be resolved in future. Board members began talking about a proposal to allow parents to submit an alternative remedy signed by a homeopathic physician as effective against smallpox. They knew this practice would probably be rejected by the state's board of health and that "in all probability, the courts will eventually be invoked and the battle fought." Nevertheless, in Santa Barbara, desperate times called for desperate measures.[45]

The 1911 Law Allowing
Conscientious Exemption

Foreseeing an upcoming battle in the state legislature, the board of health presented its own proposed bill to the legislature in January 1911. The difference between earlier attempts to repeal the law and the effort in 1911 is the degree of compromise evident among the state's health board, the Anti-Vaccination League, and school superintendents and school board members.

The board of health's proposal included two recommendations designed to appeal to the state's school leaders. First, it proposed to remove enforcement of the vaccination law from local school boards and place it in the hands of the local health boards. California's school superintendents had been advocating for this over the previous seven years, and health authorities also had a vested interest in wanting more control over the law's enforcement. Second, the board of health recommended expanding the compulsory school vaccination law so that it applied not only to the children in public schools but also to students in private schools and those not currently attending school. For years, public school boards had expressed anxiety over the enrollment loss that resulted when parents moved their children to private schools to avoid the vaccination requirement. This proposal would eliminate that problem. And of course, from the board of health's perspective, the expansion of vaccination would help in the long-standing fight against smallpox.[46]

Both of these recommendations eventually found their way into Senate Bill 655, sponsored by Senator H. M. Hurd of Los Angeles.[47] As the legislature began its debate, San Diego County Superintendent Hugh Baldwin, who had just returned from spending two weeks discussing the measure in Sacramento, proclaimed, "The question of vaccination in the public schools promises to develop into a warm fight at this session." According to Baldwin, "The bill most favored by the teachers and those connected with the schools is the one which does not make it compulsory for a child to be vaccinated before entering the school."[48] Despite the prediction of a legislative battle, S.B. 655 passed on February 22, and Governor Hiram Johnson signed it into law on March 7, 1911.[49]

With passage of the new law, California began allowing conscientious exemption from school vaccination requirements. The law applied to both private and public schools. To attend school, every student now had to submit either a doctor's signed certificate of successful vaccination, a doctor's signed statement explaining that the student was medically unable to be vaccinated, or a signed statement from the parents or guardians stating that the family was "conscientiously opposed to vaccination." Health officers retained the power to exclude unvaccinated students from schools when local communities faced outbreaks of disease—during such events, all unvaccinated students would have to leave the school until the local health board declared the epidemic to be over.[50]

As is often the case with outcomes based on political compromise, none of the groups involved in the legislation's development was entirely satisfied with the result. The state's health board described the new law as "a lonely waif": "The teachers befriended it because it relieves the schools of the serious friction resulting from the old-law discrimination between the public and the private school. The State Board of Health and the Anti-vaccination League agreed to endorse it as a fair compromise between their divergent points of view."[51]

The Movement to Repeal the Law

California's 1911 law allowing conscientious exemption from school vaccination passed because public health officials, school leaders, and state legislators feared that without it, more parents would withdraw their children from the public schools and continued anti-vaccination protests would cause ongoing turmoil and undermine the public's trust in vaccines. However, the law did not resolve these problems, and in 1921 the state's board of health decided to support its repeal.

The 1911 law did not strengthen Californians' trust in the smallpox vaccine. Over the next decade, more families took advantage of the provision allowing conscientious exemption from vaccination, and outbreaks of smallpox occurred each year. From 1917 to 1920, the number of cases increased sharply (table 4.1). In 1920, the health board reported that because of the increased use of exemptions, vaccination rates had fallen dramatically: "It is estimated that nearly 75 or 80 per cent of the children in most communities of the state are at the present time unvaccinated."[52]

The fact that smallpox no longer seemed deadly may have partly explained the reluctance of California parents to vaccinate their children. During the years from 1920 to 1925, the state's board of health received reports of 28,592 cases of smallpox, and in 1925, the US Health Service reported that there were more cases of smallpox in California than in any other state in the nation.[53] But despite the

Table 4.1. Smallpox cases and deaths in California, 1913–1925

Year	Cases	Deaths
1913	800	15
1914	677	1
1915	336	3
1916	234	12
1917	329	13
1918	1,016	3
1919	2,002	5
1920	4,492	4
1921	5,579	19
1922	2,129	20
1923	2,026	1
1924	9,445	7
1925	4,921	58

Sources: "Report of the Secretary," *Twenty-Eighth Biennial Report of the State Board of Health of California* [Sacramento, CA: John E. King, State Printer, 1924], 8; "Smallpox—California," *Twenty-Ninth Biennial Report of the State Board of Health of California* [Sacramento, CA: John E. King, State Printer, 1926], 39.

increase in cases, only a small number of people died each year, because a milder strain of smallpox—*variola minor*—had become far more prominent than the older, more virulent strain, *variola major*.[54]

But perhaps the most important factor in parents' disinclination to vaccinate their children was the ease of obtaining exemption certificates. According to one principal, "A parent brings a child to enter him in school, and I tell her that the child must be vaccinated. She asks if there is any way out of it, and I give her one of the 'conscientiously opposed' forms to sign." In a 1920 study of smallpox in California, U.C. Berkeley epidemiologist John Force found that because the law required school authorities to furnish the exemption forms, in some cases schools simply distributed the forms to students to take home for signatures. Parents' increasing use of exemptions seems to have arisen from indifference rather than any ideological opposition to vaccination. During a 1913 outbreak of smallpox in Berkeley, 74 percent of the parents that had signed exemption certificates quickly changed their minds and decided to vaccinate their children. The same phenomenon occurred in Berkeley during another outbreak seven years later. John Force asked, "With the trouble and expense of a vaccination on one hand, and a simple signature on the other, is it any wonder that our State board of Health has recently estimated that 80% of our school children are unvaccinated?"[55]

Protests from parents disappeared as more families took advantage of the ability to exempt their children from vaccination. Nevertheless, opposition to the 1911 law persisted in the state, not only from organized anti-vaccination groups, but also from the schools.

Public school authorities represented an ongoing source of opposition. This occurred because the new law required all unvaccinated students to remain home during outbreaks of disease, and since California distributed school funds to local districts based on students' attendance rates, this caused an enduring problem—a loss of state funding. As the proportion of unvaccinated students in the schools increased, the losses increased sharply during smallpox outbreaks. Previously, school boards had avoided this problem by simply ignoring the directives of the local health boards, but the 1910 ruling in *State Board of Health v. Board of Trustees of Watsonville* gave local health boards the legal authority to enforce the requirement, and they now did so consistently.

As the frequency of smallpox outbreaks increased and the policy of barring unvaccinated students from California classrooms became a continual source of revenue loss, superintendents and school boards began to complain, and some began to openly resist. In 1912, when Fresno's board of health ordered the quarantine of over one hundred students during a smallpox epidemic in the city, the board of education decided to defy the orders and keep the students in the schools. The school board only complied with the orders once the state's board of health threatened a lawsuit.[56]

In 1913, school superintendents participated in a legislative hearing to consider overturning or revising the law after four hundred unvaccinated students were excluded from Sacramento's schools. Sacramento educators complained that schools were annually losing considerable sums of state money through their support of the law, "which automatically throws out of school children who are not vaccinated when smallpox breaks out in the neighborhood."[57] News of the events in Sacramento appeared in newspapers across the state, and educators in other towns began to speak up. The press reported that an upcoming legislative hearing would consider reports from school superintendents and health officers and that "the general opinion expressed is that some change should be made." However, despite educators' concerns, nothing came from the hearing, and the law remained on the books.[58]

The issue of enrollment loss continued to cause tension between local school boards and health boards. The influenza epidemic of 1918 was deadlier and more widespread than smallpox, and in 1919, numerous outbreaks of both diseases led hundreds of schools to close their doors for so long that they failed to meet the state's legal requirement requiring classes be maintained at least 120 days per year. According to State Superintendent of Public Instruction William C. Wood, "Between 200 and 300 district schools in California are threatened with closing during the next school year . . . for the failure of their trustees to obey the provisions of the constitution and the law."[59]

An anti-vaccination group called the Public School Protective League leveraged the issue of school enrollment loss in a campaign to overturn the 1911 school vaccination law, arguing that the financial and educational cost of lost school enrollments during epidemics was too high. The league, which first appeared in Los Angeles in 1917, embraced the concept of medical liberty—defined as the parents' right to determine their children's medical treatment and "the right of unvaccinated children to attend the public schools."[60]

Dr. Lewis P. Crutcher, the league's founder and president, was a director of the National League for Medical Freedom, a former president of the Long Beach school board, and a homeopathic physician.[61] By this date, many homeopaths had long accepted the germ theory of disease, but Crutcher rejected it.[62] He believed that homeopathic remedies could produce the best results in preventing and fighting disease, not vaccination. He was a relentless opponent of allopathic medicine. As he explained, "For a period extending over 20 years, at no little sacrifice of time and money, I have fought in season and out, the aggressions of the medical trust. I clearly foresaw that their program included the elimination of the Homeopathic School of medicine and my endearment to that cause has been the incentive that has prompted me in the fight I have made."[63] Under Crutcher's leadership, the Public School Protective League established a statewide organization with executive offices in Los Angeles and San Francisco, and by 1918 it had established offices in Oregon and Washington as well, with the goal of fighting any kind of allopathic medicine in schools.[64]

Historians have explained the rise of groups like the Public School Protective League as a populist backlash against increasing medical intervention in the public schools, not only through compulsory vaccination, but also through the practice of medical inspection. Medical inspection in the schools was not new—local public health boards had frequently conducted inspections during outbreaks of disease during the nineteenth century. The first city to implement mandatory inspections was Boston in 1894; by 1898, three other cities had followed, and by 1908 the number had risen to seventy cities.[65]

Over time the goal of such inspections broadened, from preventing disease to preventing poor hygiene, vision, hearing, and dental problems—and in some cases, recommending surgery. Public health educator and registered nurse Sally Lucas Jean described the way a school nurse, health social worker, and public health doctor collaborated in medical inspection in one Maryland school with a population of 925 children. Because three-fourths of absences at the school were caused by illness, the school became "the health center of the community." The nurse visited the school each day, received reports of absences, and conducted follow-up visits in students' homes. The social worker examined every child returning to school before allowing entry to the classroom. Cases of children with parasites, poor vision, hearing loss, and recurring throat infections were referred to the doctor, who arranged for treatment free of charge for those unable to pay. According to Jean,

> [W]hen the child requires attention, such as removal of
> tonsils and adenoids, the mother is sent a polite personal
> note asking her to come to school and see the worker about
> her little boy or girl. She always comes! And she usually
> agrees to do the thing you ask her to do. When she does
> not at once, we know it is because she does not know us
> well enough to trust to our judgement, and it is the business
> of the worker to gain her confidence."[66]

But not all parents had confidence in such treatments, and those who believed in alternative methods of healing found such interventions particularly galling. In some areas, the practice of medical inspection in the schools was so unpopular that it sparked school boycotts from parents outraged, not only over vaccination, but also over the intrusion of medical inspectors into their children's health. They found an advocate for their concerns in the Public School Protective League.[67]

In the fall of 1919, the Public School Protective League announced its plan to submit a proposition to amend the state constitution to repeal the vaccination law.[68] The league collected enough signatures to place its proposition on the ballot—if it passed, Proposition 6 would prohibit vaccination as a "condition for admission to or attendance in any public school, college, university, or other educational institution in this state." Lewis P. Crutcher composed the "Argument in Favor," claiming, "If vaccination has all the merits which are claimed for it no compulsion should be necessary on its behalf. If, on the contrary, vaccination does not protect against smallpox and is, according to many reputable medical authorities, not only valueless but the cause of cancer, tuberculosis, syphilis and death, any compulsion in its behalf is criminal."[69] Many parents who refused to vaccinate their children agreed with the Pubic School Protective League. For instance, in Mill Valley, a town just north of San Francisco in Marin County, smallpox epidemics had broken out three years in a row, and school attendance was reduced to 68 percent because so many children were exempted from vaccination. The local paper reported, "The loss of revenue thus might mean one less teacher the coming year."[70]

Nevertheless, despite strong support for the measure to prohibit vaccination requirements in places like Mill Valley, the Protective League's ballot proposal did not pass. Although Crutcher had informed his followers that "80 percent" of Californians were opposed to vaccination, 57 percent of Californians voted it down.[71] Those opposed to the state's vaccination law would have to wait one more year.

By 1921, those seeking to overturn the law included the state's board of health. A decade of protest and rising rates of unvaccinated students had convinced the board that the vaccination law allowing conscientious exemption was an utter failure. As Walter M. Dickie, the board secretary, explained to the Senate's Public Health and Quarantine Committee, "The present law has failed in its purpose and the State Board of Health asks its repeal. . . . The present law was aimed to encourage vaccination. It has not done so." That year, the California State Board of Health endorsed Senate Bill 408, which proposed to repeal the 1911 law.[72]

The participation of California's health authorities in overturning the state's compulsory vaccination law reflected a national trend among health officials. As historian James Colgrove has shown, across the country, public health departments had grown weary of the never-ending battles over vaccination and were ready for a new approach, one that emphasized persuasion over compulsion.[73] According to Charles-Edward A. Winslow, founder of Yale Medical School's Department of Public Health, "Public health conceived in these terms will be something vastly different from the exercise of the purely police power which has been its principal manifestation in the past."[74]

In his comments supporting the law's repeal, Walter M. Dickie highlighted the concerns of school authorities: "Children are being kept out of school, yet permitted to visit moving picture theaters with no restriction upon their movements whatsoever." According to Dickie, "With repeal of the present law and proposed amendment substituted upon the statute books, the controversy over vaccination which has been going on in California for years will stop."[75]

The state legislature found these arguments very persuasive. On May 26, 1921, the 1911 Vaccination Act was repealed. The new ruling stated, "The control of smallpox shall be under the direction of the State Board of Health, and no rule or regulation on the subject of vaccination shall be adopted by school or local health authorities." Under this ruling, school authorities could not make any rules requiring smallpox vaccination for admission to school, but health authorities still retained the power to exclude unvaccinated students from school during outbreaks of disease.[76] The repeal of the 1911 law eliminated all forms of compulsory school vaccination in California for decades.

The Aftermath

Anti-vaccination activity in the state waned after the law's repeal, although it had already been declining during the previous decade (see chart 4.1). Scholars have identified several factors contributing to the decrease of anti-vaccination protest during these years: the public's growing awareness and acceptance of the germ theory of disease, the greater safety of vaccines as a result of the federal government's increased regulation and oversight, and a shift among public health authorities toward policies that emphasized persuasion over coercion.[77]

In California, three additional developments had an influence. First, the state's health textbooks began including more information about immunization and germ theory. Second, schools started cooperating with local health boards in encouraging voluntary vaccination. And third, a deadly form of smallpox broke out in 1926.

In 1910, the year after the report from the state's board of health on the spread of misinformation about vaccines, the state's board of education began carefully reviewing publishers' health and hygiene textbooks. The board asked some authors to add language to directly counter false claims before including their books in its California

State Series for public schools. Authors who wanted their books listed in the Series complied. For instance, one revised text added information to counter the widespread belief that cleanliness was an effective deterrent against contagious disease: "Many persons have not yet realized that it is germs, and not dirt and disorder that cause disease.... Let us be neat and clean by all means, but let us remember that the home of disease germs is in the human body; that it is germs, and not dirt we must keep in mind when we would prevent disease."[78] Biologist John W. Ritchie's *Primer of Sanitation* argued against the age-old idea of blood purity. He acknowledged that many people believed that having "pure" blood would protect from contagious disease, but he stated that this idea was incorrect. "A person's blood may be as pure as any flowing in the veins of man, and yet that person will fall a victim to smallpox germs," he explained. "Therefore, when any one begins to tell you that health consists in keeping the blood pure, and that vaccination is contrary to the principles of health because it introduces into the body matter from a cow that will cause the blood to be impure—when any one talks to you after this fashion, pay no attention at all to him."[79]

Providing valid information in textbooks designed for upperelementary students may have helped both teachers and students counter misinformation. Additionally, it may also have had a longrange impact on public attitudes regarding contagious disease and vaccination. Eventually, those students grew up, and many became parents with children of their own to protect.

The attitudes of educators also began to change. After the repeal of the vaccination law in 1921, more school officials came to accept that it was in their best interest to encourage immunization. Since vaccination was no longer required, parents ceased protesting and threatening lawsuits, but local health boards retained the power to exclude unvaccinated students during smallpox outbreaks. The only way for a school to avoid financial losses during an epidemic was to ensure that few students became ill. In 1924, when the number of smallpox cases in California rose to around eight thousand, San Luis Obispo's health officer took the unusual step of cooperating with the superintendent of schools to open a free voluntary vaccination clinic on school grounds.[80] It had become clear—in San Luis Obispo, at least—that boosting the percentage of vaccinated students was an effective way to save money by reducing the number of students too sick to attend school.

During the late 1920s and 1930s, doctors employed by local school districts joined health board officials in publishing editorials and articles urging citizens to vaccinate their children. A search of California newspapers during this period reveals scores of news articles describing these efforts.[81] "If you had once seen the horrible picture of a patient suffering from a severe case of smallpox, I am sure your conscience would not allow you to sign a protest," urged one Santa Rosa school physician during an outbreak. "What real objection can you have? The vaccination is not painful. I have vaccinated over 11,000 children in our schools, and hardly any of them has even whimpered, and I have not had a single infected arm."[82]

The involvement of public health nurses in teachers' professional development and in school health campaigns also helped turn the tide. A 1902 experiment in New York City showed that bringing public health nurses to work in the schools could dramatically reduce incidents of absenteeism. Lillian Wald, the founder of the Henry Street Nurses Settlement, pressured New York's public school system to hire Lina L. Rogers, a Henry Street nurse, for a thirty-day trial period. During this time, Rogers made 137 home visits, treated 893 students, and helped sick children recover and rejoin their classes.

The experiment was highly successful, and soon afterward, New York City's board of health hired its first group of twelve nurses to work in the schools. Within a year, school absenteeism fell by 90 percent.

News of this successful outcome soon spread among health officials and educators across the country, and by the 1920s, school nurses had become a regular feature in California's public schools. In some areas, nurses employed by public health departments met with teachers during professional development conferences focused on sanitation and immunization; in other areas, Red Cross nurses conducted visits to the schools to examine students and talk with teachers about the prevention of communicable diseases.[83]

Once an antitoxin against diphtheria became widely available in the 1920s, nurses employed by local school districts also began publishing notices encouraging parents to immunize their children against the disease. For instance, Mary Newbold, Colusa County's public school nurse, published a notice in the local newspaper urging parents to protect their children against "one of the most deadly and virulent of children's diseases. Before this anti-toxin process was perfected, children died by the thousands. . . . In the latter part of the 19th century, the hospitals of Berlin and Paris were crowded to overflowing with little babies. . . . Five out of every ten cots sent their occupants to the morgue. Vaccination has changed all that."[84] Such public messaging may have alleviated some parents' concerns about immunization.

Another reason organized opposition to vaccination declined in California is that a deadly form of smallpox returned. During the early 1920s, outbreaks of smallpox had risen dramatically across the state, but because these were of the mild *variola minor* strain, few people had died. However, when the more dangerous *variola major* strain reemerged in 1926, it quickly killed 236 people. Once they learned that the worst form of smallpox was threatening their communities, Californians abandoned their complacency, rolled up their sleeves, and submitted to vaccination, bringing their children in tow. That year the state's board of health reported, "It has been found, in many cities and counties of California, that the opposition to vaccination is actually not so strong as many have heretofore believed." After that year, the Public School Protective League disappeared from view in the state's newspapers.[85]

Although anti-vaccination protest dwindled, Californians soon reprised their former ambivalence regarding the smallpox vaccine. Few people died from the milder strain of smallpox that persisted in the state throughout the 1930s, but most of those deaths were among the unvaccinated. As Giles S. Porter, director of the state's board of health explained, "In 1930, out of a total of 3,139 persons who suffered from smallpox, 2,931 had never been vaccinated. . . . In 1931, out of 1,524 individuals who suffered from smallpox, 1,326 had never been vaccinated."[86]

Ongoing complacency regarding vaccination also made it difficult to fight diphtheria. Children seated closely together for hours in crowded classrooms were particularly susceptible to the disease, which commonly killed about 12 percent or more of its victims. When the antitoxin used to inoculate against diphtheria became available in the United States, health officers recommended it to parents. In New York City, the percentage of deaths from diphtheria fell significantly as a result of voluntary immunization programs.[87] Impressed with these results, the California State Board of Health announced, "By such a procedure, 95 percent of the diphtheria in our country could be wiped out."[88]

Voluntary immunization programs in California, encouraged by school nurses, physicians, and health departments, helped to reduce the number of diphtheria cases over time (table 4.2), but the fatality rate among young children remained high. During the 1920s, thousands of children died from what had become a preventable disease.

Alarmed by diphtheria's high fatality rates in 1927 and 1928, Walter M. Dickie, director of the state's health board, urged Californians to immunize their children. "Until such time as all California cities and counties develop practical programs for the immunization of all children within their respective territories, we must expect to have a high morbidity and a higher mortality from this much-to-be dreaded disease."[89]

When he wrote those words, California's health authorities had no authority to enforce the immunization of children against diphtheria or any other disease. Nor could they expect any help from the state legislature—no politician had the political will to try to resurrect compulsory vaccination. In the new era of persuasion, many

Table 4.2. Diphtheria in California: Cases, deaths, and fatality rate, 1921–1931

Year	Cases	Deaths	Case Fatality Rate [%][a]
1921	9,464	644	6.8
1922	8,709	599	6.9
1923	9,532	640	6.7
1924	11,109	695	6.3
1925	5,575	266	4.8
1926	6,129	291	4.8
1927	6,412	306	4.8
1928	4,741	273	5.8
1929	3,022	185	6.1
1930	3,071	193	6.2
1931	3,421	175	5.1
Total	71,185	4,267	Mean = 5.8

Sources: Thirty-First Biennial Report of the Department of Public Health of California [Sacramento, CA: Superintendent of State Printing, 1929], 3; Thirty-Second Biennial Report of the Department of Public Health of California [1931], 23.
[a] Case fatality rate percentages are rounded up to the nearest tenth.

people rejected proposals to make immunization against diphtheria a requirement for school. As one doctor attending the White House conference on Child Health and Protection explained in 1932, "Making immunization compulsory will arouse and prejudice a large group of people against health work and organize this group to active opposition, thus interfering with other important health activities."[90]

Conclusion

The disputes between California's school and health authorities, like similar disputes elsewhere in the country, reflected differences in their professional priorities and responsibilities. Health officials sought to protect schools and communities from smallpox, and they believed that increasing the number of vaccinated adults and children was the best means of achieving that goal. Educators believed their first duty was to educate students, and effective education required adequate finding to hire staff and keep the schools open and running smoothly. Because state funding was tied to school enrollments, any policy that reduced student attendance threatened the mission to educate. From the perspective of California's school leaders, any law that required the exclusion of unvaccinated students interfered with this core mission.

Did ideological differences play a role? There is no way to know how many school board members and superintendents may have subscribed to the ideas of the anti-vaccinationists—that vaccination was ineffective, caused other diseases, and poisoned the blood. What is certain is that over the decades, school leaders came to better understand the importance and value of vaccination in protecting students from contagious disease. Once vaccination became purely voluntary, and angry parents no longer thronged school boardrooms, a policy of collaborating with local health officials to encourage vaccination made sense—after all, fewer ill students meant more students attending their lessons in school.

California's 1911 law allowing conscientious exemption had pleased no one—not the school authorities who had wished to stop enrollment loss, not the anti-vaccination groups who wanted to end immunization altogether, and not the public health authorities who had hoped that allowing exemptions would lead to more vaccinated children. The law had failed to restore the public's trust in vaccination, and the 1921 law eliminating compulsory vaccination altogether had not improved matters. Too many children were still dying.

For better or worse, persuasion became the health board's last remaining tool. During disease outbreaks, people came willingly to be vaccinated, but at other times, persuasion seemed a futile enterprise. "In too many communities of the state," wrote Walter Dickie in 1929, "absolutely no action whatsoever is taken for immunizing the children of the community."[91]

Three decades would pass before Californians would again consider compulsory vaccination. It would take a polio epidemic to usher in a sea change.

PART II

A Sea Change
From Persuasion to Compulsion
in the Quest for Herd Immunity

5

Schools and the Campaign against Polio

Polio most often struck children between the ages of one and fourteen. Severe cases could leave victims without the use of a limb or completely paralyzed. The worst cases were heartbreaking. Thirteen-year-old Richard Dagget woke up one morning in California with pain in his neck and back. His parents took him to the doctor, who sent him to the hospital for testing. When paralysis spread throughout his body and he could no longer breathe on his own, the hospital staff enclosed him in a respirator tank known as an "iron lung," which forced air into his lungs (figure 5.1). His parents visited him in the hospital each day. It was incredibly difficult. "Imagine entering a room filled with these huge metal tanks," Richard wrote. "The tanks are making their whooshing sound. All you can see are heads sticking out one end of each tank, and you know that one of these heads belongs to your child."[1]

Poliovirus attacks nerve cells and the nervous system. It spreads through fecal matter in contaminated food or water and through droplets sprayed into the air when infected people cough or sneeze. The disease remains uncurable. Although poliomyelitis was often

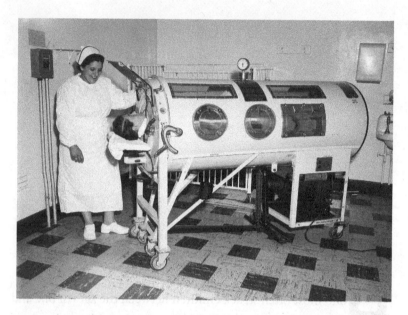

Figure 5.1. Nurse caring for a victim of a Rhode Island polio epidemic inside an Emerson Respirator ("iron lung"), 1960. *Source*: CDC, Public Health Image Library, phil.cdc.gov, ID# 12009.

called "infantile paralysis" during the early twentieth century, the name was misleading, because the disease did not always lead to permanent paralysis, and although it most commonly struck children, adults could also become infected.[2]

Public health officials first documented poliomyelitis in the United States in a small outbreak in West Feliciana, Louisiana, in 1841. Gradually, episodic outbreaks grew larger.

During the 1940s and early 1950s, the number of polio cases rose in both rural and urban areas across the country, frequently striking children and young adults and prompting school closings to prevent the spread of disease.[3] Mary Duncan, a Red Cross nurse employed by the Kentucky state health department to work in the schools from 1942 to 1963, recalled the sudden increase of polio in rural Wayne

County: "All the time during my training years, I never saw polio. I'd heard of it. But I thought it was such a rare thing. But suddenly, in Wayne County, every spring and summer, there were cases of polio. . . . That was the age where you could see children in braces and crutches, things like that, all over the place."[4] In California from 1948 to 1951, polio erupted in every county of the state but one, and the percentage of cases showing weakness or paralysis ranged from 68 to 73 percent. In 1948 alone, more than six thousand Californians fell victim to the disease, most of them children.[5] Across the United States in 1952, there were 3,145 deaths and more than 21,000 cases of polio resulting in permanent paralysis.[6]

The nationwide effort to prevent polio culminated in a mass voluntary vaccination campaign in the 1950s. In later years, many Americans would remember the speed of that campaign. As one California letter writer to the *San Jose Mercury News* recalled, "Once Jonas Salk discovered a cure the reaction of America was swift and sure. In my junior high school, we were told on a certain Tuesday school would be closed for mass inoculation. All students, teachers and parents, about 2,000, lined up at 8 a.m. and marched in the front door of the nurse's office, needle time 30 seconds, out the back door and home—start to finish about six hours. Called again the greatest generation for a reason."[7]

This *Mercury News* writer recalled the polio vaccination campaign as "swift and sure," but as historians have shown, the success of that campaign was years in the making. Some authors have focused on the scientists who developed the vaccines. Others have highlighted the efforts of public health officials in specific areas of the country, the public relations campaign championed by the March of Dimes, or the political maneuvering in federal and state legislatures that supported the vaccination campaign.[8] It was not all smooth sailing. Significant challenges and setbacks included inequitable access to polio prevention and treatment, critical vaccine shortages, and a deadly contamination of the vaccine supply.[9]

Despite the setbacks, the campaign against polio ushered in a sea change in American attitudes about vaccination. In contrast to the earlier era of hostility toward the perceived intrusions of doctors and public health officials, once the polio vaccine became available, local communities in both rural and urban areas welcomed vaccination on school grounds. The schools themselves had a critical role in this development.

Refining the Art of Persuasion: The National Foundation for Infantile Paralysis

When he was a young politician, Franklin D. Roosevelt became the most famous polio victim after surviving a 1921 outbreak that left him paralyzed from the waist down. In 1937, the National Foundation for Infantile Paralysis, a private, nonprofit organization founded with President Roosevelt's help, began raising funds for prevention of the disease.[10]

The National Foundation's campaign marked a turning point in American attitudes toward scientific medicine and vaccines. By this point, the leaders of the former national anti-vaccination societies had either passed away or given up their activism, and the era of organized opposition to allopathic medicine and vaccination was over. Moreover, the public's trust in vaccines was growing, thanks not only to their increased safety but also to public health policies that had emphasized persuasion over coercion since the late 1920s.

Basil O'Connor, the foundation's president, reached out to radio and television celebrity Eddie Cantor and other media personalities for help in developing a public relations campaign. During a meeting on November 22, 1937, with Warner Brothers and Metro-Goldwyn-Mayer executives, Cantor said, "I am sure that all of the national radio programs originating in Hollywood would devote 30 seconds to this great cause! We could call it the March of Dimes." His idea was that if every American could donate a dime, and if a million people sent only one, the total would be $100,000.[11] The first year, the program collected over two and a half million dimes, and President Roosevelt expressed his thanks via radio: "In all the envelopes are dimes and quarters and even dollar bills—gifts from grownups and children—mostly from children who want to help other children to get well."[12]

The March of Dimes campaign widely publicized the need for a vaccine, and to an extent never seen before in American public life, many individuals, families, communities, and students came together to support a voluntary immunization campaign. From the very start, schools began educating students about polio and publicizing the fight against the disease. This occurred through the curriculum, student-led fund-raising activities, and school outreach to local communities. The National Foundation for Infantile Paralysis supported this effort by providing publications free of charge, and its pamphlets and booklets became an important source of information for teachers who wanted to be able to answer questions about polio from students and parents.[13]

Curriculum and Campaigns in Schools

Polio entered the official school curriculum shortly after the March of Dimes campaign began. Although few elementary texts ever mentioned either the germ theory of disease or vaccination at the start of the twentieth century, by 1940 every book aimed at grades 4 through 12 covered the subjects (chart 5.1), and some were beginning to discuss polio.[14]

Then, on December 7, 1941, the Japanese attacked Pearl Harbor. As the shocked nation began mobilizing in response, newspaper and radio announcements issued patriotic calls to Americans to buy Liberty Bonds and support the Red Cross. Uncertain how to proceed, Basil O'Connor wondered whether the foundation should suspend its outreach and fund-raising drive during the war effort. But in a note to O'Conner, President Roosevelt opposed any interruption of the campaign, describing it as a key part of the nation's struggle and "one of the front lines of our National Defense." This presidential endorsement gave the foundation the impetus it needed to move forward, and with the nonpartisan slogan, "Polio Wears No Party Label," the March of Dimes ramped up its fund-raising through the placement of collection boxes at movie theaters.[15] In his annual radio broadcast appeal for the foundation in 1944, President Roosevelt expressed his thanks to the nation. "The generous participation of the American people in this fight is a sign of the healthy condition of our Nation," he said. "It is democracy in action." He aligned participation in the March of Dimes campaign with America's

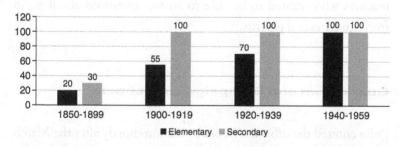

Chart 5.1. Elementary and secondary health schoolbooks mentioning germ theory and vaccination, 1850–1959 (in percentages). *Note*: N = 139. These results do not include data from texts developed for students in the primary grades 1–3. *Source*: Cubberley Library Textbook Collection, Stanford University.

wartime efforts: "The unity of our people . . . in protecting the welfare of our young, in preserving the eternal principle of kindliness—all of this is evidence of our fundamental strength—the strength with which we are meeting our enemies throughout the world."[16]

During the mid-1940s, as the March of Dimes campaign was in full swing, the Bobbs-Merrill Company included a section on "the dreaded polio" in a text for upper-elementary students, explaining, "In view of the seriousness of the affliction, people contribute large sums of money annually to care for victims in need of help and to promote research in prevention and cure."[17] As newspapers reported the ongoing quest for a vaccine, a Silver Burdett Company textbook probably raised elementary students' anxiety by reporting it had "not been proven" that any vaccine or serum was effective.[18]

At the secondary level, textbook coverage increased exponentially after Sally Lucas Jean became involved. From 1918 to 1923, she was director of the Child Health Organization of America, and she later served as a director of health education in the American Child Health Association and the National Congress of Parents and Teachers.[19] In 1943, Basil O'Connor recruited her to join the National Foundation for Infantile Paralysis as director of education service, where she took on the task of improving public education regarding poliomyelitis.[20] As part of this effort, she began to consider what students were learning about polio from their schoolbooks.

Jean conducted a study, reaching out to publishers of high school and college health textbooks "to ascertain their infantile paralysis content." Publishers provided volumes free of charge for the study, asking only that she send them the results of her analysis. In her subsequent report to the National Foundation in 1944, she claimed that out of the sample of twenty-seven textbooks, not one adequately discussed the means of spread, symptoms, or treatment of polio. No books provided any information about ongoing research, recent developments in treatment, or the movement "to prepare communities to deal adequately with epidemics." As a result, she explained, "It has been arranged to supply all publishers of school and college health texts with accurate information."[21]

The impact of this plan was dramatic—by the 1950s, prominent secondary textbook publishers were including special sections on polio, sometimes with eye-catching two-page inserts. For instance, a Harcourt, Brace and Company book included a two-page insert on "Conquering Polio" in its section on "Fighting Germ Diseases." A McGraw-Hill textbook included a similar insert with detailed information about experimental methods and development of new vaccines to provide protection against the disease.[22]

By 1950, educators had begun talking about how teachers could participate in the fight against polio. The previous year, polio had spread to almost every state in the country, with 42,375 cases reported, and the National Foundation had supported the treatment of more than 31,000 children below the age of fifteen. The foundation published a free curriculum for high schools, called *A Highschool Unit on Poliomyelitis*, which Sally Lucas Jean highlighted in an article in the National Education Association's journal. Jean urged teachers to get involved, not only by teaching students about polio but also by talking with parents to clear up any misconceptions about the disease. She also recommended teachers watch for any signs of polio among their students, saying, "[T]he teacher can serve in seeing that every child who needs it is directed to medical care. Only the teacher, aside from parents, can make a daily check on the individual child. Even the parent does not see a child with quite the same perspective as the teacher." That spring, the National Foundation distributed 30 million pamphlets on polio to schools across the country for the use of teachers, parents, and high school students.[23]

The federal government also began encouraging teachers and schools to become more involved in health education. Throughout the 1950s, the US Department of Health, Education, and Welfare published reprints of a widely used bulletin titled *Teachers Contribute to Child Health*, which proclaimed, "THE SCHOOL, as one of the significant agencies of the community, accepts its responsibilities for contributing to individual, family, and community health. . . . *Classroom teachers in their daily contacts with boys and girls are the key persons in the school health program.*" The bulletin included a section on "Prevention and Control of Communicable Diseases," which urged teachers to "assist in the development of school health policies" and help carry them out, including teaching children and parents about school vaccination policies, the kinds of immunization available, and "steps to be taken in case of epidemic."[24]

Teachers were not the only ones raising awareness about polio—with the support of their schools, students themselves also took part. In schools around the country, high school students ran March of Dimes campaigns. In Whittier, California, the local high school's student cabinet organized a penny toss to raise money. The students put up a pool in the middle of the quad with sailboats as targets for all the coins tossed by the students. Student body president Jim McKibben said, "Whether it is a hit or a miss the donations all go toward the drive to fight polio."[25] In some high schools, separate campaigns were organized by freshman, sophomore, junior, and senior classes, and the ensuing competition helped boost the yield of coins. At Routt High School in Jacksonville, Illinois, the organizers planned to showcase the final results at a school assembly where representatives from each class would line up the coins they had collected, and the class with the longest line would receive "special recognition for its work."[26] In the South, these campaigns occurred in the context of school segregation. In 1952, the segregated high school students in Rayne, Louisiana, planned to distribute coin envelopes to all the schoolchildren in town. Rayne high school's white student council aimed to distribute to white children in the K–12 schools, while the student council at St. Joseph would distribute envelopes there. According to the local newspaper, "A drive is also being organized among the Negro students of Rayne."[27]

Newspaper publicity made school polio campaigns visible not only to parents but also to entire communities. In towns large and small, local newspapers reported the totals raised by local elementary, middle, and high school students. In Alexandria, Indiana, the local newspaper announced the schoolchildren's total with a front-page headline.[28] In Nebraska, when the Comstock School student council announced the start of a March of Dimes drive in Comstock, that too became front-page news. In 1954, when the town of Perry, Georgia, announced its total fund-raising amount on the front page of the *Houston Home Journal,* it reported donations of $119 from collections taken at the Muse Theatre, $44 from the community of Henderson, $28 from the Bonaire community, and $53.05 from three Black schools: the Elko Negro School, the Oak Ridge Negro School, and the Jerusalem Negro School.[29]

The Field Trial: Operation Polio

By the mid-1950s, Dr. Jonas Salk, head of the Virus Research Laboratory at the University of Pittsburgh, had developed a vaccine against the disease, and at the start of 1954, the National Foundation sponsored a massive field trial known as Operation Polio. Foundation president Basil O'Connor announced that local assistance would be sought from "school faculties" as well as county authorities, medical societies, and volunteers. He explained the test would take place in schools in at least two counties in each state, and the counties selected would be those with a high incidence of polio, a high case rate among children, "adequate health and educational facilities," and diversity in socioeconomic factors and geography "to provide a true cross-section study."[30] Logistically, it would be a massive undertaking. As Marvin Glasser, who led the effort, recalled, "We estimated that approximately 14,000 school principals, 50,000 classroom teachers, 20,000 physicians and 40,000 nurses would be needed."[31]

Hart E. Van Riper, the foundation's medical director, explained the key part of schools in the operation. Information passed from teachers and school administrators to the community would "go far toward convincing parents of the safety and importance of this great scientific project." Providing educational experiences for the children was also important, since "even very young children can understand something about this effort . . . to free them from a dreaded disease."[32]

Schools had long served as important community centers for families, and they now helped to bring entire communities together in fund-raising to support Operation Polio. In contrast to the smallpox vaccination campaigns of the Progressive Era, this undertaking had widespread grassroots support. On February 2, 1954, some three million women across the country held a "Mothers' March on Polio," going from house to house in their neighborhoods to collect money for the March of Dimes field test. Parent-teachers associations and school mothers' clubs often organized the effort. For instance, in Healdsburg, California, where the event took place in the evening, leaders of the town's High School Mothers Club, the Union

Elementary School PTA, and the Mother's Club of St. John's Parochial School publicized the event, asking residents to "turn your porch light on for polio."[33]

During the national vaccination effort, school personnel actively promoted vaccination among local communities. Teachers who had received little or no training in the subject reached out for assistance in teaching about health and answering parents' questions. From 1954 to 1955, the School Health Bureau of the Metropolitan Life Insurance Foundation received over five thousand pieces of mail regarding its booklets and filmstrips on health. One teacher wrote, "This is a small expression of gratitude to you for the film, filmstrips and pamphlets that helped so much." Another noted, "I feel this material is coming from a very reliable and informative source, and we are in a school where library funds and books are very limited." Children sometimes wrote too. One child said, "You sent me what I wanted. Thank you." The bureau hired correspondents to answer all the mail.[34]

Teachers prepared their second-grade students for the vaccination and sent children home with the required "request to participate" forms and paperwork school nurses had prepared. State superintendents urged county and city superintendents to lend assistance to polio immunization programs. In Texas, school principals held meetings to give parents and guardians information about the required forms and talk about the three shots the students would receive in school.[35]

Some scholars have claimed that clinical settings, rather than schools, would have been more ethically appropriate for the Salk vaccine trial, because in clinical settings, parents would have felt no public pressure to participate and would have received clear and comprehensive information about the trial's experimental nature.[36] However, there is no evidence to suggest that parents would have received any different kind of messaging in clinical settings during this time period. Local and state health departments provided the information distributed by the schools. During the trial, a mix of public health doctors, nurses, and private physicians staffed the clinics on school grounds, and they were well qualified to answer parents' questions.[37] Moreover, given the intensive news coverage of the trial and the participation of civic groups in supporting it, there is no evidence that parents would have felt any less pressure to participate in a trial held only in health clinics or private doctors' offices. All the major religious organizations in the country supported the effort. Leaders of the Protestant, Jewish, and Catholic faiths held special services to mark the start of the nationwide field trial, and throughout the campaign, they urged their followers to support the effort.[38]

The Operation Polio field trial was a success. Thomas Francis Jr. of the University of Michigan oversaw the trial, which took place in schools and involved around 1.8 million children from the United States, Canada, and Finland, and on April 12, 1955, his research group announced the vaccine was "safe, effective, and potent." That same day, the US government licensed the Salk vaccine and arranged for the six licensed pharmaceutical companies to produce and distribute it to children throughout the country.[39]

The National Rollout: Setbacks and Uneven Progress

In May, Republican President Dwight D. Eisenhower announced plans for a national rollout of the vaccine, based on recommendations from the National Advisory Committee on Poliomyelitis Vaccine and the secretary of health, education, and welfare. The Salk vaccine would be administered in three doses to a priority group composed of all children ages five to nine, and the states would bear responsibility for developing plans to distribute the vaccine in free mass public vaccination programs.[40] In August, Congress passed the Poliomyelitis Vaccination Assistance Act, and Eisenhower signed it into law, allowing the states to begin drawing federal funds to cover the cost of providing the required three shots of the vaccine.[41]

Given the green light, states began developing plans to vaccinate schoolchildren. The US Office of Education's *School Life* magazine published articles to keep teachers and school officials up to date about the upcoming campaign.[42] Plans for mass inoculation often involved joint meetings of school and Red Cross officials, PTA members, health officials, and doctors. Local PTAs conducted information campaigns to inform parents and guardians about the polio vaccination, and in some communities, PTA members also helped transport children to the schools serving as vaccination centers.[43]

Almost immediately, the vaccination effort hit a major stumbling block. Within weeks of the rollout, the recommendation for polio administration was halted for a period because 120,000 doses had been contaminated with live virus at Cutter Laboratories in Berkeley, California, leading to about two hundred cases of paralytic polio and ten deaths. States suspended vaccination programs as the investigation unfolded, and Cutter took its vaccine off the market on April 27. The so-called Cutter incident was one of the worst pharmaceutical disasters in the United States. By June, the District of Columbia and nine other states—California, Idaho, Maryland, New Jersey, New Mexico, New York, Oregon, Texas, and Washington—debated whether to continue their vaccination programs during the summer, polio's peak season. Multiple senior federal officials resigned, and lowered vaccination rates in the wake of the incident provided evidence that the public had lost confidence in the vaccine.[44]

The Cutter disaster fanned lingering opposition to vaccination that still persisted in some areas of the country. Christian Scientists and the very few Americans who objected to vaccines on religious grounds remained largely silent during this period, but here and there, a few adherents of drugless forms of healing began attacking the polio vaccine in pamphlets and newspaper advertisements. During the 1950s, a chiropractor named R. G. Wilborn founded a publishing company called Health Research and began producing reprints of nineteenth- and early-twentieth-century pamphlets and books on natural hygiene and nature cures. Many of these works rejected all aspects of scientific medicine, including vaccines. His press published *The Poisoned Needle*, an inflammatory book by naturopath Eleanor McBean that recycled the arguments of earlier generations of vaccine opponents to denounce the germ theory of disease and vaccination. McBean's book, which received little attention in the press, was a compendium of misinformation. She advanced a host of assertions now well known to be false, including claims that vaccines caused cancer, syphilis, and many other diseases, including polio. "All vaccines can cause polio," she pronounced.[45]

McBean also advanced an argument circulating in some areas—that cola drinks caused polio. This idea had originated with a doctor named Benjamin P. Sandler, who specialized in nutrition. Sandler published a little book in 1951 called *Diet Prevents Polio*, in which he theorized that a diet high in protein and low in sugar could increase the body's ability to fight disease.[46] He was not against vaccines—as he explained, "a polio vaccine may some day be a reality." Until one became available, he aimed to show "how one may fortify the body through diet and thus offer protection."[47] However, some vaccine opponents seized on the idea that perhaps sugar itself caused polio.

By the mid-1950s, an activist group in southern Florida called Polio Prevention Inc. had begun a propaganda campaign based on this idea. Shampoo manufacturer Duon H. Miller led this group.[48] Miller refused to accept that polio was caused by a virus; instead, he believed it was caused by malnutrition—the result of consuming too many sugary soda drinks.[49] Polio Prevention distributed pamphlets through the mail—with titles like "The Truth about Polio," "Murder, Inc.," and "Stop This Voodooism"—urging parents not to have their children injected. On the eve of the Salk vaccine trials, one such tract warned, "thousands of little white coffins will be used to bury victims of Salk's heinous and fraudulent vaccine." Miller also provided support to other like-minded vaccine opponents. He added his name and endorsement to newspaper ads placed by Zenna H. Mills and Samuel A. Mills, two chiropractors from Burlington, Kansas, who claimed that polio could be eliminated within ninety days through manipulation of the spine. Their ads accused the National Foundation of "bleeding the public out of MILLIONS of DOLLARS while innocent little children are offered in sacrifice on the altar of GREED for the almighty DOLLLAR."[50]

In many ways, Polio Prevention's anti-vaccine campaign was similar to the propaganda of the Progressive Era anti-vaccinationists—during both periods, opponents of vaccination denied that bacteria or viruses caused disease and recommended drugless methods of prevention and cure. But there were significant differences. This was no longer a boundary quarrel over a still-disputed medical theory. Miller and his followers were not participating in legitimate discourse about the prevention of polio—they were engaged in the deliberate production of misinformation with the aim of sowing public mistrust in the Salk vaccine. The federal government recognized the difference. Whereas Progressive Era vaccine opponents had mailed their tracts and pamphlets across the country with impunity, the full weight of the US Attorney General's office came down on Polio Prevention. Viewing the anti-vaccination propaganda as a direct attack on a program of national interest, the government filed charges of mail fraud and criminal libel against Duon Miller, and he was sentenced to two years' probation.[51]

In contrast to the debates over vaccination near the end of the Progressive Era, newspapers largely ignored the relatively few voices of opposition during the polio campaign (chart 5.2). The media lined up in support of the national vaccination campaign, much as it had supported the government in the war effort several years previously. Very few papers reported anti-vaccination views, and when they did, the tone was often critical. The editor of the *Times Record* in Troy, New York, dismissed the naysayers as members of "religious and pseudo-scientific cults which cannot remain quiet when any such effort for health is attempted. They assert that health is a family matter, to be determined by each individual or parent. They claim fiercely against everything medical. Snakes may bite and only prayer may be used. Polio may be abroad and no mass remedy adopted." As the editor pointed out, most parents were so fearful of polio, they were willing to "try out anything which seems likely to limit its ravages."[52]

Yet fear of polio does not entirely explain parents' wide acceptance of the vaccine during this period. One reason for the public's favorable

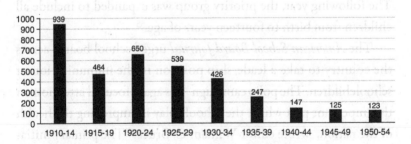

Chart 5.2. Number of US newspaper articles reporting on anti-vaccination sentiment, 1910–1954. *Source:* Data derived from a search conducted February 8, 2023, of newspapers published from 1910 through 1954 on Newspapers.com using the phrase *opposed to vaccination.*

reception is that by the mid-1950s, Americans had come to have a high degree of trust in science. A national survey of public attitudes toward science and technology conducted in 1957–58 found that a large majority of people (83 percent) believed that the world was "better off . . . because of science."[53] Americans had also come to have a great deal of confidence in allopathic medicine. The influence of alternative health practitioners had been waning for two decades. A survey of nine thousand families conducted from 1928 to 1931 revealed that alternative health practitioners treated only 5.1 percent of all cases of illness. By the time of the polio campaign, allopathic medicine had firmly established itself as the dominant form of medicine.[54]

Most parents accepted the Salk vaccine because, in contrast to the nineteenth-century smallpox vaccine, which inherently came with some adverse side effects, it was very safe. Although vaccination rates fell for a while following the Cutter disaster, after investigators determined the cause, most people seem to have understood that the incident at Cutter Labs was a rare event, one unlikely to recur. Once investigators deemed production at the other laboratories safe, polio administration resumed, and by July 1955, about six million first- and second-grade children had reportedly been vaccinated. The following year, the priority group was expanded to include all children from birth to fourteen years of age.[55]

The *American School Board Journal* urged school boards across the country to take a leadership position in the immunization of schoolchildren. The polio campaign "has again focused attention on the important part which the schools play in improving the health of the nation," wrote editor William C. Bruce. "The primary initiative and responsibility belong to the health boards, but the schools are the surest means of reaching the children and of systematizing the procedures in urban and rural communities."[56] In line with this advice, the California State Legislature passed an act authorizing school districts to "accept the volunteered services of physicians" and other members of the medical profession and "administer the vaccine to pupils" whose parents provided written consent.[57]

States varied in their approach to vaccination, however, and not every state followed this model. For example, Georgia's Department of Health delegated authority for vaccination to its local regional health offices, which organized vaccination clinics in each county and also provided some vaccine to private physicians.[58] Health offices developed varying procedures in each county. In some, officials worked with school authorities to provide vaccination at school sites, but in others, vaccination clinics were held off campus.

The national vaccination campaign began about a year after the US Supreme Court's May 17, 1954, ruling to desegregate schools in *Brown v. Board of Education.* As was common in many southern states, Georgia's schools remained segregated in the immediate aftermath of *Brown v. Board.*[59] In Houston County, beginning on April 21, 1955, doctors and public officials traveled to all the local segregated schools to administer the vaccines free to all first- and second-graders. Discrimination was evident in the timing—the first shots went to white children in all-white schools. In the town of Perry, students at "Perry White school," were scheduled to receive their shots on April 27, whereas students at the "the colored schools of the county" would receive theirs on April 29. For their children to receive an injection, parents were required to submit an approval form in advance.[60] Vaccination results varied widely from county to county. In Butts County, officials administered the vaccine off-campus at local health clinics, where white children in the city of Jackson received their shots a week before Black students received theirs. The local newspaper reported that applications from Black parents requesting vaccination were "coming in more slowly."[61] By

May 12, 1955, 85 percent of eligible white children in Jackson had received the first dose, compared with just 57 percent of Black students.[62]

Research conducted during the mass field trials of 1954 and throughout the mass vaccination campaigns concluded that such different outcomes were most often due to differences in socioeconomic status, as measured by the parents' education and the occupation of the male head of household. One study that examined the relationship between parents' socioeconomic status and children's vaccination status found that less wealthy and less educated parents were slower to consent to vaccination, with the result that their children were slower to receive polio shots. The link between socioeconomic status and vaccination status was also found in studies conducted in subsequent years.[63] However, as historians have pointed out, racial discrimination was also a factor influencing access to the vaccine. For example, in Montgomery, Alabama, Black children had to wait on the front lawns of all-white schools to receive their inoculations, unable to use the restrooms indoors.[64]

The Role of Schools in Increasing Access to the Vaccine

During the mass vaccination program in 1955, school personnel leveled the playing field in some areas of the South by taking steps to encourage vaccination among Black families. For instance, in Butler, Alabama, more Black children than white children received their first shots because J. O. Bush, the county superintendent of education, provided school buses to transport all the county's first- and second-graders to the designated vaccination centers. According to a newspaper report, by April 28, 645 Black children had received the first shot, compared with only 309 white children.[65] In Georgia too, Blacks had higher vaccination rates than whites in some areas. In 1956, sociologist John C. Belcher conducted a survey involving 701 households in Greene and Hancock counties, where non-whites were more often renters, more rural, and had lower incomes than whites. He found that a higher percentage of Black children than white children received the Salk vaccine.[66] Interview data from Belcher's study suggest that a connection with schools encouraged Black families to view vaccination positively. In interviews, whites commonly credited the county school superintendent as crucial to the success of the polio vaccination program. The superintendent reportedly arranged for school buses to bring non-white children to the local health department for immunizations. According to white respondents, bus transportation for white children was not always ensured.[67]

Schools also served as important sources of information about polio vaccination. When asked where they had first heard of polio vaccination, non-white families in Belcher's study identified the local schools as the most important source of information, followed by radio or television. In contrast, whites identified newspapers and magazines as the most important source (chart 5.3).[68] After analyzing this data, Belcher speculated that perhaps non-whites had higher rates of vaccination because they did not have much access to newspapers carrying stories about the Cutter incident, whereas white families may have read reports in the papers and become more distrustful of vaccination.[69]

For their part, the Black interviewees in Belcher's study cited the importance of schoolteachers. Many explained that they knew children could become paralyzed or die from polio, so when a vaccine became available, they accepted it. Some recalled that during the annual March of Dimes campaign, a Black teacher had driven women

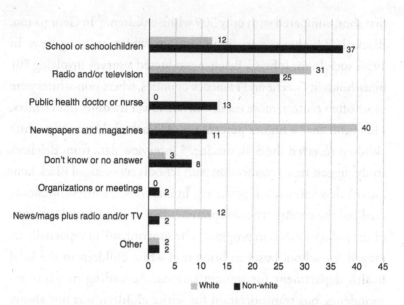

Chart 5.3. Earliest source of information regarding the polio vaccine reported by 254 Black and 191 white households in two Georgia counties (in percentages). *Source*: Chart created from data in table 14, "Source of first information regarding polio vaccine by color," in John C. Belcher, "Acceptance of the Salk Polio Vaccine," *Rural Sociology* 23, no. 2 (June 1958): 170.

from each section of one county to Tuskegee, where they witnessed firsthand the suffering children endured from polio. These women came back to their communities and spread word of the horrors of the disease. In many interviews, Black residents highlighted the efforts of Black teachers in both counties to raise awareness of the vaccination program. Black teachers informed parents about the Salk vaccine and encouraged them to allow their children to be inoculated. Some teachers took their enthusiasm to extreme levels. There were rumors that some educators, seeking to achieve 100 percent vaccination rates in their classrooms and schools, informed children they would not be promoted unless they had received their shots.[70]

Survey research conducted in California the same year also revealed the important part schools played in encouraging vaccination, particularly among non-white children. In 1956, in an effort to improve its vaccination program, California's Department of Public Health conducted a statewide survey of attitudes toward polio vaccination in collaboration with the US Census. At the time, all children below the age of fifteen were eligible to be vaccinated, but only 42 percent had received at least one shot. As a result, researchers were particularly interested to understand parents' attitudes toward vaccination. The California survey analyzed responses from 3,544 households. Of the respondents, 51 percent were female and 49 percent were male. Nearly 92 percent were white, a category that included "persons of Spanish or Mexican ancestry"; 6 percent were Black, and around 2 percent were "primarily oriental."[71]

The survey revealed that schools were important sources of information about health information for California families. When researchers asked mothers about the best way to get important information from the health department, most replied, "send the notice through the schools" (chart 5.4). Getting accurate information into mothers' hands was important, because the mother's attitude

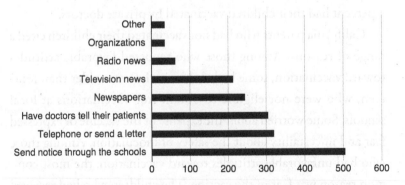

Chart 5.4. Numbers of various responses to the question: "If the health department had information it wanted to get to people, what would be the best way of being sure it got to you personally?" *Source:* Chart created from data in table 203, California Department of Public Health, *California Health Survey 1956, Vol. 1* [Berkeley: State of California, Department of Public Health, 1958), chap. 3 appendix, n.p.

toward polio vaccination correlated significantly with her children's vaccination status. Among the mothers of unvaccinated children, only 65 percent reported favorable attitudes, in contrast to 97 percent of the mothers whose children had received the vaccine.[72] Previous experience with vaccination also made a positive difference—the greater the immunization level of each child in the family below the age of six against smallpox and DPT (diphtheria/pertussis/tetanus), the greater the percentage of mothers with favorable attitudes toward polio vaccination.[73]

The survey results highlighted the importance of schools to the success of the vaccine rollout. Schools were the most frequently cited sources of polio vaccination for children between the ages of six and nine, and they were especially important for families with lower household incomes. The wealthiest group of households, those earning more than $8,000 per year, often took their children to private doctors to get the vaccine. In contrast, parents in every other group generally relied on the vaccination clinics in the schools. Schools were by far the most significant source of vaccination for families earning no more than $1,999 per year. Among this group, only 1 percent had their children vaccinated by private doctors.[74]

California parents who had not vaccinated their children cited a range of reasons. Among those who reported favorable attitudes toward vaccination, some had children who were older than fourteen, who were not eligible to obtain free vaccinations at local schools. Some worried about the expense of the vaccine or expressed fear and uncertainty about the safety of inoculation. Among those who had unfavorable attitudes toward vaccination, the most common reason was fear of the vaccine. The children who had received the defective polio vaccine from Cutter Laboratories lived in five western and midwestern states, including California—three children from Los Angeles and a girl from Riverside had been struck with paralytic polio within a week of receiving their injections.[75]

At the time of the 1956 survey, vaccination rates differed greatly between white and Black children in California. Only 23 percent of Black children between birth and age fourteen had been vaccinated, whereas 43 percent of whites had received at least one shot. Among vaccinated Black children, most (75 percent) had only received one shot, whereas among the vaccinated white children, most (81 percent) had received more than one.[76] Nevertheless, the racial vaccination gap was closing—the degree of increase among children vaccinated was much greater among Blacks than whites. Of children aged six through nine, the percentage of Black children vaccinated tripled, whereas the percentage of white children doubled. The survey's authors credited California's school-based rollout policy in this development, as it provided "a more intensive educational campaign and more readily available vaccine."[77]

The snapshots provided by the 1956 survey in California and Belcher's study in Georgia illustrate the key role of schools in providing outreach and communication to families and convenient access to vaccination. Holding vaccination clinics on school grounds, as happened in many states, and using school buses to carry students to vaccination sites, as occurred in some areas, ensured higher rates of vaccination than was achieved with preschool children, particularly for families without easy transportation to off-campus facilities. By July 1956, the priority group for vaccination included all ages under twenty years, and by 1957, the number of polio cases in the country had declined by 68 percent.[78]

By any measure, it was the most successful vaccination campaign against childhood disease ever undertaken in the United States. In 1958 alone, mass polio immunization programs reached 11,809,000 children.[79] The immunization gap between white and non-white children narrowed significantly, and cases of polio decreased dramatically across the country (chart 5.5).[80]

The Movement to Require Vaccination for School Admission

The movement to pass standing compulsory school vaccination laws began during the fight against polio. In many states, a growing sense of frustration as cases of polio began to rise in some areas led to the passage of new laws.

Despite the dramatic drop in polio cases nationwide, the goal of vaccinating every young person remained elusive. Although preschool children were among those most susceptible to paralytic polio, vaccination rates among preschoolers lagged behind those of elementary and secondary children, who had access to vaccination clinics at their school sites. For example, a survey conducted in Seattle showed that about 93 percent of all elementary schoolchildren in

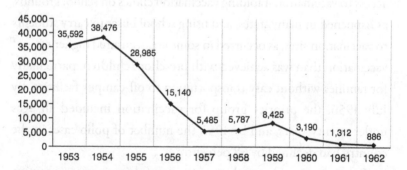

Chart 5.5. Numbers of reported cases of poliomyelitis in the United States, 1953–1962. *Source*: Chart compiled from data in US Department of Health, Education, and Welfare, *Poliomyelitis Health Information Series, No. 8: Public Health Service Publication No. 74* [Washington, DC: GPO, rev. 1963], 10. Historical Medical Library of the College of Physicians of Philadelphia.

the city had received three or more shots of the Salk vaccine. However, in the "poorest school districts," fewer than half of children entering kindergarten were protected.[81] As a result, the youngest children were often the most frequent victims of the disease. National statistics showed that more than four out of every ten cases of paralytic polio occurred among preschoolers. Adults were also susceptible to polio, and yet vaccination rates for those over the age of twenty dropped sharply. And in every region of the country and among every age group, more whites than non-whites had received shots.[82]

"Why are there so many young people in the United States who have not yet had even a single shot of the Salk vaccine?" asked the editor of *School Life*. "Plainly, education is now the major weapon in the battle against polio. The Office of Education urges school officials and teachers to direct their most persuasive efforts toward this goal: Vaccination of all persons under 40 *now*."[83]

Public health officials worried about reports of vaccine hesitancy and refusal among parents of children too young to attend school. Researchers from the US Public Health Service conducted a study of the factors influencing parents' reluctance. Their report identified four psychosocial domains influencing parents' decision to vaccinate their children: (1) susceptibility, or parents' assessment of their child's risk of getting polio; (2) seriousness, or parents' assessment of whether polio was a serious enough threat to warrant vaccination; (3) efficacy and safety, or parents' assessment of the degree to which the vaccine was safe and would work; and (4) social and institutional factors—the concerns and influences that facilitated or discouraged their decision to get their child vaccinated.[84]

These four domains mapped well with the factors that had led parents to avoid or accept vaccination during the earlier Progressive Era. As had occurred during the years of smallpox outbreaks, families living in areas with few cases of disease may have thought their children's risk of catching the illness was extremely low. And although the Salk vaccine was much safer than the earlier smallpox vaccine, parents who heard the news about defective lots of vaccine from Cutter Labs may well have feared the possibility of harm from vaccination. There were also major differences between these eras. In contrast to the smallpox vaccine, there were relatively few reports of breakthrough infections with the Salk vaccine—it was highly effective against polio. Most important, society's attitudes toward vaccination had shifted toward greater acceptance of immunization. Public health policies emphasizing persuasion had contributed to this trend, and apart from the efforts of a few groups, such as Polio Prevention Inc., no influential national anti-vaccine organization had risen to influence any widespread resistance to the polio vaccination campaign. Nevertheless, despite these positive developments, the goal of achieving universal vaccination remained elusive.

Public health officials became very concerned once it became clear that polio seemed to be returning in areas with large numbers of unvaccinated people. The number of polio cases nationwide stopped falling after 1957 and began rising. In 1958, they increased by 5 percent, and in 1959, they jumped another 45 percent (see chart 5.5).

Americans followed reports of new outbreaks with anxiety. In 1958, 874 people caught polio in Detroit. Most of the victims were unvaccinated preschool children and young adults. Nearly half of them contracted paralytic polio, and nearly 3 percent died. Black families were disproportionately infected, as were those living in lower-socioeconomic neighborhoods.[85] The following year, a similar epidemic broke out in Des Moines, Iowa, infecting 135 people and killing 15. Most of the cases (52 percent) resulted in paralysis, leading the National Foundation to ship iron lungs to the city.[86] That same year, the disease also broke out in Kansas City, Missouri, infecting 210 people and leading to 188 cases of paralytic polio and 15 deaths. In both Des Moines and Kansas City, Black families and lower-socioeconomic neighborhoods with low vaccination rates had by far the highest rates of infection. The rate of infection among Blacks in Des Moines was twenty times that of whites in high socio-economic areas and thirty-two times that of whites in similar areas in Kansas City. Most of the victims were unvaccinated children from birth to nine years of age and adults between the ages of twenty and forty. The only good news from these areas was that people who were fully vaccinated were well protected—researchers estimated the Salk vaccine to have been 80 percent effective in the Des Moines outbreak and 77 percent effective in Kansas City.[87]

Newspapers across the country urged readers to get vaccinated as soon as possible, warning about the dangers of complacency. "Don't let your community be surprised by a disrupting, disastrous epidemic," warned a California paper. "There's no basis to think it can't happen here—or anywhere." The California State Department of Health warned that a five thousand–victim polio epidemic could break out in the state if more people did not become vaccinated.[88]

One of the most effective ways to protect students was to require vaccination for admission to school. The oldest school vaccination laws related to smallpox, and some states, including Georgia, still had such laws. But anti-vaccination activism during the Progressive Era had led California and nine other states to repeal their laws, and by the 1950s, the majority of states had no such mandates. Worried that polio could return and undo the progress of the previous years, and having witnessed broad support for the polio vaccine among their constituents, lawmakers in every region of the country considered enacting school vaccination laws to keep children safe from polio.[89]

Georgia was among the first states to pass a law requiring polio vaccination for school. Although Georgia had experienced no polio epidemics, lawmakers did not want to take any chances. The legislature enacted a discretionary law in 1957 allowing the State Board of Education "to require vaccination against poliomyelitis as well as smallpox as a prerequisite to admission of students to public schools."[90]

A scientific breakthrough made it easier to convince families to vaccinate their children. A new oral vaccine against polio developed by Dr. Albert Sabin became available, requiring only several drops on the tongue or the dose administered in a sugar cube. The US government approved it for use in 1960, and within a few years, Sabin's vaccine became the predominant method of inoculation against polio.[91] As Mary Duncan recalled from her years as a Red Cross nurse in rural Kentucky, the new vaccine was a game-changer: "The [Sabin] vaccine came along . . . where you just dropped two or three drops on the tongue, that was so easy, everybody volunteered for it. And that just wiped polio completely out of Wayne County. There was no polio. That was like a magic wand."[92]

Within the next few years, more states began passing school vaccination laws. In Pennsylvania, the *Evening Times* stated, "For those who will not protect their children voluntarily, compulsory immunization may provide an effective, if unpopular, means of immunizing the population. North Carolina and Ohio and many communities now require polio vaccinations as a condition of entry into the public school system. Smallpox has been virtually wiped out in this country by such strict provisions."[93] California, which had been a hotbed of anti-vaccination activism during the Progressive Era, decided to embrace school vaccination requirements. Assemblymen Umbert J. DeLotto and William Bryon Rumford sponsored the bill. Rumford, a pharmacist, was the San Francisco Bay Area's first Black legislator and served as chair of the Assembly's Public Health Committee, and DeLotto was an engineer who had been locally active in the March of Dimes campaign.[94] In 1961, A.B. 1940 passed, requir-

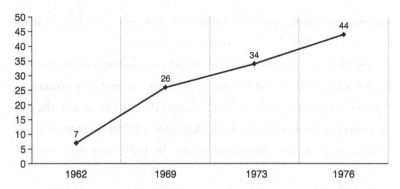

Chart 5.6. Number of states with laws requiring vaccination against polio for school admission, 1962–1976. *Sources*: US Congress, *Hearings before the Committee on Interstate and Foreign Commerce: Eighty-Seventh Congress, Second Session on H.R. 10541, May 15 and 16, 1962* (Washington, DC: GPO, 1962), 14; CDC, *Measles Surveillance: Report, No. 10, 1973–1976* (Atlanta, GA: CDC, 1977), 20; US Congress, *A Review of Selected Federal Vaccine and Immunization Policies Based on Case Studies of Pneumococcal Vaccine* (Washington, DC: GPO, 1979), 86.

ing that "no minor or adult shall be admitted to any public or private elementary or secondary school" without having been vaccinated against polio. As part of the negotiation and compromise necessary to pass the bill, California's law allowed for conscientious, or personal belief exemptions.[95] Gradually, more states followed suit, and by 1962, six states plus the District of Columbia had passed laws requiring immunization against polio for admission to school.[96]

In 1962, the federal government decided that more could be done to reach every child. Statistics collected that year showed that the racial gap in the death rate from polio had closed for school-age children from five to fourteen years old, but among children too young to attend school, the death rate of non-white children was twice that of white children.[97] Based on recommendations from the Public Health Service, President John Kennedy proposed a mass immunization program to Congress, which passed a new Vaccination Assistance Act. The act provided grants to the states for vaccination against polio and three other diseases commonly striking children: diphtheria, pertussis, and tetanus.[98]

By 1969, the number of states requiring vaccination against polio for school admission had more than tripled, and it continued to rise in later years (see chart 5.6).[99] Across the United States, the disease was gradually extinguished. During the 1970s there were fewer than ten cases in the entire country, and by 1979 there were none.[100]

Conclusion

Looking back, many Americans would later recall the polio vaccination campaign of the 1950s as "swift and sure," as did the California letter writer to the *San Jose Mercury News* in 2021. But in fact, nothing about that campaign was swift.

Compared with the smallpox vaccination campaigns of the nineteenth century, the twentieth-century operation against polio occurred during a time when most Americans held very positive views of science and allopathic medicine; nevertheless, that difference alone does not explain the success of the polio campaign. The mass polio vaccinations carried out from 1955 onward were possible because of fund-raising, publicity, and education that had been underway for two decades. During the mid-1930s, when the March of Dimes began its nationwide fund-raising campaign, students' health textbooks began to include discussion of the disease, and student clubs in middle schools and high schools across the country started organizing their own grassroots campaigns—often publicized in local newspapers—to encourage the public to support the production and deployment of a vaccine against polio. By the time a vaccine became available, these developments not only facilitated a swift mobilization to vaccinate on school grounds, but they also helped persuade large numbers of American parents to allow their children to be vaccinated.

However, swift mobilization did not lead to continuous progress. Within a year, researchers began documenting a slowdown in vaccination rates and inequitable vaccination outcomes across the country. The letter writer remembered the polio campaign of the 1950s as having been "sure," and for those born to white families in higher-socioeconomic areas with favorable attitudes toward vaccination, it probably felt that way. For others, the experience was uncertain. Inequitable access to vaccines, apathy, fear, and resistance yielded frustratingly low vaccination rates among adults and preschool children for four years after the start of the mass vaccination campaign. Nevertheless, the positive results, many associated with schools, predominated. Holding vaccination clinics on school grounds, assuring bus transportation to health clinics, and providing effective communication from schools to communities helped ensure that schoolchildren had the highest vaccination rates of any group in the country.

The critical influence of schools in the vaccination campaign illustrated how collaboration among schools, communities, and healthcare providers could help achieve high vaccination rates. As a result of that partnership, when outbreaks of polio emerged in the late 1950s, it seemed natural for state lawmakers to consider how schools could take part in protecting families and communities by requiring vaccination for admission. The campaign to defeat polio ushered in a movement to fight other long-standing childhood diseases through compulsory school admission requirements, a strategy that would become universal across all fifty states by the end of the twentieth century.

6

Schools in the Age of Eradication

During a brief address after his inauguration in 1961, President John Fitzgerald Kennedy called for a new era: "Together let us explore the stars, conquer the deserts, eradicate disease, tap the ocean depths and encourage the arts and commerce."[1] In his State of the Union message one year later, he asked Congress to pass a new mass immunization program targeting polio, diphtheria, whooping cough, and tetanus. The goal was "to take advantage of modern vaccination achievements." As a spokesperson for the administration told the press, "It is one of the disturbing things that we do have these proven vaccines, yet so many children remain without immunization."[2]

With the success of the polio campaign and the American public now seemingly on board with the idea of mass vaccination, the development of new vaccines, and more sophisticated surveillance systems to track the incidence and spread of disease, the goal appeared within reach. The idea that preventable diseases should be completely eliminated rather than simply controlled took hold during the 1960s, and thus began what some historians call an "era of eradicationism."[3] During this period, the goal of establishing compulsory school vaccination laws across the country became a cornerstone of programs and policies aiming to create a nation free from poverty and disease.

Questions and setbacks lay ahead, however. Would American parents, who had broadly endorsed the voluntary polio vaccination campaign, now support the passage of compulsory vaccination requirements? Should there be exemptions for parents who objected to vaccination on the basis of religious or personal belief? And who would enforce the laws? It fell to the states to consider these questions, and each one's answer depended on the political negotiation and compromise needed to pass the new legislation.

Two familiar roadblocks emerged during the 1970s. First, a growing sense of complacency arose in some areas, leading to new outbreaks of disease; and second, although federal and state authorities viewed schools as an important part of the eradication campaign because of their ability to teach children about health, communicate with parents, and enforce school vaccination laws, not all school districts followed through with enforcement, leading to low rates of immunization in some areas.

The 1962 Vaccination Assistance Act

Most of the proven vaccines President Kennedy mentioned in his post-inauguration address had been developed decades before the polio vaccine.

Immunization against diphtheria had been available for a very long time. Spreading quickly through families and schools with a very high fatality rate, diphtheria was one of the leading killers of children in the nineteenth and early twentieth centuries.[4] The bacterium that causes the disease creates a toxin in the body, a poison that can rapidly cause heart, nerve, kidney, and tissue damage once it enters the bloodstream.[5] In 1890, scientists in Germany discovered antitoxins capable of neutralizing the toxic proteins of the diphtheria bacteria.[6] In 1913, two physicians made groundbreaking discoveries: the Viennese doctor Bela Schick created a skin test that could reveal whether a person had immunity to diphtheria, and the German doctor Emil Behring discovered that a formulation based on a combination of diphtheria toxin with antitoxin provided long-lasting immunity. Now, physicians could immunize against diphtheria and also measure whether immunization had taken effect.[7] Despite these breakthroughs, the disease persisted in the United States for decades. During the 1920s, it killed between thirteen thousand and fifteen thousand people each year, most of them children. With the increased availability of antitoxin in the 1920s, mortality rates declined, but in 1933 nearly five thousand still died.[8]

Researchers created a vaccine against pertussis in 1913, and a vaccine against tetanus soon followed. Pertussis, also known as whooping cough, leads to violent, uncontrollable coughing, making it difficult to breathe. It is an extremely contagious respiratory disease that affects all ages and is particularly dangerous for children less than five years old. Tetanus, also known as lockjaw, is caused by spores of bacteria commonly found in dust, soil, and manure. The bacteria enter the body through punctures and tears in the skin. It causes the muscles of the jaw and throat to seize up or lock, making it difficult to swallow or open the mouth at all. The first toxoid against tetanus was produced in 1924.[9] In 1948, scientists combined the pertussis vaccine with toxoids against diphtheria and tetanus, creating the vaccine known as DPT.[10]

The era of eradication began with congressional hearings on Kennedy's call for a new mass vaccination program in 1962. With the aim of building on the momentum of the polio mass vaccination campaign, in February 1962, Abraham Ribicoff, secretary of the Department of Health, Education, and Welfare, submitted a draft of a bill to Congress to help the states carry out "intensive vaccination programs." In his cover letter, Ribicoff explained that the fight against polio was not yet over. Too many people remained unvaccinated, especially children under the age of five. He also pointed out that too many remained unprotected from other "other diseases for which effective vaccines are available—diphtheria, whooping cough, and tetanus." He urged Congress to undertake a two-stage national effort: first, a large-scale program of community vaccination campaigns across the country and second, follow-up measures to "strengthen regular ongoing vaccination programs, with particular attention to more effective coverage of the newly born each year."[11]

Congress held hearings on the proposed Vaccination Assistance Act that year. The legislation aimed to provide grants to the states for vaccination against polio and the other vaccine-preventable diseases Kennedy had called out in his address.[12]

Testimony by Dr. Russell E. Teague on behalf of the American Public Health Association emphasized the goal of eradication and the centrality of school vaccination laws in achieving it. Teague was Kentucky's commissioner of health and had extensive experience in public health at the county, state, and federal levels.[13] He pointed out that only about 38 percent of children received the DPT vaccine under the current voluntary system, and those children came from families with the financial means to pay for private pediatricians to provide inoculation. "The number of children that receive this is not enough," he explained, "so the American Public Health Association, with its 33,000 members, does endorse this bill and agree with it in principle."[14] According to Teague, "Our objective is to eradicate these four diseases, to get them so controlled that they will just be rare."[15]

Many of those working in public health during this period had come to support the goal of eradication, and the APHA's stance reflected this development.[16]

The policy of using school vaccination laws to eradicate disease came up during the hearings. By the time Teague spoke before Congress, a number of states had already passed laws requiring vaccination against the four diseases for admission to school, including Kentucky, Teague's home state. He provided the committee a list of nineteen states with compulsory laws requiring vaccination against smallpox before entry to school. Of these, six states—Kansas, Kentucky, Michigan, Missouri, North Carolina, and Ohio—were already requiring that students be vaccinated against the four diseases recommended in the proposed act.[17]

The APHA believed that if more states passed compulsory school vaccination laws, eradication would be within reach. As Teague explained to the committee, "This is enforced by entrance upon school. They are required to bring a certificate, showing that they have been immunized successfully against these four diseases and smallpox and many states are passing such laws. The Federal entrance into this field of promoting immunization would give impetus to more states taking this action and completely eradicating these diseases."[18]

The congressional hearings produced little resistance to the proposed bill. Having witnessed the success of the mass vaccination program against polio, few questioned the benefits of eliminating disease. However, concerns were expressed about the use of compulsion to accomplish this. After all, the mass vaccination against polio had been a voluntary campaign. How would Americans react to compulsory requirements to vaccinate their children against new diseases? The idea of requiring immunization against diphtheria for admission to school, as had been done for smallpox, had been unpopular for a long time. Educators had long feared that making immunization compulsory could turn "a large group of people against health work" and trigger "active opposition."[19]

Some public health officers, long retired, still recalled this opposition clearly. According to William Kelsay, who had served as a public health officer in rural Kentucky during the 1940s, parents would bring their children for voluntary immunizations against tetanus and diphtheria, but the mandatory smallpox shots required for school admission sparked hostility and resistance: "That was a mandatory procedure. . . . Some parents were opposed to any kind of immunization. That was against their practice, or against their religion, so to speak. They had several excuses or alibis. Didn't want to participate. And they would be there to see that the children did not get their shots."[20]

Voluntary immunization programs had greatly reduced disease outbreaks across the country, and although the American public had been far more supportive of medical science and vaccination throughout the polio campaign, during the hearings, some people wondered if exemptions to any new compulsory vaccination laws would be necessary. After all, not everyone was a fan of vaccination. Some health practitioners did not accept the underlying science, and others raised concerns about the safety and effectiveness of vaccines.

Several representatives of organizations opposed to vaccination spoke during the hearings. Frances Adelhardt, a natural hygienist, spoke against the Vaccination Assistance Act, explaining that natural hygienists believed health could be attained only through natural means, and that vaccination would only poison the blood and cause illness, not prevent disease. Referring to the injuries and deaths that had resulted from the use of contaminated polio vaccine in 1955, she stated, "I believe it is a crime to jeopardize the life of even one child in a vaccination program of contaminated polio vaccine that has not been proven effective nor is endorsed by the population unanimously."

Iva Purdue, president of the Natural Hygiene Society of Washington, DC, also provided a statement opposing the bill.[21]

Boroughs Stokes, a Christian Scientist authorized to appear before the committee by the Christian Science board of directors, explained that vaccination violated the religious beliefs of Christian Science. He pointed out that in many of the states with vaccination laws, "exemptions have been provided for those who object to vaccination on religious grounds." He proposed an insertion of new language in the bill: "Nothing in this section shall be construed to require a State or community to have a compulsory intensive vaccination program, or to prevent the exemption of any person, and the child, infant, or ward of any person who objects to immunization on religious grounds."[22]

Advocates of medical liberty also spoke out to express their concerns. Clinton R. Miller, representing a group called the National Health Federation, founded in 1955, outlined his group's opposition to the act, explaining that not everyone believed the recommended vaccines were effective, and some people believed the adverse effects from vaccines outweighed any potential benefit. For this reason, he argued, individuals should have freedom of choice and the ability to refuse vaccination if it was contrary to their beliefs, whether those beliefs were religious or not.[23]

The concerns of those opposed to compulsory vaccination were addressed in the final language of the Vaccination Assistance Act, which President Kennedy signed into law on October 23, 1962. Almost word-for-word, although it omitted any mention of religion, the text included Boroughs Stokes's suggested language: "Nothing in this section shall be construed to require any State or any political subdivision or instrumentality of a State to have an intensive community vaccination program which would require any person who objects to immunization to be immunized or to have any child or ward of his immunized." Adding this statement could neither force the states to allow exemptions on the basis of religion or conscientious objection nor prevent them from passing laws prohibiting exemptions from vaccination. The act simply authorized grants to the states to help pay for vaccination programs against polio, diphtheria, whooping cough, and tetanus.[24]

Nevertheless, the act's language was influential. West Virginia was the only state to never allow nonmedical exemptions. In 1905, when the state passed its first compulsory vaccination law, it had allowed only medical exemptions, and later, in the absence of any meaningful public pushback against proposals to require vaccination against measles and other diseases, the state kept its earlier language intact, adding the additional requirement that a physician must certify in writing that vaccination was not medically feasible for the child.[25] In contrast, most other states added language to their laws allowing religious exemptions from school vaccination requirements, largely in response to lobbying by Christian Scientists. By 1980, forty-eight states had school vaccination laws that allowed exemptions based on religious conviction, and some states allowed exemptions based on personal belief.[26]

Passage of the act was not only significant in providing financial support to the states and upholding their authority to determine whether to add nonmedical exemptions to their laws—it also gave the Communicable Disease Center in Atlanta (CDC) an important leadership role in vaccination programs around the country. The CDC began as a branch of the US Public Health Service and was founded to prevent malaria from spreading across the states. During the 1940s, the agency broadened its focus to include all contagious diseases. After the Vaccination Assistance Act went into effect, the CDC took responsibility for coordinating efforts of the states in developing intensive vaccination programs to eradicate the four diseases.[27]

The Shift from Persuasion to Compulsory School Vaccination Laws

As federal funding became available under the Vaccination Assistance Act, most states continued to promote voluntary immunization rather than pass new compulsory vaccination laws, but this began to change after a vaccine against measles became available. Measles, or rubeola, is a highly contagious disease caused by a virus. Often confused with the milder German measles, or rubella, measles is far more dangerous. Among children it can lead to a fever as high as 105 degrees Fahrenheit. Before the discovery of a vaccine, the general fatality rate was just over 3 percent, but the youngest and oldest victims were the most susceptible.[28] Between 1912 and 1922, about six thousand measles-related deaths occurred in the United States each year. Some survivors faced complications, because measles could also cause encephalitis, leading to intellectual disability.[29]

In 1963, researchers developed and licensed the first vaccine against measles, and two years later, under President Lyndon Baines Johnson, Congress revised and extended the Vaccination Assistance Act to support "special efforts needed to overcome the attitude that measles is a harmless childhood disease."[30] An important force behind the new law was the Joseph P. Kennedy Foundation, established to "seek the prevention of intellectual disabilities by identifying its causes, and to improve the means by which society deals with citizens who have intellectual disabilities." Eunice Kennedy Shriver directed the foundation, and at her urging, President Kennedy had prioritized intellectual disabilities in his administration.[31]

Under the Johnson administration, the effort to eliminate measles and other childhood diseases picked up speed. In 1966, the CDC sponsored a national conference in St. Louis, bringing together "some 450 physicians, laboratory scientists, health educators, and other public health workers from coast to coast" to make plans for a nationwide program to eradicate polio, diphtheria, whooping cough, tetanus, and measles."[32] In 1967, Surgeon General William H. Stewart claimed that measles could be eradicated by the end of 1968.[33] This was an ambitious timeline, but many public health officials believed it could be achieved. The health officer in Pocatello, Idaho, announced, "The goal of the 1968 January program here is to eliminate measles entirely as a threat to life and health in Pocatello." To cover his bases, he added a qualifier: "The response of each parent will largely determine whether this program is successful."[34]

Women's groups and civic organizations like the Lions Clubs joined the effort to build widespread grassroots support for the eradication campaign.[35] In California, the Junior Women's Clubs asked the state senate to pass a bill requiring students be vaccinated against measles, and when the legislature voted on S.B. 288, it passed with unanimous votes in both the Senate and the Assembly.[36] Legislative documents show only a handful letters asking Republican Governor Ronald Reagan to veto the bill. For example, the secretary of the Santa Monica Organic Garden and Nutrition Club opposed the bill on the grounds of medical freedom and the conviction that health came from good nutrition and exercise, "not from foreign substances being injected into the bloodstream with who knows what after effects in years to come."[37]

By the following year, seventeen states had passed laws requiring that students be vaccinated against measles before entering school, and the incidence of measles dropped dramatically. From about 458,000 cases and 421 deaths in 1964, measles accounted for only 22,000 cases and fewer than 100 deaths in 1968.[38]

Complacency and Increased
Outbreaks of Disease

Unfortunately, the progress achieved in 1968 did not continue over the next few years. New measles outbreaks struck a number of states that had not yet seen a need for new school vaccination policies, and governments and health officials became concerned about complacency. From 1968 to 1971, cases of measles in the United States more than tripled, from 22,231 cases to 75,290, the result of falling immunization rates.[39] Irene Kanta, a health department administrator in Idaho, summed up the problem: "In the past decade the concern of parents and physicians over such diseases as polio and measles has declined steadily. Apathy set in because epidemics were prevented and people believed the danger was over."[40] According to Dr. William H. Foege of the CDC, "Many of our younger parents have no memory of polio and the iron lungs have all but disappeared. Many of our younger physicians have never seen a case of polio in a youngster. It is unfortunate but in the absence of disease some people do become complacent."[41]

Seeking a more permanent solution to the problem of complacency, more states began to consider mandates. Each state's decision to pass a school vaccination law in the wake of disease outbreaks was shaped, not only by the severity of the outbreaks, but also by its prior history with school vaccination laws. Developments in Texas and Wisconsin illustrate this phenomenon.

Texas, whose supreme court had often upheld the state's school vaccination law, moved fairly quickly to impose a new school vaccination mandate. In 1971, Texas had the highest level of measles in five years, owing to epidemics in urban areas, including Dallas. Texas newspapers began reporting that doctors predicted that given current trends, an epidemic of measles and German measles would spread across the state in the next two years. German measles, known as rubella, was a milder disease than measles, but it posed a danger to a pregnant woman, because if infected, her newborn could suffer birth defects. "Until 1963," reported one newspaper, "measles was virtually unstoppable. Today, one dose of measles vaccine given to children 12 months or older offers almost 100 percent protection. It's the best odds a parent can find anywhere."[42]

Because school vaccination policies were already in place, in 1971 Texas quickly passed a law requiring students to receive the DPT vaccine and vaccines against polio, measles, and German measles. The law allowed medical and religious exemptions, but also gave the state commissioner the power to set religious exemptions aside "in time of emergency." By 1973, the immunization levels of Texas schoolchildren approached 95 percent, with the result that polio cases disappeared, diphtheria cases fell 92 percent, and cases of the other targeted diseases also plummeted.[43]

In contrast to Texas, Wisconsin moved more slowly. The state had long preferred the strategy of persuasion over compulsion. With relatively low immunization rates, Wisconsin had the highest rates of infection in the country in 1971.[44] During repeated outbreaks over the next few years, Wisconsin public health officials used federal funds to set up voluntary immunization clinics where, with parental consent, children could be vaccinated. Wisconsin schools cooperated in the effort by communicating with parents about the clinics and distributing the consent slips.[45]

But voluntary programs failed to produce the desired results. The immunization rate against polio fell from a high of 84 percent in 1963 to a low of 60 percent in 1973. This news made front-page headlines in Wisconsin papers, which began publishing editorials urging parents to immunize their children. "What is the most recent national epidemic you can recall?" asked one editorial. "If the source of polio during the 1950's is the only one that comes to mind don't be fooled into thinking the immunizations of the 50's and 60's have made us so safe. . . . To the contrary, immunization remains as important and as urgent as ever."[46] No one in Wisconsin wanted to see polio come roaring back amid a resurgence of deadly childhood diseases. Faced with the possibility of more outbreaks, the public's long-standing resistance to school vaccination mandates vanished. The legislature passed a Student Immunization Law in 1975 without any noticeable controversy or pushback. The law required that all children entering the state's schools and day care centers for the first time must be vaccinated against polio, DTP, and measles.[47]

Declining immunization levels among children in many states led to the creation of a federal government Childhood Immunization Initiative in 1977. Under the direction of the Department of Health, Education, and Welfare, the program aimed to immunize 90 percent of all children under the age of fifteen against polio, diphtheria, tetanus, pertussis, and measles by the fall of 1979. The initiative coordinated federal resources to promote the immunization of children in every state, including infants. An important part of the program was to enforce school vaccination requirements and to broaden those requirements to cover, not just students entering school for the first time, but students in all grades.[48] The program aimed to close the gap in immunization levels between high- and low-income areas. To achieve this, the program sought to strengthen the enforcement of school immunization laws. It had become clear that in many states with school vaccination laws, the schools were not enforcing the regulations.[49]

Schools Fail to Enforce the Laws

With the increase in state vaccination laws from 1962 onward, the legal infrastructure to prevent the spread of disease was in place, but enforcement of the laws depended on the cooperation of the schools. No teacher wanted children to contract an illness in the classroom. Sick students fell behind in their lessons, requiring additional help to make up for lost time. No principal wanted outbreaks of disease in the school, because days of recorded absence could lead to declines in funding. For educators, learning that a contagious disease at the school had resulted in a child's death was heartbreaking. However, not all schools welcomed their new role as enforcers of vaccination laws.

In many areas, public health authorities failed to notice a lack of enforcement until a serious epidemic spread across the state. Alaska's health authorities learned that the state's school immunization law was not being enforced during an outbreak of measles in Fairbanks in the fall of 1976. When health officials asked the schools for their vaccination records, they discovered that only 25 percent of schoolchildren had been vaccinated against the disease. Citing state law, the health authorities ordered all unvaccinated children to be excluded from school, forcing 11 percent of the city's students to remain at home until immunized. During the exclusion, no more cases of measles emerged, leading the authorities to enforce the school law statewide. On March 1, 1977, health authorities excluded over 8 percent of the state's K–12 students not yet immunized against polio, diphtheria, tetanus, pertussis, measles, and German measles. Just one month later, fewer than fifty-one children remained unvaccinated, and among the more than thirty-five thousand children immunized, none suffered any adverse effects from a vaccine.[50]

The same thing happened in California during a measles epidemic in Los Angeles. According to Representative Henry A. Waxman, even though state law required the schools to "see some proof of vaccination" before admitting students, it became clear during the epidemic that the "law was not being enforced."[51] Los Angeles health administrator Shirley Fannin agreed, explaining that some schools "had records that were almost impossible to audit. Some complained of insufficient time to comply."[52]

Financial concerns were one reason for the lack of enforcement in California and other states. When California's legislature passed S.B. 942 in 1977 calling for students to be immunized against diphtheria, pertussis, tetanus, polio, and measles, the language in the bill required school authorities to collect proof of students' immunization, periodically review records to ensure all students had been immunized, and exclude from school any students "who failed to obtain the required immunizations within the time limits."[53] Although the bill had originally appropriated funding for schools to cover the costs of the additional record-keeping, monitoring, and follow-up, the appropriation was deleted on the recommendation of the Senate Finance Committee, which had concluded that the money was unnecessary because "the schools should already be doing what this bill requires."[54] Educational leaders and school nurses were outraged, and many sent letters and telegrams to Governor Edmund G. Brown, asking him to veto the unfunded mandate.[55] Their efforts were to no avail. According to Dr. Eunice Turrell, health services coordinator for the Los Angeles school district, funding issues affected immunization in two ways: first, there simply was not enough money for California school districts to employ enough nurses, doctors, and other professionals to comply with the law; and second, some school officials were reluctant to exclude students, because they feared losing state funding based on student enrollments.[56]

Educators everywhere were concerned about funding tied to enrollments. This had been a persistent issue with smallpox mandates during the Progressive Era, and now as more states added new vaccination mandates, the problem took center stage once again. In Illinois, health officials encountered this dilemma during an outbreak of measles in the schools of Cook County. "The district was lax in requiring the children to have the immunizations," reported Jim Mulrooney, public health adviser with the county health department. He claimed that school districts did not want to exclude unvaccinated children from school "because state education aid for each district is based on pupil attendance."[57]

Other reasons schools failed to enforce the laws included differences in professional priorities and a lack of commitment to immunization. In Oklahoma, responses from a survey of 1,370 school superintendents and principals from every county in the state showed that only 82 percent found the school vaccination law beneficial and worth the effort.[58] In Los Angeles, some educators felt that it was not their business to enforce vaccination. As Eunice Turrell explained, "We could not always get the cooperation of the school administrator to exclude a child. They feel the primary purpose is education. As educators, they do not appreciate the need for immunizations as much as we do. Some have been very cooperative, and we have excluded children. Other administrators have not done this."[59]

New York City school administrators also viewed public health priorities as outside their purview. A review of ten schools in the city conducted by the CDC and the Department of Health, Education, and Welfare revealed a general lack of enforcement, but the problem was not a lack of money—instead, the investigators found a general lack of coordination and cooperation among the departments of health and education. According to New York University law professor Barry Ensminger, "School officials had never taken [the state law] seriously. It was seen as a public health measure—the responsibility of the Department of Health, not the Board of Education." As a result, no principal had ever faced a penalty for admitting unvaccinated students. In the wake of the review, the Board of Education resolved "to take disciplinary action against recalcitrant school officials."[60]

Some states strengthened their school vaccination laws to increase enforcement. Illinois changed its school law in 1979 after it became clear that although every school district asked parents to submit their children's immunization records, in some places, school officials were not actually checking them. Under the new law, if fewer than 80 percent of a district's students were not immunized, the state could withhold 10 percent of the district's funding. According to Richard Galati, immunization specialist for the Illinois Department of Public Health, "It was amazing how quickly school districts began to get their act together and started complying." The immunization standard was increased to 90 percent for the 1981–82 school year, and according to Galati, by 1990, "98 or 99 percent" of K–12 students in Illinois were immunized.[61]

Despite a lack of enforcement in some areas, more school districts began to comply with state requirements during the two-year Childhood Immunization Initiative that began in 1977. At the Department of Health, Education, and Welfare, Secretary Joseph A. Califano Jr. took steps to make sure that school officials understood that control of diseases in their schools was one of their most important professional responsibilities. He asked the Office of Education to "place the highest priority" on reaching out to school systems to enlist their support, emphasizing the need for schools to educate the public about the importance of immunization, cooperate with public health departments, and enforce the school immunization laws. He also urged schools to carry out "outbreak control programs" when disease was discovered.[62]

More school districts began to enforce the laws, not only in response to Califano's urging but also because new research studies showed that enforcement in the schools reduced disease outbreaks in communities. Evidence for this had been available for a number of years. A measles outbreak in Texarkana, which was divided by the Texas-Arkansas state line, revealed the effectiveness of school vaccination mandates in 1971. Whereas Arkansas required immunization against measles for admission to school, Texas did not. During the outbreak, about 96 percent of the cases in Texarkana occurred among communities on the Texas side of the border, whereas residents on the Arkansas side were much better protected.[63]

Larger studies conducted from 1977 to 1978 confirmed that for childhood diseases like measles, schools were the major site of disease transmission in the country. These studies also showed that states that strictly enforced school vaccination laws had rates of disease less than half those of the rest of the country. Alaska was a case in point. After ensuring enforcement of the law, in 1977, Governor Jay Hammond announced that immunization levels in the state had reached 95 percent and diseases among schoolchildren had plummeted, even as they were rising in other areas of the country.[64]

Of course, fewer cases of illness among children in the schools translated to higher rates of enrollment and thus higher levels of state funding. In Los Angeles, where school officials had been lax in enforcing vaccination requirements when a measles epidemic swept through the city, the L.A. County Public Health Department gave the parents of 1.6 million children a choice: Vaccinate your children within the month or keep them home. As the schools began to enforce the order, the measles epidemic, which had caused brain damage in five children and killed two, finally disappeared.[65]

School Vaccination Laws Take Hold in Every State

By the end of 1979, all fifty states had passed standing school vaccination laws allowing exemption for medical or other reasons (chart 6.1), and more than 90 percent of students in kindergarten through the eighth grade had been immunized against measles, polio, diphtheria, tetanus, and pertussis. As a result, measles cases in the country dropped 78 percent over the two-year period, and there were no reported cases of diphtheria that year. US Surgeon General Julius B. Richmond called the Childhood Immunization Program a "dramatic success."[66] By the following year, although deaths from bacterial dis-

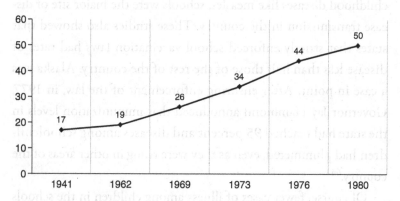

Chart 6.1. Number of states with standing school vaccination laws, 1941–1980.
Sources: Data compiled from William Fowler, "Principal Provisions of Smallpox Vaccination Laws and Provisions in the United States," *PHR* 56, no. 5 (Jan. 31, 1941): 169; US Congress, *Hearings before the Committee on Interstate and Foreign Commerce: Eighty-Seventh Congress, Second Session on H.R. 10541, May 15 and 16, 1962* (Washington, DC: GPO, 1962), 14; CDC, *Measles Surveillance: Report, No. 10, 1973–1976* (Atlanta, GA: CDC, 1977), 20; US Congress, *A Review of Selected Federal Vaccine and Immunization Policies Based on Case Studies of Pneumococcal Vaccine* (Washington, DC: GPO, 1979), 86; Wyoming Legislature, *Digest of Senate and House Journals of the* [. . .] *State Legislature of Wyoming* (Cheyenne, WY: Legislative Service Office, 1979), 70; "Idaho Statutes: Title 39, Health and Safety; Chapter 48, Immunization," Idaho Legislature, https://legislature.idaho.gov/statutesrules/idstat /title39/t39ch48/sect39-4801.

eases and viruses killed 10,441 people across the nation, school-age children were well protected—of children between the ages of five and fourteen, only 77 died from such diseases.[67]

During the 1980s, college and university campuses also began to implement vaccination mandates to achieve herd immunity against measles and other diseases. Unlike preschool, elementary, and secondary schools, institutions of higher education were largely exempt from state vaccination requirements. In 1927, only fifty-nine institutions— twenty-five public and thirty-four private—required students to be vaccinated against smallpox, and at most schools, the mandates were part of the R.O.T.C. regulations.[68] This state of affairs changed during the 1980s. In 1983, about 20 percent of measles infections in the country occurred on college campuses. College officials initially reported outbreaks at Dartmouth College, Indiana University, the University of Miami in Ohio, the University of Houston, and Louisiana State University, and before the year was out, measles cases had emerged on nineteen college campuses. CDC scientists announced that measles outbreaks, although a "disappearing childhood disease, remain a problem on American college campuses." In response, the American College Health Association adopted a policy recommending that universities and colleges require all students born before 1956 to show proof of immunization before matriculation. By 1986, the percentage of institutions with such a requirement had more than doubled.[69]

Conclusion

The success of the polio campaign gave rise to the idea that the American public might finally be ready to endorse an effort to eliminate some of the nation's deadliest childhood diseases. For decades, Americans had preferred voluntary immunization programs to lessen the impact of diphtheria, whooping cough, measles, and other illnesses. Voluntary programs reduced civil unrest by accommodating those opposed to vaccination, but the price of that accommodation was the ongoing deaths of thousands of children each year from vaccine-preventable diseases. The goal of eradication took hold during the 1960s, ushering in a two-decade effort to wipe diphtheria and other diseases off the map.

Executives at both the federal and state levels regarded schools as the linchpin of disease-eradication programs because of their ability to provide children with health information, communicate effectively with parents, and ensure compliance with school vaccination laws. But school authorities were sometimes resistant to their new responsibility for enforcement. Persistent concerns about the impact of state vaccination laws on school funding, coupled with a long-standing belief that vaccination was the responsibility of the local health department rather than the school, continued throughout this era. Nevertheless, the passage of new vaccination mandates at every level of schooling represented an enormous shift in American attitudes toward vaccination, not only among policymakers and voters, but also among school officials. During this period, schools in many areas of country came to accept that it was their responsibility to help prevent contagious diseases from spreading, and they began enforcing the laws.

Throughout the 1960s and '70s, newspapers reported the victories—first against polio, then diphtheria, pertussis, and tetanus, and finally, against measles. Rarely was there any mention of problems that occasionally surfaced during legislative hearings and public health conferences—cases of vaccine injury, lawsuits raising the issue of liability, and a growing sense among some Americans that the government was intruding too much into the private lives of citizens. But that would soon change.

7

Vaccine Hesitancy and the Rise of Personal Belief Exemptions

In 1970, the parents of eight-month-old Anita Reyes took her to a health department clinic in Texas, where a registered nurse fed her two drops of Sabin vaccine. Within two weeks, she became paralyzed and was diagnosed with polio. The family filed suit against Wyeth Laboratories, claiming that the company's vaccine had infected the child. The charges included product liability, negligence, and breach of warranty. Although Wyeth had included an insert warning of potential risk associated with the vaccine with every shipment of one hundred doses, the parents said no one had informed them of any risk, a claim corroborated by the nurse who gave Anita her inoculation. According to the nurse, the clinic staff did not regularly give any warnings to patients receiving vaccines. A Texas federal district court awarded the family damages of $200,000, ruling that even if the company could not warn the recipient directly, it had to make sure that whoever performed the immunization would do so. The US Court of Appeals for the Fifth Circuit upheld the verdict in 1974. In his ruling, the judge said that the case "raises a policy consideration scarcely less urgent than the need for mass immunization from disease; the right of the individual to choose and control what risk he will take."[1]

Unlike the lawsuits over the defective lots of Salk vaccine produced by Cutter Laboratories, the Sabin vaccine was not defective in this case. Very rarely, in around one out of every three million cases—the Sabin vaccine itself could cause paralytic polio.[2] As the families of other children with vaccine-related injuries filed suit against drug manufacturers, the size of the damages increased over time. The ensuing lawsuits raised questions and concerns about risk, liability, and compensation in cases of injury from vaccines.

Over the following decades, concerns about vaccine safety led some parents of infants and toddlers to delay or refuse some vaccines. Other factors contributed to parents' hesitancy as well. As serious outbreaks of diseases dwindled because of the herd immunity achieved through high rates of vaccination, some felt their children no longer needed the vaccines. And other parents hesitated because they had heard or read misinformation about vaccines.

Parents' hesitancy to vaccinate their children evolved along with developments in vaccine science. Scientific disputes over vaccines, and the long time it takes for the scientific community to validate or reject a claim, meant that some unfounded allegations—such as the contention that vaccines caused autism—continued to circulate on television and social media for many years, leading some parents to refuse vaccination. Additionally, as researchers discovered new vaccines and the CDC recommended them for children, some parents worried about the cumulative effect of multiple shots. Others protested against new requirements to vaccinate school-age children against diseases that were sexually transmitted and not actually contagious in schools.

The era from the late twentieth to the twenty-first century was a time of growing hesitancy and opposition to vaccines among a vocal minority. Most people still supported school vaccination policies—elementary and high school vaccination rates remained high, even as national survey data showed a rise in vaccine hesitancy among young parents. Nevertheless, more parents began applying for exemptions from school vaccination laws on the basis of personal belief, and gradually, the number of states allowing such exemptions increased.

A Growing Distrust

By the 1980s, a new movement against compulsory vaccination emerged, with roots in earlier decades. The 1960s and early 1970s were a time of civil rights protests, antiwar demonstrations, civil unrest, feminism, and environmentalism. These decades saw growing public criticism of government institutions, science, and technology.

During the 1950s, the American public had embraced the idea that a marriage of science and industry would bring forth an era of plentiful harvests, abundance on grocery shelves, and all-round "better living through chemistry," but popular reaction to Rachel Carson's *Silent Spring*, which came out in 1962, revealed a profound change in attitudes about the natural world.[3] Carson, a biologist and former employee of the US Fish and Wildlife Service, documented the way the use of the insecticide DDT to improve crop yields was threatening the existence of wildlife—including the beloved songbirds that Americans saw disappearing from their backyard feeders. As a result of the book's widespread impact, people began raising questions about the chemicals lingering on the skins of the fruits and vegetables their families consumed. By 1965, the Food and Drug Administration (FDA) and the Department of Health, Education, and Welfare (HEW) jointly sponsored a study of the use of toxic pesticides on food, and the US Congress began holding hearings to discuss public policy regarding the use of pesticides in food production. As historian Elena Conis has shown, it was not long before some Americans began talking about vaccines as artificial, unnatural, and thus potentially toxic.[4]

By the 1970s, a counterculture movement was in full swing, and young Americans joined conservation groups, took up backpacking in wilderness areas, and turned to organic gardening, vegetarianism, environmentalism, and alternative forms of healing. Newspaper coverage of articles discussing "back to nature" and "natural health" reflected this trend (chart 7.1). The growing interest in all things natural mirrored some of the published discourse from the Progressive Era, a time when many alternative health practitioners viewed vaccines as inherently unnatural.[5]

This was also an era of increasing distrust in the male doctors and scientists who were usually the ones dispensing expertise. As historian Wendy Kline has shown, second-wave feminists sought to challenge traditional, male-dominated science and medicine by arguing

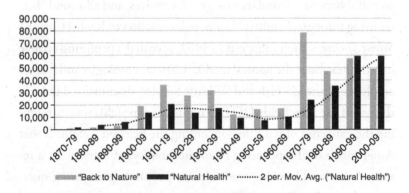

Chart 7.1. Number of US newspaper articles reporting on "back to nature" and "natural health," by decade, 1870–2009. *Note:* "2 per. Mov. Avg." = two-period moving average. *Source:* Data derived from a search conducted February 8, 2023, of newspapers published from 1870 through 2009 on Newspapers.com using the terms *back to nature* and *natural health.*

that a woman's way of knowing, based on subjective experience, was just as valid as the empirical scientific method. Health feminists viewed a mother's feelings and experience about her own child—and her child's potential risk from vaccines—as equally authoritative as the doctor's clinical assessment.[6]

As the media began carrying reports of the dangers of food additives, nuclear waste, and pollution, scientists became anxious about the apparent disintegration of American confidence in science and technology. In 1976, the National Science Board included a section about the declining level of public support for scientific endeavors in its bicentennial report.[7] Near the end of the 1950s, during the polio campaign, 83 percent of Americans had agreed with the statement, "the world is better off . . . because of science." However, only 37 percent of Americans reported "a great deal of confidence" in science in 1973.[8]

Nevertheless, scientists were not the only ones facing an increasingly skeptical public. Americans had also lost confidence in medicine, education, the press, and the U.S. Congress (table 7.1). When it came to vaccines, news reports of state and federal governments' inadequate responses to issues of risk, liability, and compensation began appearing more frequently in news media.

Table 7.1. US public indicating "a great deal of confidence" in selected institutional areas, 1966 vs. 1971–1977 (in percentages)

Institutional areas	1966	1971	1972	1973	1974	1975	1976	1977
Medicine	72	61	48	54	60	50	54	51
Education	61	37	33	37	49	31	37	41
Science	56	32	37	37	45	38	43	41
Congress	42	19	21	23	17	13	14	19
Media	29	18	18	23	26	24	28	25

Source: Table adapted from Georgine M. Pion and Mark W. Lipsey, "Public Attitudes toward Science and Technology: What Have the Surveys Told Us?," Public Opinion Quarterly 45, no. 3 (Autumn 1981): 308.

Reports of risk from vaccines kept questions of vaccine safety before the public. At what point was the risk of adverse effects greater than the risk of the disease? By the end of the 1960s, it had become clear that routine vaccination against smallpox was no longer worth the risk. Since 1949, there had been no documented cases of smallpox in the country, and yet one out of every million people vaccinated died from the procedure every year. As a result, in 1971 the US Public Health Service recommended ending the practice of routine smallpox vaccination in the country, stating, "vaccination against smallpox unnecessarily exposes a large segment of the United States public to the risk of complications resulting from vaccination—a risk greater than the probability of their contracting the disease."[9]

Doctors serving as medical experts in their communities disagreed over the recommendation. For instance, in Connecticut, where education authorities had statutory control over vaccination requirements for school admission, the state commissioner of education wrote to local school boards recommending they stop requiring proof of smallpox vaccinations. In the town of Bridgeport, the school board scheduled a meeting to discuss the issue. At the time, local doctors were divided over the recommendation.

On the one hand, Dr. Chester E. Haberlin, who had served as acting public health director during Bridgeport's mass polio vaccination campaign, told the board that it would be a mistake to discontinue smallpox vaccinations. He was not alone in this belief—many readers encountered this opinion in a nationally syndicated column, "Ask Dr. Lamb," which appeared in over seven hundred newspapers. Dr. Lawrence Lamb, an internist and former professor of medicine at Baylor College of Medicine told readers that smallpox vaccinations should continue, because it was possible that the virus could still be living in remote isolated areas and suddenly emerge.[10]

Not everyone agreed. Dr. H. Patterson Harris, Bridgeport's current director of public health, informed the school board that while there had been no reported cases of smallpox in the previous two decades, three children had died from adverse reactions to the vaccine. Ultimately, once Bridgeport's school board learned that three children had died from a vaccine for a disease that no longer existed in the United States, they voted to stop requiring it.[11]

In some areas, school boards delayed taking any action because their state legislatures were slow to revise the law. This happened in Ohio, where in January 1972, the state's department of health announced that a bill had been introduced into the state legislature to delete the smallpox vaccination requirement from the School Immunization Act, and that "all schools should discontinue requiring evidence of smallpox vaccination."[12] After this, many local doctors decided to no longer offer smallpox vaccinations. But Ohio school boards found themselves between a rock and a hard place— as the town of Piqua's board explained, "This places the parent and the school district in an untenable position, because we still must require the smallpox vaccination as well as other immunizations." Some school districts joined Piqua in maintaining the smallpox vaccination requirement until the state legislature changed the law at the end of the summer. Others went ahead and ended the practice earlier, trusting that the law would eventually pass.[13]

Issues of Liability and Compensation

Ending smallpox vaccination did nothing to abate concerns over vaccines, however. During the 1970s, fears over risk and liability for vaccine injury continued as states expanded their vaccination laws and schools added new vaccines to their admission requirements. In cases of lawsuits arising from vaccine-related injury, the awards for damages grew more substantial. For example, Mary J. Griffin became infected with a severe case of paralytic polio after taking a dose of Pfizer's Sabin vaccine. When she emerged from a coma in the hospital, she was left a quadriplegic. She and her husband sued, and in 1972 a US district court in Pennsylvania awarded the couple over $2 million in damages.[14]

School districts were very worried about liability. This became evident in New York, where ongoing measles outbreaks during the late 1970s led the state's health department to insist that schools exclude unvaccinated students and cooperate with immunization programs. It soon became evident that school authorities in Nassau County on Long Island were not complying with the order. The district's lawyers and insurance agent had advised against excluding unvaccinated students from the school, and they had also warned the district against allowing the health department to set up a vaccination clinic on school grounds without any agreement to cover the costs of the program or safeguard the school from liability. Shortly after this meeting, another district on Long Island also refused to comply with the state's immunization program unless the county would indemnify its schools against any lawsuits. Ultimately, the New York State health commissioner obtained a court order to force the districts to comply.[15]

With a new awareness of risk and liability, policymakers began raising the question of government compensation, but the US Congress failed to act. In February 1975, a meeting of the CDC, the FDA, the American Academy of Pediatrics, vaccine manufacturers, and state health representatives came to a consensus. The group agreed that the US government should pass legislation to provide federal compensation for the victims of vaccine injury. "Otherwise," the group concluded, "the United States faces a very real possibility of an immunization shortfall in the near future, as a result of manufacturers withdrawing from vaccine production." At the time, the governments of France, Japan, and Switzerland had already established vaccine-injury compensation programs. But despite their recommendation, the federal government would take no action for another eleven years.[16]

Scientific Disputes and Ongoing Controversies over Vaccines

Lawsuits over injury from vaccines were not the only cause of vaccine hesitancy during the following decades. Disputes among medical researchers over possible adverse effects from vaccines also fanned distrust in scientific expertise and resistance to vaccines. In contrast to the boundary disputes between alternative and allopathic physicians a century earlier, these disputes had nothing to do with disagreements over scientific theory. Instead, they arose during a regular and ongoing part of the scientific method—the quest to replicate researchers' findings to see if their claims are valid.[17] Unfortunately, the process of replication and verification can take many years, and by the time a false claim is finally shown to be unsupported by evidence, many people may have come to accept it as a core belief. This happened with controversies over the diphtheria-pertussis-tetanus (DPT) and measles-mumps-rubella (MMR) vaccines.

In 1979, reports of adverse effects from the DPT vaccine began to emerge as more states recommended that infants receive the shot. On March 9, Tennessee health officials informed the CDC that four infants between the ages of two and three months had died within twenty-four hours of receiving a dose of DPT vaccine. All of the vaccine came from a single tainted lot produced by Wyeth Labs. Tennessee withdrew the lot from all of its health clinics, and Wyeth removed it from the market. The government's recall of one hundred thousand doses of vaccine was widely reported in the press.[18]

By itself, the recall probably would have alleviated parents' concerns, but doctors in England had been sounding alarms about the DPT vaccine since the early 1970s, and disputes among scientists over the validity of these fears lasted for years. In 1973, John Wilson, a pediatric neurologist, told an audience at the Royal Society of Medicine that he believed the pertussis portion of the vaccine had caused neurological illnesses to about fifty patients in the Hospital for Sick Children in London during the previous decade. Although Wilson's claim was never confirmed, British health officials asked Dr. David Miller to conduct a study of DTP adverse effects. Miller launched a four-year survey of health practitioners, and in 1981, he reported a significant correlation between the vaccine and serious neurological illnesses like epilepsy and intellectual disability. He concluded that DTP caused permanent brain damage in around one out of every one hundred thousand vaccinated children.[19]

During later years, claims that the DTP vaccine caused neurological illnesses would not stand up to scrutiny. Identifying cases of epilepsy and mental disability caused by vaccines is difficult, because symptoms of these conditions often arise in the first of year of life, which is when infants receive three doses of the vaccine. Researchers later attempted to confirm Miller's findings, with no success. In 1989, the British Pediatric Association and the Canadian National Advisory Committee found no proof the vaccine caused permanent harm. During the 1990s, large-scale studies by the US Institute of Medicine, a combined University of Washington and CDC team, and other research groups also reported no evidence that the pertussis vaccine caused any permanent neurological damage.[20]

But for people reading newspapers and watching television in the 1970s and early '80s, hearing that the DPT vaccine could cause epilepsy or intellectual disability in children was a bombshell. The ongoing, complex process of replicating scientific research findings did not instill confidence in parents whose local school districts were requiring immunization against diphtheria, pertussis, and tetanus for admission to school.

In April 1982, a television station in Washington, DC, aired a documentary with the sensational title *Vaccine Roulette*, which covered cases of injuries believed to be caused by the pertussis portion of the DPT vaccine. "What we have found are serious questions about the safety and effectiveness of the shot," announced the show's producer.[21] *Vaccine Roulette* was broadcast by television stations affiliated with the National Broadcasting Company (NBC).

This was the first time a major news group had presented a documentary airing some of the same questions scientists were grappling with. The research had not yet confirmed that the pertussis portion of the DPT vaccine caused any neurological damage, but for parents whose children had experienced seizures after vaccination, the broadcast confirmed their suspicions that there were problems with the vaccine.

After the show aired, a group of parents founded a new activist group called Dissatisfied Parents Together, using the same acronym as the DPT vaccine. The founders included Barbara Loe Fisher, whose oldest son had experienced a seizure after vaccination and later developed learning disabilities and attention deficit disorder, and Jeffrey Schwartz, a Washington lawyer whose daughter had died two years after reacting with a seizure to the DPT shot as an infant.

Schwartz told reporters that in order to keep vaccination rates high, the medical profession had not adequately informed parents of the risks: "In the effort to calm parental fears they've gone overboard in minimizing the dangers," he said. Schwartz and others in the group were well aware that cases of vaccine injury were exceedingly rare, but they considered any injury unacceptable. "It's not that we're antivaccine," he said. "But from the standpoint of parents, even one child who is severely injured is too many."[22]

Two years later, a nine-month investigation conducted by two journalists for the Gannett News Service produced a report critical of US vaccine policy. The probe, which was published by newspapers across the country, identified three major problems: First, there were no incentives to induce manufacturers to produce the safest vaccines possible; second, there was no real transparency regarding vaccine safety; and third, there were no federal mechanisms in place to identify a bad batch of vaccine quickly and remove it from the market.[23]

In response to public pressure, the American Academy of Pediatrics began seeking federal legislation to develop a national compensation program to address the issue of adverse reactions to childhood vaccines. In 1985, the US Congress held hearings on two bills, one of which was coauthored by Dissatisfied Parents Together. During the next few years, representatives from concerned parent groups spoke at additional congressional hearings, and their testimony was influential.[24]

In 1986, Congress passed the National Childhood Vaccine Injury Act, and President Ronald Reagan signed it into law. The act established the National Vaccine Injury Compensation Program to provide financial compensation to those who had suffered injury or death as a result of vaccination. To protect manufacturers and medical practitioners from lawsuits, the act capped the amount of damages that could be filed against a vaccine producer or a vaccine administrator at $1,000. It also established the National Vaccine Program, which became responsible for the coordination and oversight of vaccine research, development, safety and testing, licensing, production, procurement, distribution, and the evaluation of efficacy and adverse effects.[25]

One of the goals of the vaccine injury act was to build a climate of public safety and trust regarding vaccines, but concerns over vaccination mandates did not diminish. A new scientific dispute arose over whether the MMR vaccine could cause autism. The MMR vaccine was licensed in 1971 as a combined vaccine that protected against measles, mumps, and rubella, or German measles.[26]

During the 1980s, questions about the causes of autism, and whether vaccines were responsible, led to greater controversy over vaccines. Autism, or autism spectrum disorder (ASD), is a lifelong developmental disability causing social, communication, and behavioral challenges. Symptoms emerge during early childhood, around the same time that children commonly receive immunizations. Autism became a nationwide concern in the 1980s and '90s as studies showed that cases were increasing across the country. Finding a cure or effective treatment for autism required understanding what caused it, but researchers could not agree. Some hypothesized that autism was caused by a virus. Others looked for genetic factors or sought environmental triggers, focusing on toxic waste in the environment, pesticides, plastics, or the preservatives used in foods.[27] Throughout the 1990s, some parents and doctors raised questions about vaccines.

In 1998, a study claiming that vaccines caused autism breathed life to a small but growing anti-vaccine movement. That year, the British medical journal *Lancet* published research by British surgeon Andrew Wakefield and thirteen colleagues reporting that among a group of twelve children in their practice who had been identified as having autism, all had received the measles-mumps-rubella vaccine years earlier. The authors hypothesized that the children's autism might be associated with the MMR immunization.[28] Shortly after publication, Wakefield declared at a press conference that the vaccine should be withdrawn. Almost immediately, scientists raised questions about the extremely small size of the study sample, pointing out that it was impossible to conclude from the data that the MMR vaccine had played any role in the children's autism. But their concerns were largely drowned out by a news media storm and voices of outrage from parents.[29] The press had a field day with this news, and soon headlines around the world were announcing that scientists had discovered that vaccines caused autism.

At the time, no one was aware that Wakefield's paper was fraudulent. Not until 2004 did the *Lancet* issue a statement describing a number of ethical improprieties with the research, including the fact that while he was conducting the study, Wakefield had been gathering evidence for a group of parents who believed that their children's autism was caused by vaccines. Subsequent investigations found that lawyers acting for parents involved in lawsuits against vaccine manufacturers had paid for some of the research and that Wakefield had apparently falsified some of his data. Finally, in 2010, twelve years after the publication of the article, the *Lancet* retracted the paper.[30]

During the twelve years after Wakefield's paper first appeared, many scientists conducted research to confirm a link between autism and the MMR vaccine and other vaccines, with no success. Research studies in the United States, the United Kingdom, Sweden, and Denmark found no evidence that vaccines caused autism.[31]

Those findings came far too late to prevent distrust of vaccines in the late 1990s. Concerns over autism were acute in California, which saw increases in the number of students diagnosed with autism during the 1980s. In 1999, the California Department of Developmental Services (DDS) reported that cases of autism in the state had nearly tripled, from 7.5 cases per 10,000 children in the 1983–85 birth cohort to 20.2 cases per 10,000 in the 1993–95 cohort.[32]

Researchers would later show that improvements in detection and changes in diagnosis explained much of this increase. The rise in cases diagnosed as "autism" almost exactly matched a decline in cases earlier diagnosed as "retardation." Additional research would come to show that older parents have a greater likelihood of having a child with autism, and advances in genetic research would also reveal that autism can be an inherited condition.[33]

But in 1999, people did not know any of this, and many were ready to believe that vaccines were to blame. The Internet provided parents a new source of information about vaccines and autism, and it also enabled new forms of community. As Elena Conis has pointed out, many found it empowering. Families could connect with other parents of autistic children and learn from their experiences. Worried parents went online to diagnose their own children, and they shared their personal experience with others. And the Internet provided parents with all sorts of reasons to distrust vaccines.[34]

At the same time that California officials were raising alarms about the rise of autism cases, questions arose about a preservative used in vaccines. Thimerosal, a preservative with trace amounts of ethyl mercury, was included in some multidose vaccines. In 1997, New Jersey Representative Frank Pallone, who represented a district whose constituents were concerned about environmental mercury poisoning, initiated an assessment of the FDA's products for mercury content. As a result, starting in 1998—the same year Wakefield's study came out in the *Lancet*, the FDA undertook a formal risk assessment of thimerosal in vaccines. Both the FDA and the Environmental Protection Agency had set thresholds for exposure to mercury, and of the two, the EPA's threshold was lower. The risk assessment team found that as a result of the presence of thimerosal in the CDC's recommended list of vaccines, the amount of mercury children would receive through routine vaccination would exceed the EPA's threshold. Based on this finding, the FDA invited leading vaccine advisory groups for consultation. The American Academy of Pediatrics (AAP) and the CDC issued a joint statement on July 9, 1999, stating that because of concerns regarding the EPA guidelines, "thimerosal-containing vaccines should be removed as soon as possible."[35]

Thus, everything came to a head—Wakefield's fraudulent article was circulating, leading people to believe there was a connection between vaccines and autism, and now the US government itself, by recommending the removal of thimerosal-containing vaccines, appeared to acknowledge an unacceptable level of risk in its recommended list of vaccines. The joint statement by the AAP and CDC explained that there was no evidence that the level of exposure children may have encountered in their recommended vaccines caused any harm, but not everyone was convinced. To some, this qualification seemed like backpedaling to justify former government actions in having recommended thimerosal-containing vaccines. As it happened, research would come to show that autism cases continued to increase after thimerosal was eliminated from most vaccines, indicating that thimerosal exposure did not contribute to autism.[36] But by this point, the scientific findings came too late to influence those who had become convinced that the benefits of vaccines were not worth the risk.

Americans who questioned vaccines felt the government could not be relied on to ensure the safety of children—after all, federal authorities had not considered assessing the levels of mercury in vaccines earlier; instead, it had taken a push from concerned citizens and a congressman willing to represent them to bring that assessment about. Nor had the government taken steps to ensure the vaccine against polio was safe. It had taken parent advocates to stop the use of the oral Sabin vaccine, which in rare cases could cause polio.

During the 1990s, newspaper articles reported that parents John and Kathy Salamone, whose son David had become infected with polio after receiving the Sabin vaccine, had created an organization called Informed Parents Against Vaccine-Associated Polio (IPAV). The Salamones were not anti-vaccine—their goal was to remove the Sabin vaccine from the market and replace it with the Salk vaccine, which did not transmit polio. For many years, public health officials and doctors had used the Sabin vaccine, which provided stronger protection against the disease, believing the benefits outweighed the risk. "It was like a dirty little secret," said John Salamone. "Nobody told you there were going to be sacrificial lambs."[37] As a result of IPAV's advocacy, the CDC finally switched to the Salk vaccine. John Salamone would later recall, "I think what worked was organizing families [and] getting the media involved."[38]

But for those already distrustful of government, this grassroots victory only confirmed their belief that government bureaucrats could not be trusted to ensure vaccines were as safe as possible. Nor were people more inclined to trust science, because scientists seemed to be at a loss to explain the causes of autism. Why then, should the public believe that scientists and public health officials had a good grasp of the full range of possible risks presented by vaccines?

In 2000, the CDC reported that measles had been eliminated from the United States, and four years later, the elimination of rubella and congenital rubella syndrome was also confirmed.[39] But for a small group of critics, these achievements did nothing to instill confidence in vaccines.

A 2001 *New York Times* interview with Barbara Loe Fisher, co-founder of the National Vaccine Information Center, which had been organized in 1982 under the name Dissatisfied Parents Together (DPT), revealed the depth of the skepticism. The interviewer noted that many people viewed vaccination as one of the "great medical successes of the 20th century." He asked, "Do you disagree with that assessment?" Fisher answered, "Certainly with the implementation of mass-vaccination policies in the last 40 years we've seen a decline in infectious diseases of childhood. However, we have at the same time seen a doubling of asthma and learning disabilities. A tripling of diabetes. Autism is affecting one in 500 children. We need to look at whether an intervention used with every child is perhaps contributing to the background rate of chronic disease or disability."[40]

At the time Fisher made this statement, a large majority of Americans still trusted vaccines. Results from the 2002 National Immunization Survey showed that 93 percent of parents rated vaccines as safe, 6 percent as neither safe nor unsafe, and 1 percent as unsafe.[41] But doubts grew as the unfounded claim that vaccines caused autism continued to circulate on news sites and online.

In 2008, four years after the *Lancet* had issued a statement about the ethical improprieties in Wakefield's study, Fisher appeared on NBC's *Today* show, saying, "We need to find out why so many of our highly vaccinated children are so sick. The biggest worry today is autism." A number of high-profile celebrities were also saying the same thing, including Robert F. Kennedy Jr., a nephew of President John F. Kennedy. Vaccination, he proclaimed, "poisoned an entire generation of American children. It's causing IQ loss, mental retardation, speech delay, ADD, hyperactivity." Paul Offit, then chief of infectious diseases at Children's Hospital of Philadelphia, tried to allay concerns by pointing to the findings of countless research studies: "[I]t's perfectly reasonable to be skeptical about anything you put into your body . . . and vaccines do have side effects. But vaccines don't cause autism."[42]

Unfortunately, television viewers who turned to the Internet to find some unbiased information about vaccines were likely to encounter anti-vaccination websites. By this time, about 74 percent of Americans regularly conducted online searches, where they often landed on anti-vaccination websites. One study showed that a search using the term *vaccination* retrieved many sites, of which 71 percent could be classified as "anti-vaccination."[43] Internet searches also yielded modern-day reprints of one-hundred-year-old anti-vaccination books, including *Horrors of Vaccination Exposed and Illustrated* and *Compulsory Vaccination: The Crime against the School Child*—all for sale online by Amazon and other mainstream booksellers.[44] It is hardly surprising that by 2010, one survey showed that one in four Americans believed that some vaccines caused autism.[45]

Other fears had also begun circulating. Survey research revealed that parents were anxious about the increase in the number of vaccines on the CDC's recommended vaccination schedule. A vaccine against varicella, or chickenpox, was licensed for use in the United States in 1995, and some states added it to the list of required children's vaccines. In 2001, a combination vaccine against hepatitis A and hepatitis B was licensed and added to the CDC's list of recommended inoculations. In 2005, the varicella vaccine was combined with the MMR vaccine, which was then renamed MMRV. In 2012, the CDC recommended eleven vaccines—several of them combination vaccines—for children from birth to six years of age. State laws varied in specifying which vaccines were required for admission to school, but in every state, the requirements increased.[46]

This increase led some parents to believe that exposure to so many vaccines could overwhelm the child's immune system. Others speculated that giving vaccines to children below the age of two could negatively impact their neurological development. Multiple research studies conducted between 2005 and 2018 found no evidence to support these fears, and yet concerns over the vaccination schedule persisted.[47] In 2007, pediatrician Robert Sears published an alternative schedule in *The Vaccine Book: Making the Right Decision for Your Child*, in which he suggested that parents might delay or space out some vaccines and opt out of others. The book became very popular, and the idea of spacing out vaccines took hold in some areas.[48]

In 2009, research based on survey and interview data from 11,206 parents found that among those with children between the ages of two and three, about 26 percent delayed vaccines, 8 percent delayed some and refused others, and 6 percent refused vaccines altogether. Those who delayed or refused vaccines were less likely to believe that medical professionals had their best interests at heart, and they were less likely to think that vaccines were necessary to protect their children's health. The demographic data revealed that these parents were more likely to be white, married, and living in the suburbs with above-average annual incomes. When asked why they delayed or refused vaccines, the most common reasons given were fear of vaccine side effects (53.2 percent), disbelief in the vaccine's effectiveness (52.8 percent), belief that the vaccine might cause autism (50.8 percent), and that they had "heard or read bad things" about vaccines (38.8 percent). Additionally, 78 percent stated they felt that too many shots were recommended.[49]

The parents who delayed or refused some vaccines for their infants and toddlers did not always refuse to follow school vaccination laws when their children were older. In fact, the CDC's national data showed that a large majority of parents followed state laws and had their children vaccinated for school. Nevertheless, doctors and public health officials worried about the possible reemergence of childhood diseases to which very young children were susceptible, such as whooping cough. And over time, the overall percentage of parents receiving personal belief exemptions from school vaccination requirements crept up.

The Rise of Personal Belief Exemptions

Very few Americans applied for exemption from school vaccination laws on religious grounds. Only a small number of churches practicing faith healing officially opposed the use of medicines and vaccination. For this reason, the percentage of parents filing for religious exemptions remained stable—in states allowing only religious exemptions, about 1 percent of parents submitted exemptions on religious grounds between 1991 and 2004. In contrast, states that allowed personal belief exemptions saw their exemption rate rise to 2.4 percent during these years, and in some pockets of the country, the rates were much higher. This rise was not fueled solely by individuals who opposed vaccines for secular reasons. Over the years, more Americans from conservative religious groups began to oppose vaccines on moral grounds.[50]

Why did more states start offering personal belief exemptions? Despite some erosion in the American public's trust of science, states began adding the exemptions during an era in which a large majority of parents complied with school vaccination requirements and school immunization rates remained high. In fact, these high rates made it possible for state legislatures to expand nonmedical exemptions from vaccination without triggering public controversy—no one could foresee that decades later, a rising number of exemptions would lead to new outbreaks of childhood diseases. Ultimately, a state's decision regarding whether to add nonmedical exemptions was shaped by the amount of public support or opposition to the proposed legislation, the recommendations of its public health authorities, the degree to which outbreaks of vaccine-preventable disease continued to pose a perceived threat to public safety, and the outcomes of state supreme court rulings.

Advocacy from health officials who preferred policies of persuasion over coercion influenced legislative debates. In 1959, Ohio passed a compulsory law that required students to be vaccinated against smallpox, polio, diphtheria, pertussis, and tetanus, but the law also allowed exemptions to parents who provided a written statement "objecting to the immunization."[51] The recommendations of the state's health officials likely were a factor. In 1963, a survey of state health officials found that many believed persuasive methods were effective and worried that making vaccination compulsory might discourage the idea that "preservation of health is an individual or family responsibility."[52]

In 1961, when California's legislature debated a compulsory law requiring students to be vaccinated against polio, a long-standing preference for persuasion among the state's health officials, coupled with lobbying by the National Health Federation, a medical liberty group, affected the outcome. Fred J. Hart, a farmer, radio station owner, and advocate of alternative medicine, had founded a health business, the Electronic Medical Foundation (EMF) and developed the "radioscope" to diagnose and cure all diseases through the use of electronic frequencies. After FDA scientists investigated and found the radioscope "no more capable of diagnosing disease than a juke box or a pinball machine," a US district court ruling forced the EMF to stop shipping its devices across state lines, and the foundation went out of business.[53]

In 1955, Hart established the National Health Federation (NHF) to lobby for medical freedom.[54] During California's legislative debates over A.B. 1940, Hart claimed that the justifications for the Salk vaccine were fallacious and that many children who had received the shots "will develop leukemia."[55] Don C. Matchan, publisher of *Herald of Health* magazine and a close associate of Hart's, asserted that "polio is a nutritional deficiency disease," citing Benjamin P. Sandler's *Diet Prevents Polio*. Several letter writers to the committee made this same claim. Others argued that the proposed bill would violate constitutional rights to liberty and freedom.[56]

Originally, the language in California's bill had allowed exemption on the basis of religious belief, but the word *religious* was removed as A.B. 1940 wound through the legislature. Assemblyman Umbert J. DeLotto, one of the bill's sponsors, provided a public explanation of what had occurred. "We had to drop 'religious' in order to get the bill passed," he said. "There was too much opposition from people who do not believe in medications for treatment and prevention of disease on general as well as religious grounds."[57]

Given Americans' widespread acceptance of allopathic medicine during this period, it is likely that the legislature's motivation to amend the bill had less to do with the alternative health rhetoric of the NHF and more to do with a desire to ensure widespread acceptance of vaccination through a policy of persuasion. In a letter to Bryon Rumford, chair of the Assembly's Public Health Committee, Fred J. Hart asked for the bill to be revised to allow for exemption based on the parent's "wishes." He argued that with that revision, the bill would be in keeping with the "American traditional philosophy" that "progress is best made in all things by education rather than by compulsion."[58] The state's leading public health officers agreed with this philosophy. The California Conference of Local

Health Officers, an organization of sixty legally appointed health officers, representing the state's fifty-eight counties and the cities of Berkeley, Long Beach, and Pasadena, stated that "enlightened self-interest, by voluntary and persuasive means" would be far more effective in encouraging vaccination than "law enforcement."[59]

In other states, however, the movement to add personal belief exemptions had nothing to do with public health philosophy or political negotiation and compromise. Rather, state legislatures added personal belief exemptions in response to state supreme court rulings that found exemptions on the basis of religion to be discriminatory and unconstitutional.

Some of the first lawsuits over exemptions were filed by parents who had philosophical or personal objections to vaccination but lived in states that only allowed exemption on religious grounds. Schools sometimes found themselves in a thorny position when parents submitted requests for religious exemptions. Allowing the exemption was straightforward in cases involving those belonging to religious groups whose teachings explicitly discouraged vaccination. But how was the school to evaluate a sincerely held religious belief when the parents were not members of a church opposed to vaccines?

Disputes over this issue landed school districts in the courts. For instance, in 1967, Thomas E. McCartney, a chiropractor, sued the Maine-Endwell School district in New York when it refused to grant his son a religious exemption from vaccination. Under New York's law, the exemption applied only to those belonging to "a recognized religious organization whose teachings are contrary to the practices [of vaccination]." McCartney was a Roman Catholic, but since the Catholic Church did not officially oppose vaccination, the school denied the exemption and suspended his son from school. McCartney sued, arguing that the exemption should be allowed, because even though the Catholic Church did not forbid immunization, it did require people to follow their moral convictions. The chiropractor based his argument on the fact that he had a deep moral conviction that his son should not be vaccinated. However, New York's supreme court ruled against him.[60]

Most parents seeking religious exemptions on the basis of personal beliefs lost in the courts, but not always. Defining "religion" for legal purposes was never straightforward, and in the late 1980s, a US district court ruled for the parents. In September 1987, when their son's elementary school district in New York refused to waive the vaccination requirement and admit him to school, parents Paul and Claudia Sherr sued the principal of the school and the state commissioner of education, arguing that the action violated their rights to freedom of religion and equal protection under the law. Although they were not members of any formal religious group, they argued that vaccination was against their sincerely held beliefs about the natural order: "All things are part of one intimate universe. . . . This universe includes everything good being called God. Health is the unhindered expression of life. . . . Immunization hinders life and thus is contrary to God. To deviate from this natural order would be to sin." They won their case. In its ruling, the US district court held that "there can be little doubt" that the parents' beliefs "qualify as 'religious.'" The judge held that New York's law was unconstitutional, and that under the free exercise and establishment clauses of the First Amendment, the state must extend exemption to any person holding sincere religious beliefs, whether they were members of a religious organization or not.[61]

A similar case in Mississippi led the state's supreme court to strike down Mississippi's law allowing religious exemptions. In 1979, Charles Brown, a member of the Church of Christ and a chiropractor in Houston, Mississippi, refused to permit his six-year-old son to be vaccinated for admission to elementary school, and he applied for a religious exemption. However, the school principal denied his request, because under Mississippi law, the exemption could only be granted to parents or guardians who were "members of a recognized denomination whose religious teachings require reliance on prayer or spiritual means of healing." Brown had submitted a statement signed by his minister, but the minister's statement made it clear that while the Church of Christ respected the chiropractor's convictions, the church did not teach against vaccination. After his application for exemption was denied, Brown sued the principal, and the case eventually made its way to the state supreme court. The court's ruling struck down Mississippi's law allowing religious exemption, finding the law unconstitutional because it discriminated among religions in considering those that might be exempt. The court also held that the law, by allowing nonmedical exemption, elevated individual beliefs above the welfare of the general public. In the wake of that ruling, Mississippi joined West Virginia as one of only two states prohibiting nonmedical exemptions.[62]

In some cases, legislation to allow personal belief exemptions resulted from court rulings that found the religious exemption unconstitutional. This happened in Arkansas, where parent Cynthia Boone sought a religious exemption from a requirement to vaccinate her school-age daughter against hepatitis B. The disease spread primarily through sexual contact and injection drug use, and it could pass from an infected mother to a baby at birth. At the time, critics of the vaccine argued that it should not be required for schoolchildren. Some members of religious denominations that believed in abstaining from sex until marriage opposed the mandate, finding it unnecessary and morally inappropriate for their children. Boone had based her request for exemption on religious reasons and also on "conscientious grounds which include traditional parenting concerns." However, school and health officials rejected her application, because she was not a member of a church that officially opposed vaccination. Boone sued, and in 2002, federal courts ruled in her favor and struck down the state's law, finding it unconstitutional, because it allowed officials to discriminate among various religious organizations and forms of religious belief. Two years later, the state legislature revised the school vaccination law to allow the state health department to grant philosophical or personal belief exemptions from school vaccination requirements.[63]

Over time, more states adopted personal belief exemptions. Such exemptions allowed parents who were members of religious denominations with no official policies opposing vaccines to opt out of vaccinating their children on moral grounds associated with their religious or political convictions. By 2004, some Catholics and members of other religious groups were expressing moral concerns and raising ethical questions about vaccine researchers' use of cell lines from fetuses electively aborted decades earlier.[64]

The switch from using animal cells to using fetal cells in vaccine development arose in large part from safety concerns over vaccine contamination. During the mid-1960s, Dr. Stanley Plotkin at the Wistar Institute in Philadelphia used fetal cell lines, rather than other animal cell lines, to develop a vaccine against the rubella virus, or German measles. The cells came from a fetus that had been electively aborted earlier. At the time, the use of animal cell lines was considered problematic, because such cells could carry viruses and bacteria that might contaminate the vaccine and be infectious to humans. This had occurred during the 1950s, when polio vaccines made with monkey cells were eventually found to contain Simian virus 40, or SV40. Fortunately, SV40 was found to have not harmed humans, but concerns remained about the possibility that more dangerous viruses might contaminate vaccines developed with animal cell lines.[65]

The use of fetal cell lines to improve the safety of vaccines eventually sparked a new wave of opposition based on religious and political concerns. Such considerations led some members of the Catholic church to ask for moral guidance. In a letter to Debra L. Vinnedge, director of the group Children of God for Life, Cardinal Elio Sgreccia, president of the Pontifical Academy for Life, explained that while Catholics should advocate for the development of vaccines without the use of fetal cell lines, Catholics were morally free to use the vaccines when there are no alternatives "to avoid a serious risk not only for one's own children but also, and perhaps more specifically, for the health conditions of the population as a whole."[66] At the same time, researchers noticed a growing backlash against vaccination among evangelicals and other religious groups politically opposed to abortion. On some Internet sites, abortion opponents argued that anyone accepting vaccines was morally complicit in abortion. And some sites falsely claimed that vaccines themselves included matter from aborted fetuses.[67]

During the first decade of the twenty-first century, the number of states allowing personal belief exemptions increased by a third, from fifteen in 2000 to twenty in 2010. Some states had passed laws granting personal belief exemptions decades earlier, during the vaccination campaigns of the 1970s, believing they were necessary to ensure widespread acceptance of the legislation. But by the 2010s, after plateauing for more than twenty years, the number of states passing such laws was accelerating (chart 7.2).

This was the state of affairs when a vaccine against the human papillomavirus became available, sparking a new controversy over vaccination mandates.[68]

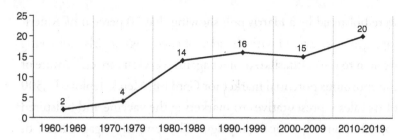

Chart 7.2. Number of states with personal belief vaccination exemption laws, by decade, 1960–2019. *Source*: Chart created from data in table 1, "States with Personal Belief Exemptions and Years Adopted," in Elena Conis, "The History of the Personal Belief Exemption," *Pediatrics* 145, no. 4 (Apr. 2020): https://doi.org/10 .1542/peds.2019-2551.

Controversy over the HPV Vaccine

A firestorm over vaccines developed when Americans learned the CDC had recommended that girls as young as eleven years old be vaccinated against a sexually transmitted disease. This time, the opposition was not primarily driven by safety concerns. Now, a much broader range of constituents opposed the vaccine, including conservative religious groups and those who supported compulsory vaccination laws in general.

By 2005, Merck Pharmaceutical Company had developed a vaccine called Gardasil to protect against human papillomavirus (HPV), the most common sexually transmitted disease in the country. HPV can cause cervical cancer in adulthood, a disease that kills about four thousand women a year.[69] The CDC's Advisory Committee on Immunization Practices recommended an initial inoculation for girls between the ages of eleven and twelve and a follow-up shot for females between the ages of thirteen and twenty-six. Researchers had field-tested the vaccine with a sample of thirty thousand women for seven years and concluded it was safe. As a result, health officials believed that its use would greatly benefit women, and their views were bolstered by a Harris poll showing that 70 percent of Americans generally agreed with the idea of encouraging girls and young women to use Gardasil to protect against cervical cancer.[70] Aware of the enormous potential market for Gardasil, Merck deployed 1,500 of its sales representatives to marketing the vaccine and bolstered contributions to political campaigns. The company engaged in a lobbying blitz, with the result that twenty-three states began considering legislation that would mandate vaccination against HPV.[71]

No one foresaw the breadth of the backlash that followed. As debates were under way in state legislatures, Barbara Loe Fisher's National Vaccine Information Center issued an inflammatory statement, speculating that young girls had died from blood clots or had become paralyzed after being inoculated with Gardasil. Fisher accused Merck of using "flawed science . . . to get it licensed." The following year, she appeared on CBS's televised *Sunday Morning* show and informed millions of American viewers, "This is an intervention that carries the risk of injury or death."[72]

After Fisher's statement on national news, and in response to growing public alarm about the vaccine's safety, the CDC undertook a long-range study of more than ten thousand reports of adverse effects to see if there was any pattern suggesting the HPV vaccine might be at fault. The research showed that seventeen people had died in the clinical trials—ten in the group that had received the HPV vaccine and seven in the placebo group, which had not received any vaccine. Among the ten people who had died after receiving the vaccine, none of the deaths was vaccine-related. Four of the ten deaths were caused by motor-vehicle accidents; one was caused by intentional drug overdose; one was attributed to cancer; two were attributed to sepsis; and two were attributed to heart conditions (one from pulmonary embolus and one from arrhythmia). The four deaths from heart conditions or sepsis matched the number of deaths in the placebo group. Overall, the proportion of deaths following HPV vaccination was consistent with the proportion of deaths in the population at large before the vaccine was available. However, Fisher refused to accept the CDC's findings. At a rally to support conscientious exemption to vaccination, she proclaimed, "The response by health officials . . . is to tell parents that, every time another child dies or regresses into poor health after vaccination, it is just a 'coincidence' while quietly writing those children off as acceptable losses."[73]

It is not possible to know how many people were influenced by misinformation regarding Gardasil's safety, but such concerns were not the only reason many people opposed adding it to the growing list of vaccines required for school. Nor were religious or secular philosophical objections to vaccination the primary driver of the opposition. In 2007, as more than twenty states considered passing legislation to mandate the HPV vaccine for school attendance, even people who accepted vaccination spoke out against it.

Some people in favor of vaccines argued that because HPV was not an epidemic contagious disease that naturally infects children in schools, mandating the vaccine was not warranted. An earlier version of this argument had been made in the late 1990s, when some doctors and parents questioned immunizing infants and young children against hepatitis B, a contagious disease that was far more likely to spread among teenagers experimenting with sex and drugs than among children in daycare centers, preschools, and elementary schools. Now, parents considering the HPV vaccine wondered why it was necessary, since their youngest children were not really in any danger from the disease. Dr. Ronald Sokol, a professor of pediatrics at the University of Colorado School of Medicine, wondered whether it was worth asking families to bear the high financial cost of the three required shots, noting, "Children are at very low risk to get this in day care—or elsewhere in this country, for that matter." Gerrit Baker, a

Colorado health official asked, "Just because we CAN vaccinate, does that mean we always should? It's a worthy public debate."[74]

When it came to the HPV vaccine, many of those in favor of vaccination spoke out against requiring it for school admission. One California mother, who supported vaccination against mumps and measles, felt the proposed legislation went too far: "Since it's not a communicable disease you can catch in a classroom setting, it's not really the school's place to tell parents that they must go out and have their children vaccinated." Some school officials agreed. In Florida, the chairman of the Collier County School Board echoed this idea, opposing the legislation because unlike tuberculosis, a highly contagious disease that schools carefully monitored, HPV was transmissible only through sexual contact. "HPV is not a health risk," he said.[75]

Some doctors and scientists also opposed mandating the vaccine. In an article published in *JAMA Journal of Ethics*, two scientists from Johns Hopkins University stated that the most compelling reason to mandate a vaccine for school attendance is when it would prevent a serious infectious disease that naturally spreads among students, which was not the case with the HPV vaccine. One of the authors was Keerti V. Shah, a virologist whose research on the connection between human papillomavirus and cervical cancer had helped pave the way for the vaccine's development. The other was Raphael P. Viscidi, a professor of pediatrics and oncology whose research focused on papillomavirus and other viruses. They also expressed concern about the possibility of rare side effects given the relatively small number of people who had been vaccinated in the clinical trials.[76]

Both liberal and conservative parents who otherwise supported vaccination spoke out against the vaccine. Among conservative parents who opposed sex education in the schools, few were happy about the idea of vaccinating their eleven-year-old daughters against a disease that spread only through vaginal, oral, or anal sex. In Texas, members of Christian groups supporting abstinence-only sex education in the schools protested Governor Rick Perry's executive order requiring the vaccination. In South Carolina, an abstinence-only group called Parents Involved in Education argued that the vaccine was unnecessary, given that a good preventative of cervical cancer already existed in the form of regular pap smears.

Among liberals, groups like Hadassah, the Jewish women's organization, also opposed any form of mandate, stating that parents should "have a frank and open discussion with health-care providers to determine if this is right for their daughter."[77] Others felt the push for a new vaccine mandate was the simply the wrong solution for the problem. "I think if state legislators really cared about the health of girls," said one mother of a ten-year-old daughter, "they would mandate comprehensive sex education for both boys and girls in the schools. That would probably save a lot more lives than the HPV vaccine."[78]

Ultimately, most legislators across the country listened to their constituents' concerns and did not mandate vaccination against HPV. By 2015, only three states had passed legislation requiring that adolescents receive the vaccine for admission to school. Other states passed bills that supported voluntary vaccination, giving parents and guardians the freedom to choose whether to have their children vaccinated.[79]

The debates over the HPV vaccine highlighted the limits of public support for new vaccine mandates in the twenty-first century. During the 1960s and '70s, the passage of compulsory school vaccination laws requiring vaccination against polio, diphtheria, and other contagious diseases had received broad support, but unlike Gardasil, each of those vaccines had targeted diseases that commonly spread through schoolrooms. In contrast, both liberal and conservative

Americans viewed adding Gardasil to the list of vaccines required for school as an overreach of state authority. Now, the number of people seeking exemptions from school vaccination requirements was rising, and it was unclear how many more vaccinations parents would tolerate. "At some point," warned officials with the Institute of Medicine, "this health promotion and disease prevention strategy could wear out its welcome with the population at large. It has already done so with some segment of society."[80]

Conclusion

Fears related to vaccine safety had been largely dormant during the campaign against polio, but they remerged in the 1960s and '70s as news coverage of vaccine injury cases and high-profile lawsuits increased. Americans learned that they had not been adequately informed of the risks of vaccination, however small. They also learned that the federal government had failed to put any mechanisms in place to quickly identify a bad lot of vaccine and remove it from the market. Although cases of serious injury and death from vaccination were extremely rare, the government had also dragged its feet in providing compensation for those few individuals who inevitably had serious adverse reactions to vaccines. The scientific community made its own share of mistakes. It did not help matters when the *Lancet* published a fraudulent study that sparked the long-standing myth that vaccines caused autism. As had happened during the anti-vaccination movement of the late nineteenth and early twentieth centuries, misinformation about vaccines circulated through print and social media well into the twenty-first century, long after the falsified claims had been shown to be completely unfounded.

Gradually, the number of states offering personal belief exemptions from vaccination requirements increased. Initially, secular concerns motivated people to seek such exemptions, including safety fears and commitments to alternative philosophies of health and healing. Later, as religious and political concerns fanned opposition to vaccines, members of religious groups that did not officially oppose vaccination began seeking exemptions. With the development of new vaccines designed to protect against diseases that commonly spread through sexual activity and injection drug use, opposition increased among some religious groups committed to other methods of prevention, such as abstinence from sex before marriage. And for those opposed to federal and state laws allowing abortion, the use of fetal cell lines in vaccine research made vaccination a morally unacceptable practice.

By the early twenty-first century, it was clear that the era of widespread, unquestioning acceptance of vaccine mandates had come to a close. A 2007 survey of international infectious disease experts revealed uncertainty and concern about the future. "If immunization rates fade, vaccine preventable diseases will be back," predicted one doctor. "And we will be able to experience first-hand what life must have been like in the early twentieth century."[81]

8

The Twenty-First-Century Effort
to Preserve Immunity in Schools

In the fall of 2007, school officials in Maryland faced a dilemma: many students had not been immunized. Maryland required students to either show they had been vaccinated or submit an exemption form before they could attend school. However, during a check of students' vaccination status in Prince George's County, authorities found that more than 2,300 lacked the required immunizations. Teachers sent notices home to parents and guardians, school nurses conducted home visits, and the district even offered free vaccinations on school grounds—something that had not happened since the polio years.

Nothing seemed to work. Parents could obtain exemptions for medical or religious reasons, but the parents of unvaccinated students had not even submitted exemption forms. Schools had to exclude students who had not provided any sort of documentation about their vaccination status, and now many had been out of classrooms for more than two months. "How can you in good conscience allow your child to miss school and their education for no particular reason?" asked John White, spokesman for the school system.[1] Determined to follow the law, school officials and county prosecutors ordered parents and guardians to appear at a special court hearing in November, where those who had not filed exemption forms would have to choose: either have their children vaccinated "on the spot" or face fines and up to ten days in jail. Newspapers reported this development as "one of the strongest efforts made by a U.S. school system to ensure its youngsters receive their shots."[2]

Despite protests and a rise in applications for exemptions, most parents supported the get-tough measure. "The kids need to have their shots," said the father of a high school student. "Parents have known. They sent letters home, everybody knows. It's on the news. Get your child shots."[3] But a small group of highly vocal anti-vaccine activists, some from outside the state, portrayed the school district's actions as an infringement of individual freedom and the right to make an informed choice about vaccination. Joining protestors outside the county courthouse, Barbara Loe Fisher, head of the National Vaccine Information Center, denounced the order: "It is terrorizing parents. When you have the threat of going to jail, it is hard to make an informed decision." Despite the protests, the stiff penalties had the desired effect. Within a week, most of the unvaccinated students had received their shots, and the others had submitted the required exemption forms. School officials breathed a sigh of relief, as did many parents. Bob Ross, the head of a local high school PTA, said, "Parents are going to have to set aside some time. Parents have a responsibility to help protect the public health."[4]

The issue of exemptions from vaccination appeared often in the news at this time because some serious childhood diseases had begun to reappear. Measles, which had been eradicated in the United States just seven years earlier, was now back. So was pertussis, or whooping cough—although it had never been eradicated, the number of reported cases had increased nearly fivefold from 1990 to 2005.

Both diseases spread rapidly wherever children congregated, and outbreaks were noticeably larger in areas where greater numbers of parents filed for religious or philosophical exemptions from school vaccination.[5]

How large could the exempt minority become before everyone's immunity was threatened? As more people began asking this question, they started to consider ways to stem the small but growing tide of unvaccinated students.

States used a variety of strategies in the twenty-first century to raise vaccination rates in the schools. As outbreaks increased, some states strengthened the enforcement of existing mandates or tightened the requirements for nonmedical exemptions. Others eliminated nonmedical exemptions entirely. The debates over vaccination differed markedly from those of the late nineteenth century, when controversy centered on the smallpox vaccine during a time when smallpox outbreaks still sometimes killed 25 percent or more of those infected. Now the debates took place in the absence of visible outbreaks, or in places where the number of cases were small—the result of effective school vaccination policies over decades. In the context of relative safety from contagious disease and ongoing concerns over vaccines, questions of risk, freedom of choice, and the child's right to education took center stage, and by 2015, the votes in many state legislatures divided along partisan lines.

Growing Concerns over Nonmedical Exemptions

The percentage of parents nationwide seeking nonmedical exemptions doubled from 1991 to 2004, and in states allowing personal belief exemptions, the increase was even greater.[6] By 2014, the nationwide median vaccination rate of kindergartners against measles, mumps, and rubella was 94.7 percent, but some states were well below the 93 to 95 percent level required for herd immunity.[7]

Outbreaks of vaccine-preventable diseases brought the issue of nonmedical exemptions to the forefront in the twenty-first century. Scientists had known for decades that disease outbreaks tended to occur in areas with high rates of exemptions. Researchers began tracking the phenomenon during a series of measles outbreaks during the 1980s and '90s. One study concluded that students who were unvaccinated on religious and philosophical grounds were thirty-five times more likely to be infected with measles than vaccinated children.[8] Another study of measles outbreaks from 2000 through 2015 showed that most of the cases were among unvaccinated individuals, and that vaccine refusal was associated with a higher risk of measles and pertussis.[9]

Doctors and public health officials worried about the rise in laws allowing personal belief exemptions, but many believed they were necessary to avoid a public backlash against vaccination. As one doctor put it, "Laws that do not allow some degree of conscientious exemption can further inflame anti-vaccination groups, leading to increased resistance to these laws."[10] Some argued that abolishing exemptions would be unjust. Some believed that allowing a small portion of the population to be exempt from vaccination requirements could still maintain adequate levels of herd immunity.[11]

Some people believed it would be impossible to abolish exemptions. Recent court rulings had expanded religious exemptions to include personal beliefs. For instance, in 2007, the Wyoming Supreme Court ruled that when a family submitted a request for a religious exemption, the Department of Education did not have the authority to evaluate whether the request was based on religious belief. As a result, any person in Wyoming could obtain a religious exemption by simply asking for one.[12] As one legal scholar concluded, pointing to cases like the one in Wyoming, "Unfortunately, given this nation's current political climate and several recent judicial decisions, it is not likely that state legislatures or the judiciary will eliminate or limit these harmful exemptions."[13]

Yet as outbreaks increased, more people began to wonder whether the slow but growing numbers of unvaccinated students in the schools were putting their communities at risk. In some areas of the country, they began to consider increasing enforcement of school vaccination laws, as had been done in Prince George's County, Maryland.

Strengthening Enforcement and Tightening Requirements

The story about the get-tough policy in Prince George's County made national news in 2007 because at the time, few other school districts were taking similar action to raise school vaccination rates. Several years earlier, researchers had found that in many states, it was far easier for parents to obtain an exemption than to have their child vaccinated. Additionally, few states had policies requiring that parents seeking exemptions be informed of the risks of not vaccinating their children.[14]

School administrators prioritized safety at school, but in an era when dangerous epidemics were few and far between, the emphasis now was on keeping children safe from bullying and violence.[15] It had not always been this way. During the polio campaign of the late 1950s and '60s, schoolbooks had increased their coverage of vaccination, adding special inserts describing the effort to find a vaccine against polio, and schools had conducted information campaigns to raise awareness as well. During the federal Childhood Immunization Initiative in the late 1970s, the Department of Health, Education, and Welfare had encouraged educators to strengthen the enforcement of school vaccination laws, and as a result of that program, health and school authorities in many areas of the country had implemented get-tough policies, ordering unvaccinated children to be excluded from schools until immunized.[16] But such efforts had long passed out of memory.

By the twenty-first century, when school administrators thought about their school health programs, the topic of vaccines was far from a top priority; other topics of social and cultural concern were front and center. In 2000, the US Department of Health and Human Services had identified the following priorities in a report called *Healthy People 2000*: physical activity, nutrition, tobacco, alcohol and other drugs, family planning, mental health and mental disorders, violent and abusive behavior, and educational programs. When immunization was discussed, it was described as a "preventive service" rather than a topic requiring promotion. In 2007, the CDC's published list of priority topics for health education was identical.[17]

No one seemed to feel that immunization needed to become a health education priority. Despite a growing awareness of anti-vaccine sentiment, many people seemed to assume that families would just continue to have their children vaccinated. However, cases like the one in Maryland revealed that large numbers of students could enroll in school without having received the required vaccines. Some entered on probationary status with the understanding that they would be immunized later. In schools with lax oversight and follow-up policies, fairly large numbers of nonexempt students might thus remain unvaccinated.

North Dakota faced this situation in 2015. The state's immunization rates had been declining, from 95 percent of kindergarteners in 2000 to 89 percent in the 2014–15 school year, then among the lowest in the country. Survey data showed that about 7 percent of students were not accounted for in school immunization records— no one knew whether they had received the vaccines but just had no record on file, or whether they had never been immunized. State law required that any students who were not fully immunized when they entered school had thirty days to receive missing immunizations, and if the children were still not vaccinated after the deadline, they had to be excluded.

To understand why the state's schools were not complying with the law, North Dakota researchers conducted a survey of school officials. Survey responses showed that administrators understood that they bore responsibility for enforcing the immunization requirements, but many felt that excluding children from school "presented a philosophical conflict for them as educators." Few educators wanted children to miss school, not only because they would fall behind in learning, but also because their schools would lose state funds tied to enrollment. Soon afterward, the state's assistant attorney general reviewed North Dakota's immunization policies with the school superintendents, calling particular attention to the fact that the State Department of Public Instruction could withhold money from any school that allowed unvaccinated children to attend. After the presentation, more school districts began enforcing the law, with the result that North Dakota's immunization rates rose to 94 percent by the 2016–17 school year.[18]

Other states that took steps to ensure all nonexempt students were vaccinated also saw increases in overall vaccination rates. In Colorado, local school districts took the initiative. Colorado's legislature had tried and failed to pass a bill that would have required parents to apply in person for exemptions. At the time, the state had nearly the lowest vaccination rate in the country. In 2016, the Brighton

School District began strict enforcement of its vaccination requirements. According to Haley Jouchens, a nurse who worked with four of the schools in Brighton, the first year was difficult. After the deadline passed and their families had still not submitted the required forms, the district excluded unvaccinated students from classrooms. Nearly three hundred students sat in the hallways, waiting to be picked up by their parents. "Obscenities were flying," she recalled.

In 2019, the public schools in Littleton began sending e-mails and letters and phoning the families of unvaccinated students who had never submitted exemption forms. By late October, there were still a hundred students on the list. The district set Friday, November 1, as its final deadline, and on that day, any students who were without exemptions or vaccinations were sent to the district's office, where their parents picked them up. The Boulder Valley School District, which had the highest rate of exemptions in the state, set a similar deadline. The district had started the school year with 4,900 students out of compliance, a number that months of reminders had whittled down to about 1,000 by the end of November.[19]

Eventually, the get-tough policies in these and other Colorado school districts had a significant effect. The percentage of Colorado children receiving the vaccine against measles, mumps, and rubella (MMR) increased from 87.4 percent in 2018–19 to 91.1 percent the following year. In the same period, similar policies in Illinois, North Carolina, and South Carolina all increased their MMR vaccine coverage to at least 95 percent—the level required for herd immunity against measles.[20]

Another strategy that states pursued was to tighten the requirements for obtaining exemptions. Studies showed that states that easily granted exemptions had higher rates of exemptions than states with more restrictive requirements.[21] Between 2011 and 2013, Oregon,

Washington, and California passed legislation requiring parents to have a conversation about the benefits of vaccines and the risks of disease with a healthcare provider or a county health department before they could obtain an exemption. Although anti-vaccine groups opposed the legislation in these states, the bills passed because most people perceived them as increasing access to information rather than taking away parents' choice.[22]

Between 2015 and 2016, ten states proposed legislation tightening the requirements for obtaining an exemption: Colorado, Florida, Illinois, Michigan, Minnesota, New Jersey, New York, Oklahoma, Pennsylvania, and Utah.[23] As was shown in Michigan, such strategies could be very effective. In response to high nonmedical exemption rates, Michigan's state legislature approved a change to the law—now parents would be required to attend an education session at their county health department as a condition of obtaining the waiver. After the law went into effect, the number of new requests for nonmedical exemptions fell 39 percent, and in some areas, the requests fell by more than 50 percent.[24]

Although some people protested, strategies to enforce existing law or to tighten the requirements for exemptions were generally accepted by the public and received bipartisan support. But the same could not be said for efforts to eliminate nonmedical exemptions altogether.

Eliminating Nonmedical Exemptions in California

From 1979 to 2015, only two states—Mississippi and West Virginia—prohibited nonmedical exemptions, and both had very high vaccination rates.[25] During the 2014–15 school year, 99.2 percent of kindergarteners in Mississippi were vaccinated, the highest rate in the nation. In West Virginia, 97.6 percent of kindergarten students were immunized. As a result, both states remained largely free from preventable childhood diseases. There had been no cases of measles in Mississippi since 1992 and none in West Virginia since 1994.[26]

No US court had ever ruled that states were constitutionally required to allow religious or personal belief exemptions from vaccination—state legislatures were free to pass laws prohibiting them.[27] The most important case bearing on the issue was a 1944 US Supreme Court case called *Prince v. Massachusetts*.[28] The court ruled that parents "cannot claim freedom from compulsory vaccination for the child. . . . The right to practice religion freely does not include liberty to expose the community or the child to communicable disease or the latter to ill health or death."[29]

By 2016, California had joined Mississippi and West Virginia in prohibiting nonmedical exemptions. Several factors contributed to this development, including the state's recurring experience with outbreaks of vaccine-preventable diseases, the effective mobilization and advocacy of pro-vaccine parents, and a successful grassroots communications campaign that reframed the issue of school vaccination to focus on one's responsibility to the children of others.

It all began with an emergence of measles in December 2014 at Disneyland Resort Theme Parks in Anaheim. Within two months, the outbreak was responsible for the infection of 147 people in seven states, Mexico, and Canada. Within six months, there were thirty-six cases in fourteen California counties, with about 20 percent requiring hospitalization. Many of those affected were not vaccinated.[30]

When measles broke out, the number of California parents seeking exemptions from vaccination was soaring. California allowed exemption on the basis of personal belief, including religious belief.[31] Between 2000 and 2012, the number of personal belief exemptions submitted for school entry tripled. At the time of the outbreak in 2014, the exemption rate had risen to 3.15 percent, but in some areas it was much, much higher. California's Senate Committee on Education reported, "In certain pockets of California, exemption rates are as high as 21%, which places our communities at risk for preventable diseases."[32]

Many California parents had become anxious over the rising number of exemptions after an outbreak of pertussis killed ten infants in 2010. There were over 9,100 reported cases in the state that year, and although the resurgence was due to a waning immunity of the vaccine, researchers also found that the cases clustered in areas where a high number of parents had exempted their children from vaccination. In response to this surge, the state passed a bill requiring those seeking to exempt their children from vaccination to meet with a healthcare practitioner to learn about the "benefits and risks of the immunization and the health risks of specified communicable diseases." Despite the tightened requirements, in 2014, two infants died during another pertussis recurrence. Thus, when measles began spreading in early 2015, many parents feared the possibility of more deaths among children.[33]

The parents of schoolchildren who could not be vaccinated were very concerned. In Marin County, where only 84 percent of schoolchildren had all their required vaccinations, Carl and Jodi Krawitt worried about protecting their son. Seven-year-old Rhett Krawitt was in remission from leukemia. Because his immune system was compromised as a result of chemotherapy he endured, he could not be vaccinated, and he was very susceptible to a highly contagious disease like measles. Carl Krawitt reached out to the Reed Union School District superintendent and asked if he would bar unvaccinated students from school to protect Rhett. However, Superintendent Steven Herzog could do nothing to help him. Such an order could only be made by the Marin County health officer, and although measles eventually appeared there, at the time of their conversation, there were no cases in Marin.

The Krawitt family decided to appeal to their local school board, and they contacted the news media as well. On February 10, young Rhett Krawitt stood on a footstool to reach the microphone and asked the Reed Union School Board to support legislation to eliminate personal belief exemptions from vaccination. After listening to him speak, the board unanimously agreed to support any such proposed legislation. The Krawitt family's story appeared on local and national news media, including NPR, CNN, MSNBC, and Al Jazeera, raising awareness of the situation in California. In response, many people in Marin County decided to vaccinated their children. "Since this story came out," said Steven Herzog, "all the districts in Marin County have seen an increase in documentation of vaccinations. We even heard there were lines of people trying to get immunized at Kaiser."[34]

By this time, other parents across the state had begun contacting legislators and starting petitions to overturn the exemptions. Hannah Henry, a parent from Napa, California, started one of the first petitions to abolish the personal belief exemption. Two and a half years earlier, she had discovered that her children's Waldorf school had a very high percentage of unvaccinated students. In 2013, it was 40 percent. "It's at 51 percent now," Henry said in early 2015. "When the measles outbreak happened," she explained, "I became really concerned for parents who might not know [about] the risk of these diseases." After signing a petition to remove the personal belief exemption, Henry decided to start her own MoveOn.org petition. As news of the measles flare-up spread across the media, the number of people who signed the petition quickly shot up, "from around 900 signers to about 18,000 signers" almost overnight.[35]

Renee DiResta, whose son was born in December 2013, had been worrying about the possibility of an outbreak for several months in the fall of 2014. When she began trying to get her son on a preschool waiting list in San Francisco, she had noticed that vaccination rates in some of the schools were extremely low, in some cases, "at 38 to 40 percent." "I called my congressman," she said. "I've never done that before, but I called, and I said, 'You know, this seems really unsafe. Why is this the way it is?' And he said, 'You know, anytime anybody tries to introduce legislation to change it, there's a huge, huge public outcry by the anti-vaccine movement, and it's just really hard to get anything done." After the outbreak in Disneyland, DiResta joined forces with other parents interested in proposing a bill to do away with personal belief exemptions in the state.[36]

Leah Russin, a lawyer turned full-time parent, joined with DiResta and others to form Vaccinate California, a nonprofit advocacy group. When measles broke out in California, Russin's son was about fourteen months old. "There were all these places where people were congregating with babies—in mommy-and-me classes, music classes, in parent and baby yoga—and vaccines weren't being required," she said. Headlines began to appear in local papers, warning of "measles exposure at Whole Foods" or "measles exposure on BART." She felt frustrated. "I wanted to change the law. I felt that basically, the legislature had let me down by not protecting my kid—by not putting in place laws that protected children."[37]

Vaccinate California came together quickly. Russin reached out to the office of State Senator Richard Pan, a pediatrician who had sponsored an earlier bill, S.B. 2109, that required parents to talk with a licensed healthcare practitioner before submitting an application for a personal belief exemption. "When I called, the person who answered was Pan's chief of staff. She said, 'Wait a minute—you're a mom, and you support vaccines? It's really nice to hear from you!

Mostly we hear from doctors. Can I connect you with some of the other moms that have been calling?' And I said, 'Sure!'"

Soon Russin and the other parents came to a decision: "We would start an organization called Vaccinate California, which would sponsor the bill. And Senator Pan and others would author legislation that would eliminate nonmedical exemptions for childhood vaccine requirements for school." The group formed on February 3, 2015. Vaccinate California's cofounders included two other parents: Renee DiResta, and actress Tisha Terrasini Banker. Russin became Vaccinate California's executive director. "Then we picked up some other people as we got rolling," she said. One of these was communications professional Jennifer Wonnacott. Another was Hannah Henry. A visual artist, Henry created the group's website and directed her MoveOn .org petition to Senator Pan's office and Vaccinate California.[38]

Vaccinate California's position was that it was "unfair and unreasonable for a small minority to put the rest of us at risk. . . . Those who can vaccinate their children but refuse are jeopardizing their own children as well as the rest of us. . . . We ought to be able to send our kids to daycare and school without fear they will come home with measles or whooping cough."[39]

Parents took front and center stage during the campaign to pass S.B. 277, the bill to eliminate nonmedical exemptions. Russin described this as a novel approach in the history of school vaccination legislation. "Until Vaccinate California, a lot of the groups pushing for vaccination around the country were medical, or medical-adjacent—school nurses, cancer survivors' groups, the American Academy of Pediatricians. It wasn't moms. You'd have a group of people in white coats saying, 'The science says . . .' and on the other side, you'd have all these vaccine hesitant or vaccine resistant moms saying, 'How dare you force me to do anything with my child?'" In contrast, she explained, "We really centered moms. Moms who were saying, 'I want legislation that means that I can send my kid to school without being afraid of a preventable disease.' "[40]

Vaccinate California's primary role was "to make it really easy for people who support vaccines to make their voices heard," but in a new era of online manipulation, this was not an easy task.[41] According to Renee DiResta, as the bill wound its way through the legislature, congressional polling data showed that about 85 percent of Californians were supportive, but the conversation on Twitter told a different story. "We would go to look at the conversation on Twitter, and we would see that it was overwhelmingly negative, 99 percent negative. . . . A lot of threats, a lot of harassment. We were saying, 'Where is this coming from?' "

To find out, DiResta teamed up with Gilad Lotan, vice-president and head of data science for BuzzFeed and adjunct professor at New York University. Their research showed that just a few groups were encouraging people to create automated accounts to push as many messages as possible, so that when people searched for information about S.B. 277, the first thing they encountered were posts and tweets against the bill. This coordination occurred simultaneously across multiple platforms. DiResta explained that people were creating extra accounts specifically for this purpose: "They created extra accounts, so there were fake people, and a lot of the conversation was being run to look like they were a much bigger group than they really were." On Twitter, a large number of voices from outside California were participating in the discussion. DiResta and Lotan shared their findings with the legislators, who began to understand that most of the opposition they were seeing on social media was not actually coming from their constituents in California.[42]

Despite the anti-vaccine pushback, S.B. 277, coauthored by Senators Richard Pan and Ben Allen, received broad support in California. A range of constituents signed Vaccinate California's online petition. In addition to the parents of infants and school-age children, supporters included government groups, including the California State Association of Counties, more than two dozen state health and medical associations, and many other political and civic organizations, including the Junior Leagues of California, California Disability Rights, and the National Coalition of 100 Black Women Sacramento Chapter, to name a few.[43]

California's education leaders supported the bill. The state's superintendent of public Instruction, Tom Torlakson, stated that the dramatic increase in the rate of personal belief exemptions of children entering kindergarten during the previous fifteen years placed other children, their families, and local communities, at risk of illness or death. In his opinion, the amended bill gave parents opting not to vaccinate the reasonable choice of educating their children through school-supported independent study and homeschooling. Statewide organizations supporting the bill included the California School Boards Association, the California State PTA, the School Nurses Organization, the Association of California School Administrators, the California School Employees Association, and numerous school districts.[44]

Opponents included national anti-vaccine organizations with deliberately innocuous names, including as the National Vaccine Information Center (NVIC)—by then the largest anti-vaccine group in the country—and a Tucson-based group called the Association of American Physicians and Surgeons (AAPS). The AAPS was a medical liberty group that rejected all forms of regulation and mandates in medicine and had begun spreading fears about the measles vaccine.[45] In submitted testimony, the NVIC's Barbara Loe Fisher claimed S.B. 277 violated the "human right to informed consent to medical risk taking and denies equal protection and education to children in California."[46]

Opponents also included two anti-abortion groups: the California ProLife Council, a political action committee, and the California Right to Life Committee, an organization founded in 1981 to educate the general public about the "sanctity and intrinsic value of each human life."[47] Over the years, the anti-abortion movement had grown in influence. The first March for Life event to protest the US Supreme Court ruling in *Roe v. Wade* was held in Washington, DC, in 1974 with about twenty thousand people in attendance. On the fortieth anniversary of the ruling in 2013, nearly a half-million people joined a March for Life in Washington to protest outside the Supreme Court building. By that time, the March for Life campaign had become a well-organized political powerhouse, encouraging citizen lobbying and organized anti-abortion marches around the country.[48] Such groups pointed out that the rubella component of Merck's MMR vaccine was developed using fetal cell lines. In response, Merck issued a statement saying that there was "currently no alternative" to protect against rubella, and "major religious groups have accepted use of the vaccine." Nevertheless, some anti-abortion parents were now refusing the vaccine on moral grounds.[49]

Fisher did not acknowledge the California parents who supported the bill; instead, she described the legislation as the result of lobbying by "wealthy and powerful medical trade and public health associations."[50] She claimed that "liability-free doctors" were "using very small groups of immune compromised individuals as an excuse to eliminate all non-medical vaccine exemptions" in a move to "blackmail virtually every American into playing vaccine roulette."[51]

But Fisher was wrong. Throughout history, opponents of vaccination laws commonly presented their struggle as a David-versus-Goliath effort, depicting themselves as ordinary citizens battling the bureaucratic forces of allopathic doctors, state legislatures, and public health departments. Similarly, historians have rarely documented the grassroots efforts of parents in support of vaccination. To some extent, this is because studies focused on developments in public health have often placed doctors, scientists, and public health officials at the center of the story. But the large, silent majority of Americans who supported vaccination was never completely silent and inactive. Parents had led a grassroots movement to impel the Massachusetts legislature to pass the nation's first state vaccination law, and in every state, parents had provided homegrown support to the polio vaccination campaign for many years. Now, the same thing was happening in California. A large majority of California voters supported the legislation, as would later be revealed through referendum.

As S.B. 277 wound through the legislature in the spring of 2015, legal debates over the bill centered on civil rights—specifically, the right to education, the right to equal protection under the law, and the right to safety in California's schools. The American Civil Liberties Union (ACLU) sent the legislature a letter of concern, stating, "Unlike other states, public education is a fundamental right under the California Constitution. Equal access to education must therefore not be limited or denied unless the State demonstrates that its actions are 'necessary to achieve a compelling interest.'" The ACLU's letter quoted from *Serrano v. Priest*, a case about equity in school finance that had spanned three California Supreme Court decisions from 1971 to 1977. *Serrano* was based on two principles: First, that education in the public schools is a fundamental interest or right, and second, that equal access to education must not be limited or denied unless the state can demonstrate a compelling interest under the law. In the ACLU's opinion, "the bill should be amended to explain specifically what that interest is, where it exists, and under what conditions and circumstances it exists."[52]

California's compelling interest under the law was based, not only on the state's constitutional authority to protect the public from contagious disease, but also on the right of California children to be safe in their public schools. As Dorit Rubinstein Reiss, a professor at U.C. Hastings College of Law, explained in her testimony before the Senate Judiciary Committee, the right to education in California was not violated by S.B. 277. The protection of the public's right to be free from contagious disease falls under the police power of the state. Starting with California's supreme court ruling in *Abeel v. Clark*, which the US Supreme Court had cited in *Jacobsen v. Massachusetts*, the courts had always upheld the right of the states to require vaccination to protect the public health. More important, in *Zucht v. King*, the US Supreme Court had upheld the right of states to require vaccination for school attendance.[53] Also speaking before the committee, Senator Ben Allen explained that low rates of vaccination created safety risks for children who were unable to be vaccinated for medical reasons. As a result of California's 1985 School Safety Act, the legislature recognized "the inalienable right" of students to attend safe public schools. But as Allen pointed out, by making it relatively easy for parents to obtain personal belief exemptions, the state had made schools less safe for such children.[54]

Opponents of vaccination often argued on the basis of freedom of choice, but as Reiss noted, "That argument cuts two ways." The parents of children who could not be vaccinated for medical reasons had no choice. Without the protection of vaccination, their children were very vulnerable to infection during any outbreak of a vaccine-preventable disease. "The barrier to access is not of their making, and not one about which they have a choice," Reiss explained. On the other hand, the parents who chose not to vaccinate on the basis of personal belief did have freedom of choice. They could choose one of the options available under S.B. 277—they could educate their children at home, either alone or with a group of other families in a private homeschool, or they could enroll their child in an independent study program offered by their local school. Or, they could choose to vaccinate their children. S.B. 277 did not violate California children's right to education. Instead, as Reiss explained, it reinforced that right "by protecting schoolchildren from disease, which is a precondition to receiving the education to which they are entitled."[55]

Ultimately the Judiciary Committee's statement of compelling interest under the law emphasized the right of California students to safety in their schools. The committee noted that students in the state's public schools not only had a right to education, they also had a right to attend schools that were safe. "A safe school for many children is a school with a high level of community immunity which would protect them from known diseases. This legislation provides the most comprehensive measure to ensure high vaccination rates—by limiting the presence of those who are not vaccinated from a campus where children mingle and may be at risk of exposure to vaccine-preventable diseases."[56]

Under the provisions of S.B. 277, parents who chose not to vaccinate their children would still have access to education, either by establishing private homeschools or having their children follow a school-sponsored independent study program. Students with an Individual Educational Program (IEP) were also exempted from the immunization requirement, and the law would be implemented gradually—children would have to provide proof of immunization upon entry to preschool or daycare, at kindergarten, and at seventh grade. The law would apply to children in both public and private schools.[57]

California's legislature passed S.B. 277, and Governor Jerry Brown signed it into law on June 30, 2015. After it went into effect on January 1, 2016, the number of kindergartners with nonmedical exemptions dropped significantly in every county. The law increased the state's overall kindergarten vaccination rates from 92.8 percent in the 2015–16 school year to 95.6 percent in 2016–17.[58]

It was not long, however, before anti-vaccination activists sought to overturn the bill. Parents and advocacy groups filed four lawsuits, each of which had to overcome two major hurdles. First, plaintiffs had to prevail against the state's compelling interest in abolishing nonmedical exemptions, and second, they had to overcome a long history of federal and state court rulings that had supported school vaccination mandates, detailed in the appendix of this book.[59]

None of the lawsuits succeeded. In *Whitlow v. California Dept. of Education*, which was filed in federal court by seventeen parents and four advocacy groups, plaintiffs lost their case when the court ruled against them, stating, "There is no question that society has a compelling interest in fighting the spread of contagious diseases through mandatory vaccination of school-aged children. All courts, state and federal, have so held either explicitly or implicitly for over a century."[60] In a second case, *Torrey-Love v. State Dept. of Education*, parents and an anti-vaccination group called A Voice for Choice argued that S.B. 277 was unconstitutional because it forced parents and children to choose between different rights—the child's right to education, the right to privacy, and the parents' right to make medical decisions for their children. However, this suit also faced numerous hurdles from the start, because the US Supreme Court and California courts had previously ruled that states had the right to set the conditions for school attendance, including the requirement that students be vaccinated. As for the right to privacy, California's court of appeals ruled against them, finding that it was "no more sacred than any of the other fundamental rights that have readily given way to a State's interest in protecting the health and safety of its citizens, and particularly, school children." The other two lawsuits failed on similar grounds.[61]

Opponents of S.B. 277 also sought to overturn the law through referendum. Just one day after Governor Jerry Brown signed the bill into law, Tim Donnelly, a conservative talk show host and a former Republican assemblyman and gubernatorial candidate, filed paperwork for a referendum to repeal the law. "Gov. Jerry Brown signed away a parent's right to choose what's best for their child," he posted on Facebook. "This is a victory for leftists bent on absolute control. No more choice, no informed consent, only compliance or else!" Shortly afterward, anti-vaccination activists also launched a recall effort to unseat pediatrician and State Senator Richard Pan.[62] Ultimately, however, both efforts failed for lack of support.

What these attempts revealed, however, was the beginning of a partisan divide over the issue of vaccination. S.B. 277 had passed with bipartisan support, but only two Republicans had joined with Democrats in endorsing the bill.[63] Among the groups that had written in support of the bill during the debates were some local Democratic Party headquarters, including those from Santa Cruz and Marin counties, areas with high rates of personal belief exemptions. In contrast, no Republican Party group wrote to support the bill.[64] Now Donnelly, a well-known Republican, was decrying the bill as a leftist victory. This was a very different political landscape from the late twentieth century, when members of both parties had supported legislation requiring school vaccination. As Leah Russin of Vaccinate California explained, "The anti-vaccine movement, five or ten years ago, people would have said it's this weird, unique space where the far left meets the far right. In my view, the portion of the far left that was anti-vaccine has shrunk. Meanwhile, the anti-vax stance on the far right has expanded."[65]

Traces of this shift could be seen in 2015. As legislation over exemptions was under way in other areas of the country that year, a partisan divide appeared in the way state legislatures voted.

Political Polarization over School Vaccination Mandates across the Country

In 2010, researchers noticed that political party membership was associated with an individual's stance on vaccination. Analysis of survey results from the 2009–10 H1N1 flu pandemic showed that those identifying as members of the Democratic Party were more willing to become vaccinated than were Republicans or independents, and that political party membership was more closely associated with one's attitude toward vaccination than whether one identified as liberal or conservative.[66]

By 2015, discussion of a partisan divide over vaccination had spilled into mainstream news media. Analysts from Pew Research found that between 2009 and 2015, although income, education, or gender made little difference in people's views, there were now some differences along political party lines. In 2009, 71 percent of both Democrats and Republicans were in favor of requiring vaccination for school attendance. But now, 76 percent of Democrats—in contrast to 65 percent of Republicans and 65 percent of independents—said vaccines should be required.[67] Other surveys drew similar conclusions.[68] Based on data from the Cooperative Congressional Election Study, the *Washington Post* reported that those who identified as politically conservative were more likely to believe the unfounded claim that vaccines caused autism. The *Post*'s researchers also found a link between one's trust in government and one's likelihood of believing the claim. They concluded that "anti-vaccination attitudes appear concentrated among conservatives and those who distrust government."[69]

By 2013, anti-abortion advocates had gained a significant foothold in the Republican party—a survey by Pew Research Center found that around half of Republicans wanted to outlaw nearly all abortions. Among religious groups seeking to overturn *Roe v. Wade*, white evangelical Protestants were the only group in which a majority favored completely overturning the decision, and over the next decade, polls would show that vaccine skepticism had spread among Protestant evangelicals worried about a connection between vaccines and abortion.[70]

Christian evangelicals had supported scientific advancement and vaccination during the polio campaign, but over the following decades, many had changed their views. Parents concerned about the effects of secular humanism, science, and technology in mainstream US culture began leaving public school systems and enrolling their children in Christian day schools. They also began homeschooling their children. By the late 1980s, Protestant evangelicals and a small number of conservative Catholics represented nearly 90 percent of families engaged in homeschooling.[71] During the 1980s, they also gained a powerful political action group in Moral Majority, a political and lobbying organization founded by Baptist minister Jerry Falwell Sr. that was closely associated with the Republican Party.[72] Although none of the major Protestant denominations officially opposed vaccination, by the early twenty-first century, the ideology of Christian nationalism, a cultural framework seeking to privilege Christianity in US national identity, public policies, and civic culture, had also become strongly associated with opposition to vaccination mandates.[73]

As vaccine skeptics from both ends of the political spectrum protested laws curtailing exemptions, they found "unexpected allies" among conservative Republicans. In Maine, Republicans mounted an effort to oppose the elimination of nonmedical exemptions, and in Minnesota, no Republicans joined an effort to make it harder to avoid vaccinating children. Colorado Republicans shut down a proposal to require parents to obtain a doctor's approval if they wanted to exempt their children from vaccination.[74]

The issue of exemptions from vaccination spilled into the upcoming 2016 presidential election as well, with some Republican Party candidates expressing their support for exemptions. New Jersey Governor Chris Christie stated in public that parents "need to have some measure of choice" when it came to vaccinating their children. Shortly afterward, his office issued a clarification, stating, "The Governor believes vaccines are an important public health protection and with a disease like measles there is no question kids should be vaccinated."[75] Kentucky senator Rand Paul took the position that parents should definitely have the power to refuse vaccinating their children. "The state doesn't own your children," he said on CNBC news. "I think vaccines are one of the greatest medical breakthroughs that we've had . . . but for most of our history, they have been voluntary, so I don't think I'm arguing for anything out of the ordinary."[76]

During the Republican debate on September 16, 2015, candidates Donald Trump, Rand Paul, and Ben Carson all stated their opinion that parents should have the right to refuse vaccines for their children. Trump claimed a connection between vaccines and autism by telling a moving story about an employee whose baby had fallen ill with a fever after being vaccinated. Later, according to Trump, the child developed autism. Carson and Paul both raised concerns about the vaccination schedule. At the time, the notion of spacing out some vaccines and opting out of others was promoted by California pediatrician Robert Spears, but the practice had never been based on any research. According to Carson, "We have extremely well-documented proof that there's no autism associated with vaccination, but it is true that we are probably giving way too many in too short a period of time." Paul agreed with Carson: "I'm for vaccines, but I'm also for freedom. . . . I ought to be able to spread my vaccines out a little bit, at the very least."[77]

Why had school vaccination become a partisan issue? In seeking explanations, some commentators pointed to the media. According to Matthew A. Baum, the relatively limited news sources of the 1950s and '60s had created an information commons, where Americans encountered nonpartisan reporting of public health issues. In contrast, by the twenty-first century, the growing availability of news sources on the Internet and via social media had created a much more fragmented media marketplace catering to specific interests, a market in which people selectively sought news information likely to reinforce their existing beliefs and political leanings.[78] Some scholars pointed to a common media phenomenon in which, simply through the act of reporting both sides of a story, the voices and influence of the anti-vaccinationists appeared far larger than they actually were. After all, despite the rise in nonmedical exemptions, the vast majority of American parents still chose to vaccinate their children in 2015. Unfortunately, this large, silent majority was not always proportionally represented on social media and in mainstream news reports. Journalists' efforts to provide balanced reporting inadvertently resulted in skewed news stories that gave equal air time to what was, in fact, a small minority group.[79]

Although the media may have amplified minority views, the media alone did not cause political polarization. It is unlikely that Republican presidential candidates would have begun talking about giving people choice in deciding whether to accept vaccines if Democrats had not been behind proposals to remove long-standing nonmedical exemptions in 2015.

Partisan divisions over vaccination exemptions became evident in state legislative debates in 2015 and early 2016, when twenty-two state legislatures introduced bills regarding exemptions from vaccination requirements. In 2015, Republicans controlled both chambers in thirty states, Democrats controlled both chambers in eleven states, eight states had divided legislatures, and one state (Nebraska) was unicameral. With the exception of West Virginia, whose legislature considered a bill to add exemptions, all the states in table 8.1 considered bills proposing to tighten or increase vaccination requirements, either by removing one or more exemptions or by adding requirements to the exemption process. Among Democratic-controlled legislatures, 73 percent proposed such bills, and among the states with split legislatures, 63 percent proposed such bills. In contrast, only 30 percent of Republican-controlled legislatures proposed such bills during this period.

All the proposed bills to abolish exemptions faced uphill battles, and in none of the Republican-controlled legislatures did they succeed. In 2015, among the Democratic-controlled or split legislatures, such bills succeeded only in California and Vermont, which banned personal belief exemptions.

By 2021, three more states had passed laws eliminating all nonmedical exemptions, bringing the total number to six. In 2019, Maine became the fourth state to overturn the exemptions. As had happened in California, partisan differences emerged during the legislative debates. At the time, an outbreak of whooping cough had spread through three counties, giving Maine the highest rate of whooping cough cases in the country, and about half of the state's kindergarten children did not meet the 95 percent herd immunity threshold needed to protect against more flare-ups.[80] Democratic representative Ralph Tucker proposed legislation to remove the nonmedical exemption, but Republicans disliked the idea, even though

Table 8.1. Proposed state legislation regarding nonmedical vaccine exemptions, 2015 and 2016

States (N = 22)	Partisan legislative composition in 2015	To eliminate nonmedical exemptions	To eliminate personal belief exemptions	To add requirements for exemptions	To add exemptions	Did the bill pass?
California	Democratic	S.B. 277 (2015)				yes
Colorado	Split			S.B. 163 (2016)		yes
Connecticut	Democratic			H.B. 6949 (2015)		yes
Florida	Republican			S.B. 646 (2016)		no
Hawaii	Democratic	H.B. 1722 (2016)				no
Illinois	Democratic			S.B. 1410 (2015)		yes
Maryland	Democratic	H.B. 0687 (2015)				no
Michigan	Republican			H.B. 5361 (2016)		yes
Minnesota	Split			H.B. 393 (2015)		no
New Jersey	Democratic			S.B. 1147 (2015)		no
New Mexico	Split	H.B. 522 (2015)				no
New York	Split	A08329 (2015); S01536 (2015)		A07016 (2015)		no
North Carolina	Republican	S.B. 346 (2015)				no
Oklahoma	Republican	S.B. 830 (2015)		H.B. 3016 (2016)		no
Oregon	Democratic	S.B. 442 (2015)				no
Pennsylvania	Republican		H.B. 883 (2015)			no
Utah	Republican			H.B. 221 (2016)		yes
Vermont	Democratic		H.B. 98 (2015)			yes
Virginia	Republican	H.B. 1342 (2016)				no
Washington	Split	H.B. 2009 (2015)				no
West Virginia	Republican				H.B. 2556 (2015–16)	no
Wisconsin	Republican	A.B. 924 (2015)				no

Sources: Created from data on state legislative websites and Wendy Underhill, Dan Diorio, and Kae Warnock, "State Vote: 2015 State Elections," National Conference of State Legislatures, Nov. 4, 2015, https://www.ncsl.org/research/elections-and-campaigns/statevote -2015-elections.aspx.

they expressed support for vaccination. As Republican representative Deborah Sanderson explained, "If you're going to mandate that a parent do something that philosophically they are opposed to, that's a tremendous overreach of government." Maine's Senate voted eighteen to seventeen to end the exemption, with all Republicans voting against the bill.[81] The same year, during the largest measles outbreak in the United States in three decades, New York's legislature also banned all nonmedical exemptions, and in 2021, Connecticut followed suit.[82]

This is not to say that partisanship affected every debate over vaccination policy. Despite deep disagreements over the question of exemptions, in some states, politicians on both sides of the aisle supported other forms of legislation designed to strengthen public health. For instance, in Illinois, Republican senator Christina Radogno presented a proposal to require daycare employees working with children age six and younger to be vaccinated with the MMR vaccine or show proof of immunity against measles, mumps, and rubella. Radogno sought to protect children but also wanted to avoid antagonizing families opposed to vaccination. "It's a very delicate issue when you're talking about immunizations in children," she said. "So the approach that I've taken hopefully has not drawn any criticism."[83] The bill, S.B. 0986, easily passed the senate and assembly with the amendment that employees must also receive the vaccine against diphtheria, tetanus, and pertussis.[84] In Montana, in response to a bill proposed by House Democrat Margaret McDonald, the Republican-controlled legislature revised the school law to require students entering kindergarten to have two doses of varicella (chicken pox) vaccine and receive a booster of pertussis vaccine at the seventh grade. The requirements were intended to reduce the incidence of both diseases, since Montana's rates were high at the time.[85]

Across the country, the laws passed during these years, coupled with efforts to strengthen enforcement, stopped the decline in vaccine coverage in many areas. School districts that began enforcing the laws raised the overall vaccination rates of children who had not submitted exemptions, and in states that had eliminated nonmedical exemptions, rates also rose.

Because of these efforts, national vaccination rates stabilized in the 2019–20 school year, as did the percentage of families seeking nonmedical exemptions. According to CDC researchers, the percentage of entering kindergartners with nonmedical exemptions increased by more than a third during the three-year period from the end of the 2015–16 school year through 2018–19 (table 8.2). Without a widespread push to raise vaccination rates during those three years, overall immunization levels in American schools would have declined below the level required for herd immunity. Instead, because of improvements in enforcement and the elimination of exemptions in some states, immunization levels remained high. This success was thanks to the efforts of elected state legislators, parent advocacy groups, local school districts, and public health departments.

Unfortunately, this success would soon be imperiled by a global pandemic.

Table 8.2. US vaccination coverage and exemption rates for selected vaccines among children in kindergarten, from the 2015–16 school year through the 2019–20 school year (in percentages)

School year	MMR (measles, mumps, rubella)	DTaP (diphtheria, tetanus, pertussis)	Medical exemptions	Nonmedical exemptions	All exemptions
2015–16	94.6	94.2	0.2	1.6	1.9[a]
2016–17	94.0	94.5	0.2	1.8	2.0
2017–18	94.3	95.1	0.2	2.0	2.2
2018–19	94.7	94.9	0.3	2.2	2.5
2019–20	95.2	94.9	0.3	2.2	2.5

Sources: Table created from data in Renee Seither et al., "Vaccination Coverage with Selected Vaccines and Exemption Rates among Children in Kindergarten—United States, 2015–16 School Year," *MMWR* 65, no. 39 [Oct. 7, 2016]: 1057–64; Seither et al., "Vaccination Coverage with Selected Vaccines and Exemption Rates [. . .] 2016–17 School Year," *MMWR* 66, no. 40 [Oct. 13, 2017]: 1073–80; Janelle L. Mellerson et al., "Vaccination Coverage with Selected Vaccines and Exemption Rates [. . .] 2017–18 School Year," *MMWR* 67, no. 40 [Oct. 12, 2018]: 1115–22; Seither et al., "Vaccination Coverage with Selected Vaccines and Exemption Rates [. . .] 2018–19 School Year," *MMWR* 68, no. 41 [Oct. 18, 2019]: 905–12; Seither et al., "Vaccination Coverage with Selected Vaccines and Exemption Rates [. . .] 2019–20 School Year," *MMWR* 70, no. 3 [Jan. 22, 2021]: 75–82.
[a] The apparent discrepancy is due to differences in reporting methods.

When the COVID-19 pandemic began in 2020, forty-nine states, the District of Columbia, Puerto Rico, and the US Virgin Islands had laws or regulations in place regarding how schools or school districts should respond to a disease outbreak. Although they varied by state, most statutes required schools to notify the public health department when a student was believed to have a contagious disease, and most included authorizations to exclude students from school. Most statutes also authorized the closure of schools during an epidemic.[86] Although state laws made no mention of masks, most had language giving schools broad latitude during epidemics. For instance, California's statute authorized school and public health authorities to take "measures necessary for the prevention and control of communicable diseases in school age children."[87]

During the pandemic, partisan politics came to affect the implementation of mask mandates in the schools. In late July 2020, the CDC recommended that all schools require students, teachers, and visitors to wear masks to prevent the spread of COVID-19. Mask wearing was a strategy dating from the great influenza epidemic of 1918–19, but few Americans were familiar or comfortable with the notion of wearing masks themselves or placing masks on their children. In many areas of the country, protests emerged over mandates to wear masks.[88]

By the summer of 2021, only ten states had passed laws requiring mask wearing in schools, and eight states had passed laws forbidding them. Among the ten states requiring masks, nine had legislatures under Democratic control, and one had a legislature that was evenly divided between the two parties. In contrast, all of the eight states forbidding masks had legislatures under Republican control. Thirty-two other states left the decision up to local schools and school districts.[89]

The pandemic dramatically changed education in the country. Given the absence of a vaccine against COVID-19, nearly every school in the United States closed its doors and switched to some form of remote learning to complete the school year in the spring of 2020.[90]

The federal government, with a Republican majority in the Senate and Republican president Donald Trump in the White House, threw its support behind vaccine development and manufacturing. Under the program Operation Warp Speed (OWS), the government invested $10 billion to create and deploy vaccines. New vaccines were developed and field-tested with unprecedented speed, with the result that the Food and Drug Administration (FDA) authorized two vaccines for emergency use just eleven months after OWS began. The first person immunized against COVID-19 in the United States received an injection on December 14, 2020. Two weeks later, the CDC reported that 4.2 million people had received their first dose.[91]

Operation Warp Speed was very effective, but the responsibility for distribution of the vaccines at the local level fell to individual states, where the vaccine rollout was slower than expected. Some states experienced storage and delivery problems. Others simply did not have enough vaccines to meet the demand.[92] Despite the roadblocks, the distribution problems and supply shortages were soon resolved. In February 2021, after Democratic president Joseph Biden took office, his administration purchased an additional 100 million doses of COVID-19 vaccines from Pfizer and Moderna Inc. to meet the demand and ease supply shortages in the states.[93]

Public health officials hoped that the increased supply would quickly lead to high vaccination rates, but in many areas, people hesitated to be vaccinated. Political party affiliation had come to define one's stance on vaccination, with more Republicans than Democrats refusing COVID-19 vaccines. A Gallup poll found that in September, only 56 percent of Republicans had received at least one COVID vaccination, in contrast to 92 percent of Democrats.[94]

On September 9, 2021, aiming to increase vaccination rates to the level required for herd immunity, President Biden took the unprecedented step of signing an executive order requiring all federal employees to be vaccinated against the disease, and he called on employers to do the same.[95] In November, the Biden administration announced two more policies to "drive even more progress and result in millions of Americans getting vaccinated, protecting workers, preventing hospitalization, saving lives, and strengthening the economy." These included a new Occupational Safety and Health Administration order for private employers with one hundred or more employees to require their employees to be vaccinated, a rule that covered 84 million employees. Additionally, the federal Centers for Medicare and Medicaid Services announced that healthcare workers at facilities receiving federal funding would have to be "fully vaccinated." This rule affected over 17 million workers.[96]

Republicans in the US Congress attacked the orders, accusing Biden of "overstepping his authority." Protests against the new rules deepened existing partisan divisions over vaccination, and lawsuits soon followed. More than two dozen Republican states sued the president over the order affecting employees in private companies.[97] Ultimately, a case made its way to the US Supreme Court, which allowed the federal mandate affecting healthcare workers to stand but blocked the vaccination requirement affecting employees in private companies.[98]

Although the federal mandates outraged many Republicans, they also increased the rate at which American adults rolled up their sleeves to receive a COVID-19 shot. As a result, adult vaccination rates far exceeded the rate at which adults had been vaccinated during the polio campaign of the 1950s. Six years after the polio vaccine became available in 1955, only 77 percent of people below the age of forty had received one dose.[99] In 1964, government and public health officials carried out "Stop Polio" campaigns across the country to vaccinate American adults who had never received a single dose. For example, in Wake County, North Carolina, officials celebrated when adult vaccination rates finally rose to 83 percent that year.[100]

In contrast to the polio era, by the end of 2021, just one year after the first vaccines against COVID-19 became available, the CDC reported that about 85 percent of adults over the age of eighteen had received a first dose. Vaccination rates were highest among the elderly, which constituted the group most at risk from COVID-19. And although a US Census Bureau survey found that about 6 percent of unvaccinated Americans said they "don't trust the COVID-19 vaccine," once vaccines received emergency use authorization from the FDA, most parents saw that their children received a first injection.[101]

Nevertheless, the political battles over vaccination policy took a terrible toll. By the fall of 2021, demographers had documented the inevitable and tragic outcome of the growing political polarization: more people in predominantly Republican areas had died from COVID-19 than those living in Democratic areas.[102]

That year, the CDC pointed out another disturbing trend— school vaccination rates were falling. This circumstance, as it turned out, had nothing to do with political partisanship. The decline was a worldwide phenomenon.

The Decline of School Vaccination Rates during the COVID-19 Pandemic

In 2022, the CDC reported that during 2021, orders for routine childhood vaccines against diseases like polio, diphtheria, and measles were about 7 percent lower than they had been before the pandemic began. A joint statement from the World Health Organization and UNICEF described the decline as a global problem, explaining that the COVID-19 pandemic had triggered a backslide in routine vaccinations. "This is a red alert for child health," announced Catherine Russell, UNICEF's executive director. "We are witnessing the largest sustained drop in childhood immunization in a generation."[103]

Some researchers attributed the drop to a general reluctance or inability to visit medical offices and hospitals for routine care during the pandemic.[104] Others thought the decline was caused by concerns about the COVID-19 vaccines. When the first vaccines to protect children became available, many parents were hesitant to allow their children to receive a vaccine that the FDA had authorized only for emergency use. Some feared the development of the vaccine had been rushed. Others worried about the possibility of adverse side effects and wondered whether vaccination was worth the risk.[105] Disruptions caused by school closures during the 2020–21 academic year may also have led parents to forgo routine vaccinations.

Misinformation also played a role. Anonymous posters on social media sites made scores of false statements, including claims that the vaccines themselves caused coronavirus, that they contained tissue from aborted fetuses, or that the new vaccines altered human DNA.[106] One anti-vaccine website claimed that President Biden had announced a policy denying government food stamps to people who refused vaccination. A British YouTuber claimed that the COVID-19 vaccine caused infertility. Video clips and memes on the Internet announced that the AstraZeneca vaccine would turn people into chimpanzees—this claim was promoted in countries where Russia aimed to market its own vaccine, leading some observers to conclude that its authors worked for the Russian government.[107]

By 2021, some people were beginning to believe conspiracy theories about COVID-19 vaccines. That year, millions of people logged onto their devices to view TikTok videos proclaiming that the federal government was placing microchips in the vaccines to track people's movements. Afterward, a survey of 1,500 Americans found that 5 percent thought the theory was true and another 15 percent believed it was "probably true."[108]

When the CDC reported that that many children were not up to date with the shots they had missed during the pandemic, doctors, and nurses began raising concerns that preventable diseases from the past could once again reappear in US schools.[109] Their concerns seemed to be validated when poliovirus was found in London sewage in June the following year. This discovery marked the first time the virus had been seen in the United Kingdom in about forty years. Health authorities there declared an emergency and urged everyone in the country to be vaccinated immediately.[110] Just one month later, health officials in New York announced the discovery of a case of polio in an unvaccinated person in Rockland County. The victim developed paralysis. No treatment exists for polio, but the disease can be prevented by vaccination. Jennifer Nuzzo, a pandemic researcher at Brown University, told a news reporter that the case should be a wake-up call for those who are not vaccinated against polio. "If you haven't gotten your kids vaccinated," she said, "it's really important that you make sure they're up to date."[111]

If a disease like polio were to reemerge, would it be possible to launch a successful, nonpartisan vaccination campaign to defeat it, as an earlier generation did? By this point, the partisan divide in the United States made it hard to imagine.

Conclusion

By the end of 2019, despite the resistance of highly vocal anti-vaccine organizations, efforts across the country to preserve immunity in the schools appeared to have succeeded. Through a combination of tougher enforcement policies in some states and the elimination of nonmedical exemptions in others, overall vaccination rates in public and private kindergartens reached the level required for community protection.

Nevertheless, there was no guarantee that the rate at which families were seeking exemptions would hold steady in future years. In states that disallowed exemptions, more parents might decide to homeschool their children to avoid vaccination. And many states left parents free to select the curriculum of their choice when they homeschooled. In California, for instance, the state's grade-level standards and adopted curriculum materials did "not apply to students schooled at home."[112] Would parents opposed to vaccination decide to teach their children the germ theory of disease and the science behind vaccination? There was no assurance that they would. In states without vaccination requirements for homeschooled children, it could be extremely difficult to encourage immunization among children learning "off the grid."[113] Allowing nonmedical exemptions has been most successful when most people have trusted their local and federal institutions and pulled together to protect their communities from contagious disease. But by 2020, that trust had eroded. It was no longer certain that Americans would be able to maintain a consensus about school vaccination policies in a new era of political polarization.

The campaign against COVID-19 resulted in historic achievements, but it also brought serious setbacks. Vaccines were developed and deployed with unprecedented speed. At the same time, disruptions caused by school closures, social distancing, and quarantine rules led to protests against public health mandates in some areas, and existing political divisions deepened. One of the most disturbing developments was a decline in routine vaccinations against other childhood diseases.

A political party skeptical of vaccines could easily undo the years of effort it took to develop herd immunity against some of the worst childhood diseases in history. Herd immunity takes decades to achieve, and maintaining it requires a commitment on everyone's part. As Marin County parent Hannah Henry explained during California's 2015 measles outbreak, "This shield has been built up over generations. [Now] the shield has a hole in it, and the hole is enlarging.... This is exactly how infectious diseases enter a society." That invisible shield we all take for granted is always there—"until it's not."[114]

Conclusion

The research for this book began with three questions: How have Americans understood the place of schools in the transmission and prevention of contagious disease? How have schools reconciled what appear to be conflicting civil rights—the child's right to an education versus the child's right to be safe from disease in school? Why does anti-vaccination activism persist?

As this volume has shown, it took more than a century for most Americans to fully understand how contagious diseases spread. Childhood diseases circulate easily through crowded schoolrooms. A child from an infected family can spread infection to classmates, who may then carry the infection home to their families, friends, and neighbors. From neighborhoods, diseases can spread easily along travel routes to other towns and cities. In the past, people may have understood this process intuitively, but the research documenting the phenomenon was not published until the 1870s. Long before they understood the underlying causes of contagious diseases, educators were well aware of the importance of maintaining healthy conditions in their schools. Rumors of sickness spreading through a school could lead parents to withdraw their children. During serious epidemics, students could die. However, the schoolbooks most students encountered throughout much of the nineteenth century provided no information about the role of bacteria and viruses in transmitting disease.

Acceptance of vaccination preceded understanding and acceptance of the germ theory of disease. Smallpox was terrifying. During the early nineteenth century, it reportedly killed one in four victims, and during severe outbreaks, the death rate could be much higher. When a vaccine became available, Americans welcomed it. However, once outbreaks subsided, and smallpox disappeared for a generation or more, people were less willing to bare their arms for the vaccinator. Their resistance was understandable. The vaccine came with adverse side effects. Additionally, vaccine lots were not always properly prepared and stored, and not all doctors administered the dose safely. It took the threat of a serious epidemic for people to seek vaccination.

States began passing school vaccination laws during the second half of the nineteenth century, when smallpox outbreaks began to reemerge in many areas. The rise of compulsory school vaccination laws, along with the establishment of state public health departments, drew more attention to the need to protect schoolchildren from smallpox outbreaks. But protecting children was not the only reason states passed such laws. As more people came to understand the nature of contagion, they began to view school vaccination policies as a way to prevent recurring cycles of epidemics. Although nineteenth- and early-twentieth-century legislators rarely used terms like *herd immunity* or *community protection* in their debates, their goal was similar. Essentially, they hoped to achieve a level of immunity that would stop future outbreaks and shield everyone from illness.

It would take many years to achieve this goal. In the late nine-teenth century, alternative physicians began speaking out against vac-cination, and many Americans found their arguments persuasive. A growing anti-vaccination movement made it difficult for states to pass laws like those of the twenty-first century, which require vac-cination for school even in the absence of disease. By 1927, only eleven states had such laws. Most required vaccination for admis-sion to school only during an outbreak, or when smallpox was spreading nearby. Such laws made it possible for families to avoid vaccination for long periods, but they also virtually guaranteed that smallpox outbreaks would return. The patchwork nature of vacci-nation laws across the country ensured that it would take nearly a century to eliminate smallpox in the United States.

Throughout history, school officials sometimes struggled to bal-ance their duty to educate with their responsibility to keep students safe from contagious disease. No one questioned the importance of keeping students healthy in school. But enforcing vaccination man-dates posed challenges.

On the one hand, schools across the country played an important part in protecting students' health. To improve children's safety, nineteenth-century educators emphasized the importance of clean-liness and fresh air in classrooms. During smallpox outbreaks, many teachers and principals excluded unvaccinated students from school. Schools also supported vaccination at critical moments, especially during campaigns against specific diseases. This was especially true during the voluntary vaccination campaigns against diphtheria and polio. During the polio era, holding vaccination clinics on school grounds and using school buses to transport students to health clin-ics helped school-aged children achieve the highest vaccination rates of any demographic group in the country. The critical role of schools in the polio campaign revealed how effective collaboration among schools, communities, and healthcare providers could be. As a result, it was natural for state and federal policymakers to consider the how schools could help in enforcing vaccination against polio and other diseases through admission requirements, and by 1980, using this strategy to protect against childhood diseases had become universal across the country.

But on the other hand, not all schools complied with the vaccination laws. Some educators felt that enforcing them interfered with their mission. Excluding unvaccinated students meant that fewer children would be sitting in classrooms and learning their lessons. Because state funds were tied to enrollment, it also meant less money to keep schools running smoothly. Some schools failed to enforce the laws for these reasons. From a legal standpoint, school boards often found themselves caught between two civil rights—the child's right to education and the child's right to protection from contagious disease. News of lawsuits against school districts alarmed many. Could schools be successfully sued for excluding unvaccinated students when state law required all children to attend? Some of the most important school vaccination cases before 1922 bore directly on this question.

Given their responsibility to keep children safe from contagious disease, schools historically have fallen short in two areas: enforcement and curriculum. Lack of enforcement has been an intermittent but persistent problem. During the 1970s and '80s, when states began passing new laws requiring vaccination against polio and other vaccine-preventable diseases, it became evident that once again, schools were not enforcing the regulations in all areas. Lack of enforcement continued in the twenty-first century, as revealed during efforts to raise vaccination rates in 2015–16.

Despite the schools' long experience with vaccination, with the exception of the polio era, vaccination has remained a relatively marginal topic in the school curriculum. Nineteenth- and early-twentieth-century schools taught students to protect their health, but textbooks generally focused on abstinence from alcohol, physical education, and sanitation—few provided adequate discussion of contagion and vaccination. This changed during the campaign against polio, largely thanks to the efforts of the National Foundation for Infantile Paralysis, which provided materials to teachers and persuaded publishers to include information about the polio vaccine in secondary textbooks. However, once concerns about polio passed away, attention shifted away from vaccination.

In the twenty-first century, researchers have pointed out that other topics have taken priority in US schools. In 2021, the subject of immunization did not even appear in the Next Generation Science Standards, the national science teaching guidelines many states follow.[1] Nor is it clear that public health leaders understand the significant influence that schools could have in countering misinformation about vaccines. In 2015, the CDC's National Advisory Committee issued a report with recommendations on how to increase confidence in vaccines, but it never mentioned education in pre-college schools.[2] This needs to change. Given the proliferation of anti-vaccine rhetoric and misinformation in the twenty-first century, now more than ever, schools can take the lead in ensuring that students have access to valid information about vaccines. They should have the knowledge to recognize and question misinformation when they encounter it.

Why does anti-vaccination activism persist? As this book demonstrates, sincerely held beliefs and safety concerns have consistently fueled opposition to vaccination. Opposition to vaccines will always persist among those whose religion prohibits vaccination. Opposition will also persist among those who do not accept the germ theory of disease, reject the idea of contagion, or hold other sincere beliefs about health and healing that are at odds with scientific medicine. In contrast to earlier eras, in the twenty-first century, only a very small percentage of the American population opposes vaccines on the basis of sincere belief. In contrast, fear of injury from vaccines has been a long-standing factor in vaccine resistance.

Fear of vaccines has not been constant—it has waxed and waned throughout history. In the past, concerns have been triggered by rare but serious mishaps with vaccine production, such as the tainted lot of smallpox vaccine that caused a serious outbreak in North Carolina in 1821, or the tainted lots of polio vaccine that infected people with paralytic polio during the 1950s. At times, the federal government's blunders have also undermined the public's trust. For example, keeping the more convenient but also more dangerous Sabin oral polio vaccine on the market when the safer Salk vaccine was available was an unconscionable decision. When Americans learned that the Sabin vaccine itself would infect the patient with polio in one out of every three million doses, their outrage was understandable.

At various times in US history, the activists who have raised concerns about adverse effects from vaccines have provided important impetus for reforms leading to improvements in safety. But not all such concerns have been based on evidence. Warnings about vaccines based on misinformation have done great harm in undermining the public's trust in vaccines and antitoxins capable of preventing some of the most dangerous childhood diseases. In the nineteenth century, unsupported claims included statements that vaccines cause cancer and poison the blood, that good nutrition or fresh air can cure any disease, or that germ theory is completely false. In the late twentieth and early twenty-first centuries, unsupported claims have included statements that vaccines cause blood poisoning, or autism, or that following the CDC's recommended vaccine schedule will harm children.

Cases of serious injury and death from vaccination are extremely rare. Nevertheless, they do occur. Whether such cases trigger widespread fears of vaccine safety depends largely on the cause of the injury and the extent to which misinformation circulates and is believed by the public. During the Progressive Era, when a number of national anti-vaccination societies were active, safety concerns continued for decades, fueled by messaging based on unfounded claims. Many people believed them because they aligned so well with the sanitary content of the health textbooks they had encountered in school. In contrast, during the polio vaccination campaign, publicized cases of vaccine injury had far less effect on parents' willingness to vaccinate their children, not only because the CDC and local newspapers clearly explained the cause of the injuries, but also because schools provided students and parents with information about the polio vaccine, and there were few well-established anti-vaccination groups active to keep anti-vaccine messaging campaigns alive.

Misinformation damages our society. As the nineteenth-century anti-vaccination movement demonstrated, messaging based on false statements can have a very long shelf life, causing mistrust of vaccines to spread. It can linger long after it has been corrected, sometimes for decades. As one writer put it, "We're only as good as the information we get. Only as grounded, as enlightened, as capable of forming rational opinions ... and making intelligent decisions about our lives. If we're fed lies, we're lost."[3]

The long duration of misinformation is evident in the nation's court records. During the Progressive Era, parents who sued school districts over vaccination requirements often based their arguments on the propaganda of the national anti-vaccination societies: that the smallpox vaccine caused a host of other diseases, that sanitation alone would protect against smallpox, and that vaccine serum would poison the blood. When such arguments failed, plaintiffs refined their strategies to focus on constitutional arguments they thought were likely to succeed. Some argued that no state could pass a law that would impinge on the individual's right to liberty. Others argued that a child's constitutional right to education meant that no unvaccinated student could be denied admission to a public school. However, the courts commonly gave short shrift to such arguments.

In rulings dating back to 1830, state and federal judges have clarified the proper reach of the state's police power, the nature of individual liberty in a democracy, and the responsibility all people bear to protect—not only their own children—but also the entire community from disease. Compulsory vaccination laws are an infringement on personal liberty. Nevertheless, as the courts have ruled over and over again, liberty is not absolute in a democratic society. Society's interest in protecting everyone from outbreaks of contagious disease outweighs the individual's interest in exercising personal choice. We each bear responsibility not only for ourselves but also for the communities in which we live.

The courts have also made it clear that there exists no conflict between a state's compulsory education laws and its compulsory vaccination laws. A child's right to education is not an absolute right—it can be suspended if the child or the child's guardians refuse to follow school regulations, including regulations requiring vaccination. Multiple rulings have established the precept that safe schools are a precondition to education. It is well within the state's interest to require vaccination as a condition of attendance to ensure the safety of all students from contagious disease.

Despite a long history of legal support for school vaccination laws, a growing partisanship over vaccination represents a new threat to the continued immunity of children in American schools. For more than half a century after Congress passed the first federal Vaccination Assistance Act and Republican president Dwight D. Eisenhower signed it into law, politicians from both sides of the aisle generally supported school vaccination policies. However, that bipartisan collaboration began to erode in the twenty-first century. Efforts to raise vaccination rates from 2015 to 2020 took place at a time when the Internet provided easy access to a vast array of misinformation about vaccines, and during a year when presidential hopefuls courted voters by signaling their stance on a host of political topics, including the controversial issue of eliminating nonmedical exemptions.

At the start of 2020, no one knew that a COVID-19 pandemic would soon spread across the world, but in many ways the battle lines for the political conflicts to follow had already fallen into place during the previous decade. "No man ever steps in the same river twice, for it's not the same river and he's not the same man."[4] These words, spoken by the Greek philosopher Heraclitus in 544 BC, apply to human encounters with contagious disease. No society ever experiences the same epidemic twice. Neither the epidemic nor the society is ever the same the second time around. Each epidemic differs, because viruses and bacteria evolve—different strains emerge, some milder and others more virulent. With each epidemic, the geographic spread of infection varies as well. In a first outbreak, the disease may spread through schools, infecting children and young families, whereas a second outbreak may skip over those who have natural immunity from the previous infection and spread in new areas, affecting different demographic groups.

The society itself changes with each epidemic. A mild outbreak may lead people to believe the disease is nothing to worry about and to neglect vaccination the next time an outbreak appears. On the other hand, a severe epidemic with a high fatality rate may convince those who had previously resisted vaccines to seek immunization. A society's experience with public health mandates can also influence people's attitudes and behavior in future epidemics. As occurred during the smallpox era, and more recently during the COVID-19 pandemic, quarantine mandates that shutter businesses, throw people out of work, and lead to economic losses can trigger widespread opposition to public health policies, including those involving school vaccination.

The COVID-19 pandemic led to the most protracted imposition of public health mandates in US history. These included prolonged mandates to close businesses and schools, rules requiring people to wear masks in crowded areas, and orders requiring federal employees and hospital staff to be vaccinated. These regulations came at a time when American society already was experiencing a partisan divide over vaccination, a division that had been deepened by state legislative efforts during the previous five years to strengthen vaccination requirements in K–12 schools.

It is not possible to draw a direct line from the anti-vaccinationists of the nineteenth century to the vaccine opponents of 2021. There are similarities, but there are also important differences.

Continuities between then and now fall into four areas: safety fears, beliefs, personal freedom claims, and misinformation. In both eras, those opposed to vaccines have raised concerns about vaccine safety. During the campaign against polio, deaths caused by tainted lots of vaccine led many parents to refuse vaccination for their children. Similarly, during the coronavirus pandemic, reports that some COVID-19 vaccines could cause inflammation of the heart or other side effects in rare cases led to fear of immunization.[5]

Throughout US history, some people have opposed vaccines because they subscribe to religious or philosophical beliefs at odds with the theories and practices of scientific medicine. Surveys conducted in 2021 revealed that one in ten Americans stated that

COVID-19 vaccinations conflicted with their religious beliefs, and some studies have indicated that a lack of support for vaccination persists among some alternative health practitioners, including chiropractors.[6] From the Progressive Era up to the lawsuits over California's 2015 legislation removing nonmedical exemptions, vaccine opponents also have advanced constitutional arguments about their personal right to liberty and freedom in efforts to prevail in the courts.

Finally, in all eras, vaccine opponents have spread misinformation in efforts to win the hearts and minds of followers to their cause. During the smallpox era, false claims included statements that vaccines would poison the blood or that exposure to sunlight or hydrotherapy could cure smallpox. Misinformation about COVID-19 vaccines has included claims that vaccines will transmit the disease or change a person's DNA, or that the US government is tracking people's movements with microchips placed in COVID-19 vaccines.[7]

Despite the similarities, there are important differences between earlier eras and the twenty-first century. These fall into three categories: education, risk, and partisan politics. Despite the marginal place of health education in many of the nation's public schools, improved information in school textbooks and public health education programs has given many Americans a better understanding of the germ theory of disease and the way high vaccination rates can provide protection for the entire community. This understanding is reflected in the nation's 2020 school vaccination rates, which were high enough to maintain herd immunity.

A second difference relates to the concepts of risk. Unlike earlier anti-vaccination activists, few twenty-first-century vaccine opponents advocate abolishing vaccination altogether. Now, many vaccine opponents base their objections on the ethics of risk, arguing that parents should be able to refuse consent for some or all vaccines based on their beliefs about the risk of rare adverse side effects.

Finally, one of the greatest differences between earlier and later eras is the emergence of partisan politics in debates over vaccination. Among the religious conservatives who have found a home in the Republican Party, some members of the anti-abortion movement oppose vaccines that have been developed with the use of fetal cell lines. And in some quarters, vaccine resistance has become a populist movement—out of all demographic groups, resistance to vaccination is now highest among evangelicals and Christian nationalists, despite attempts by Christian leaders to persuade their followers to accept COVID-19 vaccines.[8]

The danger of political polarization over vaccines is great. Researchers estimate that between 1994 and 2013, vaccines prevented over 300 million cases of illness and more than seven hundred thousand deaths among children in the United States.[9] Nevertheless, if views about vaccines were to become as partisan as views about climate change, fewer families might decide to immunize their children, and common childhood diseases could reemerge. As happened in previous eras, school vaccination laws could also be overturned. Today's laws will remain in place only as long as Americans judge them valuable in protecting their children and communities from contagious disease. In our democratic society, education and political candor free from partisanship will be crucial in ensuring that everyone has valid information on which to base such a judgment.

Every child should be safe from contagious disease in school. Unfortunately, that safety is threatened when a growing number of others remain unvaccinated. The decision to vaccinate is often portrayed as an individual, personal decision, but it is not. In 2015, seven-year-old Rhett Krawitt, unable to receive vaccines because of a long battle with cancer, stood on a footstool to address his local school board about the importance of school vaccination laws. Six years later, a journalist interviewed him about the vaccination campaign against COVID-19. Now healthy and vaccinated, Krawitt explained it simply. "People don't understand that it is not just their personal choice for them," he said. "It's that their personal choice has an impact on the lives of others."[10]

Appendix

Selected Court Cases and Rulings Cited in the Text, 1830–2021

Year	Case	Ruling
1830	*Hazen v. Strong*, 2 Vt. 427 [1830]	The selectmen of any town may prevent the spread of smallpox by providing inoculation among those exposed, and the town's citizens may vote for a tax to defray the expense.
1879	*Reynolds v. United States*, 98 U.S. 145	Federal law prohibiting polygamy does not violate the free exercise clause of the First Amendment, because Congress has the authority to regulate actions that subvert the common good. [Cited in subsequent vaccination cases.]
1890	*Abeel v. Clark*, 84 Cal. 226	The school board has the authority to prohibit unvaccinated children from attending school, because California's school vaccination law is a constitutional exercise of the police power of the legislature.
1894	*Bissell v. Davidson*, 65 Conn. 183	Under state law, the school board has the authority to prohibit children unvaccinated against smallpox from attending school during an outbreak of smallpox.
1894	*Duffield v. School Dist. of Williamsport*, 29 A. 742, Pa.	Under state law, the school board has the authority to prohibit children unvaccinated against smallpox from attending school during an outbreak of smallpox.
1895	*Re Rebenack*, 62 Mo. App. 8	The municipal charter of St. Louis gives the city school board the authority to require children be vaccinated as a condition of school attendance.

(continued)

Year	Case	Ruling
1897	*State ex rel. Adams v. Burdge*, 95 Wis. 390	In the absence of any law making vaccination a condition of admission to the public schools, the state board of health has no valid authority to exclude unvaccinated students from the schools.
1897	*Potts v. Breen*, 167 Ill. 67	Without specific authority from the state legislature, it is unreasonable for a state board of health to require vaccination for admission to school when smallpox poses no danger to the community.
1900	*Blue v. Beach*, 155 Ind. 121	The school board has the authority to prohibit children unvaccinated against smallpox from attending school during an outbreak of smallpox.
1904	*Viemeister v. White*, 84 N.Y.S. 712, aff'd, 72 N.E. 97	The New York State Legislature has the authority to impose any type of reasonable regulation, including vaccination requirements, on public education.
1905	*Jacobson v. Massachusetts*, 197 U.S. 11	It is within a state's power to enact a compulsory vaccination law. Individual liberty is not absolute, being subject to the police power of the state to act for the common good.
1906	*Stull v. Reber*, 64 A. 419 Pa.	The state's school vaccination law is a valid use of the state's police power, and the state's interest in preserving public health outweighs the privilege of students to attend school.
1916	*Commonwealth v. Aiken*, 64 Pa. Super. 96	Parents who withhold children from school to avoid vaccinating them may be convicted of violating the compulsory attendance law.
1918	*City of New Braunfels v. Waldschmidt*, 109 Tex. 302	The personal liberty guaranteed by the federal and state constitutions is not invaded by public regulations in the interest of health. Admission to public schools is a privilege rather than a strict right, and requiring children be vaccinated as a condition of admission is constitutional.
1919	*Rhea ex rel. Rhea v. Board of Education*, 41 N.D., 171 N.W. 103	In the absence of any law making vaccination a condition of admission to the public schools, neither a board of health nor a school board has authority to exclude unvaccinated children from the schools where smallpox is absent or non-threatening.
1922	*Zucht v. King*, 260 U.S. 174	States can delegate to municipal governments and local health and school boards "broad discretion required for the protection of health," including the discretion to require vaccination as a condition of school attendance.
1927	*Cram v. School Bd. of Manchester*, 136 A. 263, N.H.	A father's claim that his daughter should not be vaccinated because the vaccination involves injecting a poison into the blood and would endanger her health is rejected based on *Jacobson*.

Year	Case	Ruling
1944	*Prince v. Massachusetts*, 321 U.S. 158	The rights of religion and parenthood are not beyond limitation. The state may restrict the parent's control by requiring school attendance and compulsory vaccination. The right to practice religion freely does not include the liberty to expose the community or child to communicable disease.
1951	*Seubold v. Fort Smith Special Sch. Dist.*, 237 S.W. 2d 884, Ark.	School vaccination requirements do not deprive individuals of liberty and property interests without due process.
1964	*Cude v. State*, 377 S.W. 2d 816, Ark.	Parents do not have the right to violate the compulsory school law by keeping their children out of school to avoid vaccination, even if their objections are based on sincere religious belief.
1965	*Wright v. DeWitt Sch. Dist.*, 385 S.W. 2d 644, Ark.	A compulsory vaccination law with no religious exemption is constitutional, because the right to free exercise of religion is subject to reasonable regulation for the common good.
1971	*Dalli v. Board of Education et al.*, 358 Mass. 753	Massachusetts law allowing the exemption from vaccination on religious grounds cannot apply only to those who are members of recognized churches or denominations.
1979	*Brown v. Stone*, 378 So. 2d 218 Miss.	One person's beliefs cannot be elevated above the public welfare. Mississippi law allowing nonmedical exemptions is unconstitutional, because it violates Fourteenth Amendment rights to equal protection under the law.
1985	*Hanzel v. Arter*, 625 F. Supp. 1259, S.D. Ohio	The children of parents who object to vaccination based on "chiropractic ethics" are not exempt from school vaccination laws, because Ohio does not allow exemption for philosophical beliefs.
1987	*Sherr v. Northport-East Northport Union Free Sch. Dist.*, 672 F Supp. 81, E.D.N.Y. 1987	New York's school vaccination law requiring that an individual belong to a bona fide religious organization to be exempt, violates the Establishment Clause of the Constitution.
1988	*Mason v. General Brown Cent. Sch. Dist.*, 851 F.2d 47, 2d Cir.	The parents' belief that immunization is contrary to the human "genetic blueprint" is not a religious belief, and so the school requirement that their children be vaccinated does not violate the Establishment Clause.
2001	*Bowden v. Iona Grammar School*, 726 N.Y. S2d 685, App. Div.	Parents who are members of the Temple of the Healing Spirit are entitled to a religious exemption from New York's vaccination requirements, because state law does not qualify which religions are eligible.
2002	*Boone v. Boozman*, 217 F. Supp. 2d 938, E.D. Ark.	Arkansas's law allowing religious exemption from vaccination requirements is unconstitutional because it benefits only those belonging to religious groups recognized by the state.

(continued)

Selected Court Cases and Rulings Cited in the Text, 1830–2021

Year	Case	Ruling
2018	*Brown v. Smith*, Cal. Ct. App. B279936	California's law eliminating personal belief exemptions is constitutional.
2021	*F.F. v. State of New York*, 194 A.D.3d 80	Upholds earlier supreme court ruling, finding New York's law eliminating religious exemptions from vaccination is constitutional and does not violate plaintiff's rights to freedom of religion, freedom of speech, or equal protection.
2021	*John Does 1–3 et al. v. Janet T. Mills, Governor of Maine, et al.*, 595 U.S. 21A90	Upholds Maine's law eliminating religious and philosophical exemptions from vaccination.

Notes

Abbreviations

AMA	American Medical Association
APHA	American Public Health Association
ASBJ	*American School Board Journal*
AVLA	Anti-Vaccination League of America, 1879–85
AVLA2	Anti-Vaccination League of America, 1908–ca. 1929
AVSA	Anti-Vaccination Society of America, 1885–1906
BMSJ	*Boston Medical and Surgical Journal*
CDC	Centers for Disease Control and Prevention
CDPH	California Department of Public Health
CSA	California State Archives
CSBPH	California State Board of Public Health
FDA	US Food and Drug Administration
GPO	US Government Printing Office
HEW	US Department of Health, Education, and Welfare
HHS	US Department of Health and Human Services
HMLCPP	Historical Medical Library of the College of Physicians of Philadelphia
JAMA	*Journal of the American Medical Association*
JPHP	*Journal of Public Health Policy*
KHS	Kansas Historical Society, Topeka, KS
LOC	Library of Congress, Washington, DC
MMWR	*Morbidity and Mortality Weekly Reports*
NARA	National Archives and Records Administration, College Park, MD

NEA	National Education Association
NEJM	*New England Journal of Medicine*
NIH	National Institutes of Health, Bethesda, MD
NLM	National Library of Medicine, NIH
PHR	*Public Health Reports*
RBCWL	Rare Books Carolina Collection, Wilson Library, University of North Carolina, Chapel Hill
RHCOHP	Rural Health Care Oral History Project, Kentucky Historical Society
SDHC	San Diego History Center
SHC	Southern Historical Collection, Wilson Library, University of North Carolina, Chapel Hill
SL	*School Life: Official Organ of the United States Bureau of Education*
VSUS	*National Vital Statistics Reports*
WHO	World Health Organization

Introduction

1. World Health Organization, "WHO Director-General's Opening Remarks at the Media Briefing on COVID-19—11 March 2020," https://www.who.int /director-general/speeches/detail/who-director-general-s-opening-remarks -at-the-media-briefing-on-covid-19---11-march-2020.

2. Erika Edwards, "5-Year-Old Is First Child Death from COVID-19-Related Inflammatory Syndrome Reported in U.S.," NBC News, May 8, 2020, https://www.nbcnews.com/health/kids-health/boy-5-dies-covid-19-linked -inflammatory-syndrome-n1203076.

3. Office of Governor Gavin Newsom, "California Becomes First State in Nation to Announce COVID-19 Vaccine Requirements for Schools," Oct. 1, 2021, https://www.gov.ca.gov/2021/10/01/california-becomes-first-state-in-nation -to-announce-covid-19-vaccine-requirements-for-schools. Melissa Gomez and Howard Blume, "Parents in California Protest Student COVID-19 Vaccine Mandate, Keep Kids Home," *Los Angeles Times*, Oct. 18, 2021, https://www .latimes.com/california/story/2021-10-18/california-protests-student -vaccination-mandate.

4. CBS News, "Hundreds Protest COVID Vaccine Mandates outside New York City Hall," CBS News New York, Aug. 25, 2001, https://www.cbsnews.com /newyork/news/nyc-covid-vaccine-mandate-protest. Madeline Will, "Some Teachers Won't Get Vaccinated, Even with a Mandate: What Should Schools Do about It?," *Education Week*, Sept. 27, 2021, https://www.edweek.org /leadership/some-teachers-wont-get-vaccinated-even-with-a-mandate-what -should-schools-do-about-it/2021/09.

5. The quote is from a video posted to Twitter by freelance journalist Oliya Scootercaster, in Thomas Kika, "Anti-Vax Rally Speaker Warns Schools Will

'Burn to the Ground' if Mandates Persists [*sic*]," Newsweek.com, Oct. 31, 2021, https://www.newsweek.com/anti-vax-rally-speaker-warns-schools-will-burn -ground-if-mandates-persists-1644340.

6. Martin Kaufman, "The American Anti-Vaccinationists and Their Arguments," *Bulletin of the History of Medicine* 41, no. 5 (Sept.–Oct. 1967): 463–78; John Duffy, *A History of Public Health in New York City, 1866–1966* (New York: Russell Sage Foundation, 1974), 152.

7. Michael Willrich, *Pox: An American History* (New York: Penguin Books, 2011); James Colgrove, *State of Immunity: The Politics of Vaccination in Twentieth-Century America* (Berkeley: University of California Press, 2006); Robert D. Johnston, *The Radical Middle Class: Populist Democracy and the Question of Capitalism in Progressive Era Portland, Oregon* (Princeton, NJ: Princeton University Press, 2003); Elena Conis, *Vaccine Nation: America's Changing Relationship with Immunization* (Chicago: University of Chicago Press, 2015).

8. Exceptions include William J. Reese, who emphasizes class conflict in the confrontations between anti-vaccinationist immigrant parents and the health inspectors who sought to vaccinate their children. See Reese, *Power and Promise of School Reform: Grassroots Movements during the Progressive Era* (New York: Teachers College Press, 2002), 186–213; and Colgrove, who provides a variety of anecdotes describing school officials' responses to vaccination mandates in *State of Immunity*, 24–25, 78–79, 200–208, 239.

9. In 1900, a survey conducted by the US Census found that contagious diseases played a large role in childhood mortality, accounting for nearly half of the deaths among children from birth to age fourteen. See "Table 1.1: Leading Causes of Death among Infants and Children: U.S. Death Registration Area, 1899–1900," pp. 3–4 in Samuel H. Preston and Michael R. Haines, "The Social and Medical Context of Child Mortality in the Late Nineteenth Century," in *Fatal Years: Child Mortality in Late Nineteenth-Century America*, ed. Samuel H. Preston and Michael R. Haines (Princeton, NJ: Princeton University Press, 1991), 3–48.

10. David H. Dejong, " 'Unless They Are Kept Alive': Federal Indian Schools and Student Health, 1878–1918," *American Indian Quarterly* 31, no. 2 (Spring 2007): 256–82; Heard Museum, Phoenix, AZ, "Away from Home: American Indian Boarding School Stories," https://heard.org/boardingschool/health, accessed Feb. 3, 2022.

11. Anti-vaccination authors have commonly portrayed legislation this way, as discussed in chapters 2 and 8. So too have some historians, who describe the conflict between those who support and those who oppose vaccination as a conflict with state and public health bureaucrats on the one side, and citizen groups opposed to vaccines on the other, e.g., Johnston, *The Radical Middle Class*, 177–220; Conis, *Vaccine Nation*.

12. Johnston makes this argument in *The Radical Middle Class*, xii; 220. See also Nadja Durbach, *Bodily Matters: The Anti-Vaccination Movement in England, 1853–1907*; Elena Conis, "Vaccination Resistance in Historical Perspective," *American Historian* (2015): https://www.oah.org/tah/issues/2015/august/vaccination-resistance.

13. See Thomas F. Gieryn, "Boundary Work and the Demarcation of Science from Non-science: Strains and Interests in Professional Ideologies of Scientists," *American Sociological Review* 48, no. 6 (Dec. 1983): 781–95; Aaron Panofsky, *Misbehaving Science: Controversy and the Development of Behavior Genetics* (Chicago: University of Chicago Press, 2014), 7–9.

14. August W. Steinhilber and Carl J. Sokolowski, *State Law on Compulsory Attendance* (Washington, DC: GPO, 1966), 3. As of 2014, twenty-two states recognized education as a fundamental right. See Trish Brennan-Gac, "Educational Rights in the States," American Bar Association, April 1, 2014, https://www.americanbar.org/groups/crsj/publications/human_rights_magazine_home/2014_vol_40/vol_40_no_2_civil_rights/educational_rights_states.

15. David Jones and Stefan Helmreich, "A History of Herd Immunity," *Lancet* 396, no. 10254 (Sept. 19, 2020): 810–11.

16. Andrew Kwong and Emily M. Ambizas, "Measles and the MMR Vaccine," *US Pharmacist* 44, no. 7 (July 2019): 8–13; Tom Kovitwanichkanont, "Public Health Measures for Pertussis Prevention and Control," *Australian and New Zealand Journal of Public Health* 41, no. 6 (2017): 558.

17. Robert N. Proctor coined the term *agnotology* to denote the study of ignorance-making. See Proctor, *Agnotology: The Making and Unmaking of Ignorance* (Stanford, CA: Stanford University Press, 2008). For applications in education, see A. J. Angulo, ed., *Miseducation: A History of Ignorance-Making in America and Abroad* (Baltimore, MD: Johns Hopkins University Press, 2016).

Chapter 1. The Rise of School Vaccination Laws

1. CSBPH, "Smallpox." *Tenth Biennial Report of the State Board of Health* (Sacramento: J. D. Young, 1888), 45, 121; "Health of the State: Record of Deaths during January—Recommendations, Etc.," *Press Democrat* (Santa Rosa, CA), Feb. 14, 1888, 3; "Prevailing Ills: Abstract of the Monthly Report of the State Board of Health," *San Jose Mercury News*, Nov. 14, 1887, 1.

2. "The Yellow Flag," *Los Angeles Herald*, Dec. 30, 1887, 1.

3. "Smallpox at San Francisco," *Los Angeles Herald*, Jan. 1888, 2; "Health of the State," 3.

4. A house of pestilence, or "pest house" was a shelter to quarantine the ill during an epidemic. "Prevailing Ills"; "The Yellow Flag," 1.

5. "An Awful Story," *Santa Rosa Daily Democrat*, March 25, 1888, 2.

6. "Health of the State," 3.

7. William Squire, "Periods of Infection in Epidemic Diseases," *Half-Yearly Abstract of the Medical Sciences: Being a Digest of British and Continental Medicine* 57 (Jan.–June 1873): 32–35; William Squire, "On the Preventive Influence of Our Increased Means of Isolation in Infective Fever," *Collected Essays in Preventive Medicine* (London: J. & A. Churchill, 1887). In the United States, Squire's research was reported in Arthur H. Nichols, "School-Children and Communicable Diseases," *BMSJ* 94, no. 12 (March 23, 1876): 319–23.

8. "Health of the State," 3.

9. CSBPH, "Smallpox," 121–26.

10. California Legislature, *Appendix to the Journals of the Senate and Assembly of the Twenty-Eighth Session* (Sacramento CA: J. D. Young, 1889), 40.

11. William Fowler, *Smallpox Vaccination Laws, Regulations, and Court Decisions* (Washington DC: GPO [US Public Health Service], 1927), 3–5.

12. Samuel Bayard Woodward, "The Story of Smallpox in Massachusetts," *New England Journal of Medicine* 206, no. 23 (1932): 1181–91.

13. Michael A. Willrich, *Pox: An American History* (New York: Penguin, 2011), 21–26; CDC, "Smallpox: Transmission," https://www.cdc.gov/smallpox/transmission/index.html.

14. Willrich, *Pox*, 21–26.

15. Kristine B. Patterson and Thomas Runge, "Smallpox and the Native American," *American Journal of the Medical Sciences* 323, no. 4 (April 2002): 216–22.

16. William R. Swagerty, "Introduction" to Francis A. Chardon, *Chardon's Journal at Fort Clark, 1834–1839*, ed. Annie Helouise Abel (Lincoln: University of Nebraska Press, 1997), ix–x. Based on tragic accounts such as this, some speculated that whites deliberately spread smallpox among the tribes, but according to Clyde D. Dollar, documentary evidence suggests this was not the case at Fort Clark, where the disease appears to have been introduced by an infected deckhand on an incoming steamboat. See Dollar, "The High Plains Smallpox Epidemic of 1837–38," *Western Historical Quarterly* 8, no. 1 (Jan. 1977): 15–38.

17. Julia Louisa Lovejoy to the *Democrat*, April 29, 1857. Letters of Julia Louisa Lovejoy, KHS.

18. Journal of John Hawkins Clark, May 10, 1852, KHS.

19. Willrich, *Pox*, 24, 30–32.

20. Colin McEvedy, "The Bubonic Plague," *Scientific American* 258, no. 2 (1988): 118–23; Nicola Twilley, Geoff Manaugh, *Until Proven Safe: The History and Future of Quarantine* (New York: Farrar, Straus and Giroux, 2021).

21. "An Act to Prevent the Spreading of Any Contagious or Infectious Sickness in This State," in *The Public Laws of the State of Rhode Island* (Providence, RI: Miller and Hutchens, 1822), 265. For Progressive Era arguments against quarantine, see Willrich, *Pox*, 246–84.

22. Lawrence O. Gostin, *Public Health Law: Power, Duty, Restraint* (Berkeley: University of California Press, 2008), 423–24; Stephen K. Williams, "Gibbons v. Ogden," *Cases Argued and Decided in the Supreme Court of the United States* (New York: Lawyers Cooperative Publishing Co., 1882), 72.

23. "Smallpox in San Juan," *Santa Cruz Weekly Sentinel*, Nov. 14, 1868, 2.

24. "Small-Pox in Santa Cruz," *Daily Alta California* (San Francisco), Nov. 25, 1868, 1; John Hibble, "Aptos Bridges," Aptos History Museum, https://aptoshistory.org.

25. "Letter from St. Louis," *Sacramento Daily Union*, June 8, 1859, 4.

26. "Smallpox in San Juan."

27. See Samuel Bayard Woodward, "The Story of Smallpox in Massachusetts," *NEJM* 206, no. 23 (1932): 1181–91; D. Hopkins, *Princes and Peasants: Smallpox in History* (Chicago: University of Chicago Press, 1983); O. Winslow, *A Destroying Angel: The Conquest of Smallpox in Colonial Boston* (Boston: Houghton Mifflin, 1974); J. B. Blake, *Public Health in the Town of Boston, 1630–1822* (Cambridge, MA: Harvard University Press, 1959).

28. Elizabeth A. Fenn, *Pox Americana: The Great Smallpox Epidemic of 1775–82* (New York: Hill and Wang, 2001); Frank Fenner et al., *Smallpox and Its Eradication* (Geneva, Switzerland: World Health Organization, 1988), 217, 245–58.

29. Abijah Perkins Marvin, *The Life and Times of Cotton Mather, D. D., F. R. S.* (Boston: Congregational Sunday-School and Publishing Society, 1892), 480.

30. Edward Jenner, *An Inquiry into the Causes and Effects of the Variolae Vaccinae: A Disease Discovered in Some of the Western Counties of England, Particularly Gloucestershire, and Known by the Name of the Cow Pox* (London: Sampson Low, 1798); Edward Jenner, *On the Origin of the Vaccine Inoculation* (London: G. Elsick, 1863). Also see Fenner et al, *Smallpox and Its Eradication*, 258–73.

31. Benjamin Waterhouse, *A Prospect of Exterminating the Small-Pox; Being the History of the Variolae Vaccina, or Kine-pox, Commonly Called the Cow-Pox, as It Has Appeared in England; With the Account of a Series of Inoculations Performed for the Kine-Pox, in Massachusetts* (Cambridge, MA: William Hilliard, 1800); Blake, *Public Health in the Town of Boston*, 178–83.

32. Thomas Jefferson to John Vaughan, Nov. 5, 1801, in "History of the Introduction of Vaccination in the State of Maryland," in *The Vaccine Inquirer; or, Miscellaneous Collections Relative to Vaccination by a Society of Physicians* (Baltimore, MD: n.p., 1822–24), 17–19, RBCWL.

33. Waterhouse, *A Prospect of Exterminating the Small-Pox*; Blake, *Public Health in the Town of Boston*, 178–83. The report of Boston's board of health is reproduced in *Massachusetts Association of Boards of Health* 4 (April 1894): 3–5, National Institutes of Health—Library of Medicine Archives. The quote is on p. 5.

34. A survey of US newspapers in Chronicling America and Newspapers.com reveals no organized protests over the smallpox vaccine until the second half of the nineteenth century.

35. Alan D. Watson, "Combating Contagion: Smallpox and the Protection of Public Health in North Carolina, 1750 to 1825," *North Carolina Historical Review* 90, no. 1 (Jan. 2013): 26–48.

36. "Smallpox at Salem School in 1812," in Charles Lee Coon, *North Carolina Schools and Academies, 1790–1840: A Documentary History* (Raleigh, NC: Edwards & Broughton, 1915), 80.

37. James Smith, "Observations on Cowpox," in *The Vaccine Inquirer*, 56, RBCWL.

38. Tess Lanzarotte and Marco A. Ramos, "Mistrust in Medicine: The Rise and Fall of America's First Vaccine Institute," *American Journal of Public Health History* 108, no. 6 (June 2018): 741–47.

39. "To James Madison from James Smith, 18 June 1809," NARA, https://founders .archives.gov/documents/Madison/03-01-02-0281.

40. US Congress, "An Act to Encourage Vaccination," Feb. 27, 1813, statute II, LOC, https://www.loc.gov/law/help/statutes-at-large/12th-congress/session-2 /c12s2ch37.pdf; Watson, "Combating Contagion."

41. Watson, "Combating Contagion."

42. John F. Ward to James Smith, Dec. 29, 1821, in "The North Carolina Accident," in *The Vaccine Inquirer, or, Miscellaneous Collections*, 109, RBCWL.

43. Ward to Smith, "The North Carolina Accident."

44. Benjamin B. Hunter to John Smith, Jan. 16, 1822, in "The North Carolina Accident," 119–20.

45. Watson, "Combating Contagion"; *The Debates and Proceedings in the Congress of the United States: Seventeenth Congress—First Session, December 3, 1821 to March 8, 1822* (Washington DC: Gales and Seaton, 1855).

46. "Dan Hazen vs. David Strong," in Vermont Supreme Court, *Reports of Cases Argued and Determined in the Supreme Court of the State of Vermont*, vol. 2 (St. Albans, VT: J. Spooner, 1830), 427–34. The quotes are on pp. 428 and 429, respectively; italics are in the original.

47. Lanzarotte and Ramos, "Mistrust in Medicine"; José Esparza et al., "Early Smallpox Vaccine Manufacturing in the United States: Introduction of the 'Animal Vaccine' in 1870, Establishment of 'Vaccine Farms,' and the Beginnings of the Vaccine Industry," *Vaccine* 38 (May 2020): 4773–79.

48. Esparza et al., "Early Smallpox Vaccine Manufacturing in the United States."

49. Sharon E. Frey et al., "Clinical Responses to Undiluted and Diluted Smallpox Vaccine," *NEJM* 17 (April 25, 2002): 1265–74; CDC, "Side Effects of Smallpox Vaccination," https://www.cdc.gov/smallpox/vaccine-basics/vaccination-effects .html, accessed Oct. 4, 2022.

50. Jonathan E. Henry, "Experience in Massachusetts and a Few Other Places with Smallpox and Vaccination," *BMSJ* 185, no. 81 (Aug. 25, 1921): 221–28.

51. "Miscellaneous," *Niles' Weekly Register* (Baltimore, MD) 28, no. 712 (May 7, 1825): 149; "Chronicle," *Niles' Weekly Register* 28, no. 668 (May 29, 1826). The

quote is from p. 216. Donald R. Hopkins, *The Greatest Killer: Smallpox in History* (Chicago: University of Chicago Press, 2002), 85–90.

52. *Polynesian* (Hawaii), May 10, 1862, 2. For the rise of complacency, see John Duffy, "School Vaccination: The Precursor to School Medical Inspection," *Journal of the History of Medicine and Allied Sciences* 33, no. 3 (July 1978): 344–45.

53. Henry, "Experience in Massachusetts and a Few Other Places with Smallpox and Vaccination."

54. *First Annual Report of the State Board of Health, State of Kansas, from Its Organization April 10, 1885 and Ending December 31, 1885* (Topeka, KS: T. D. Thacher, State Printer, 1885), 62–63.

55. "Medical Police: Vaccination of the Poor," *Medical Intelligencer* 4, no. 48 (April 17, 1827): 577–80. Also see Edward Hartwell Savage, *A Chronological History of the Boston Watch and Police: From 1631 to 1865* (Boston: E. H. Savage, 1865), 67; Duffy, "School Vaccination."

56. Article 4, in *Constitution of the Infant School Society of the City of Philadelphia* (Philadelphia Infant School Society, 1827), Library Company of Philadelphia. Lowell, MA, passed a school vaccination law in 1840. See "School Regulations," *Common School Journal* 2, no. 16 (August 15, 1840): 260. The town of Lynn, MA, followed in 1850. See Lynn City Council, *The Municipal Register, Containing the City Charter, with Rules and Orders of the City Council [...] of the City of Lynn for 1850–51* (Lynn, MA: H. J. Butterfield, 1850), 76.

57. For school attendance laws, see Oriana Bandiera, Myra Mohnen, Imran Rasul, and Martina Viarengo, "Nation-Building through Compulsory Schooling during the Age of Mass Migration," *Economic Journal* 129, no. 617 (Jan. 2019): 62–109.

58. August W. Steinhilber and Carl J. Sokolowski, *State Law on Compulsory Attendance* (Washington DC: GPO, 1966), 3.

59. See Duffy, "School Vaccination"; James G. Hodge and Lawrence O. Gostin, "School Vaccination Requirements: Historical, Social, and Legal Perspectives," *Kentucky Law Journal* 90, no. 4 (Dec. 2000): 850; Gostin, *Public Health Law*, 379.

60. William Squire, "On the Preventive Influence of Our Increased Means of Isolation in Infective Fever," 18.

61. See Hodge and Gostin, "School Vaccination Requirements," 851.

62. Duffy, *The Sanitarians: A History of American Public Health* (Urbana: University of Illinois Press, 1992).

63. William Fowler, "Principal Provisions of Smallpox Vaccination Laws and Regulations in the United States," *PHR* 56, no. 5 (Jan. 31, 1941): 169. Alaska, the District of Columbia, and Puerto Rico also had such laws. "Compulsory Attendance vs. Vaccination," *Pennsylvania School Journal* 45, no. 9 (March 1897): 423–26. For the passage of the school vaccination law in Massachusetts, see Francis Dewitt, *Fourteenth Report to the Legislature of Massachusetts, Relating to the Registry and Returns of Births, Marriages, and Deaths in the Commonwealth for*

the Year Ending December 31, 1855 (Boston: William White, Printer to the State, 1857), 193. For the 1860 school vaccination law in New York, see "Report of Committee on Vaccination," *Transactions of the Medical Society of the State of New York for the Year 1859* (Albany, NY: Charles Van Benthuysen, 1859), 252–53; New York [State], "An Act to Encourage and Provide for a General Vaccination in this State," *Journal of the Senate of the State of New York, at Their Eighty-Third Session* (Albany, NY: Charles Van Benthuysen, 1860), 219, 973.

64. This petition failed. See *Journal of the Senate of the Nineteenth General Assembly of the State of Iowa, January 9, 1882* (Des Moines, IA: F. M. Mills, State Printer), 33.

65. See chapter 2 in this volume.

66. Hodge and Gostin also make this point in "School Vaccination Requirements," 850–51.

67. Dewitt, *Fourteenth Report to the Legislature of Massachusetts*, 193.

68. Commonwealth of Massachusetts, "Vaccination," *Report of the Commissioners on the Revision of the Statutes, Vol. 2. Chapters 26–68* (Boston: W. White, Printer to the State, 1858), 9.

69. *Fifth Annual Report of the State Board of Health of Illinois* (Springfield, IL: H. W. Rokker, State Printer, 1883), 485; Illinois Department of Public Health, "121 Years Ago in Public Health," http://www.idph.state.il.us/webhistory2.htm.

70. Philip L. Frana, "Battling Smallpox: State and Local Boards of Health," *Iowa Heritage Illustrated* 86 (Summer 2005): 61–66.

71. *Journal of the Senate of the Nineteenth General Assembly of the State of Iowa, January 9, 1882*, 33; "Decisions of the Attorney General," *Legislative Documents Submitted to the Twenty-Third General Assembly of the State of Iowa, January 13, 1890, Vol. 4* (Des Moines, IA: G. H. Ragsdale, State Printer, 1890), 149–51.

72. "Precautions to Use against Small-Pox," *Daily Evening Bulletin* (Marysville, KY), Dec. 1, 1883, 2. J. W. Kerr, *Vaccination: An Analysis of the Laws and Regulations Relating Thereto in Force in the United States*, Public Health Bulletin No. 52 (Washington DC: GPO, 1912), 6.

73. H. S. Orme, "Smallpox in Los Angeles in 1887," *Tenth Biennial Report of the State Board of Health of California*, 126.

74. Orme, "Smallpox in Los Angeles in 1887." The quotes are on pp. 124 and 121, respectively.

75. California Legislature, *Appendix to the Journals of the Senate and Assembly of the Twenty-Eighth Session of the Legislature of the State of California, Volume 6* (Sacramento CA: J. D. Young, 1889), 47.

76. California Legislature, *Appendix to the Journals* [...] *Volume 6*, 40.

77. Fowler, *Smallpox Vaccination Laws*, 3–5. The eleven states were Arkansas, Kentucky, Maryland, Massachusetts, New Hampshire, New Mexico, New York, Pennsylvania, Rhode Island, South Carolina, and West Virginia. The District of Columbia and Puerto Rico also had such requirements.

78. Fowler, *Smallpox Vaccination Laws*, 3–5. The six states with discretionary laws in 1927 were Connecticut, Georgia, New Jersey, North Carolina, Ohio, and Oregon. With the exception of North Carolina, school authorities in these states had the power to impose the requirement.

79. Fowler, *Smallpox Vaccination Laws*, 4. The ten states were Kansas, Louisiana, Minnesota, Montana, Nebraska, New York, North Dakota, Washington, West Virginia, and Wisconsin.

80. "Report of Committee on Vaccination," 252–53; Faculty of the Law School of the University of North Carolina, "A Survey of Statutory Changes in North Carolina in 1939," *North Carolina Law Review* 17, no. 4 (1939): 361, https://scholarship.law.unc.edu/nclr/vol17/iss4/1.

Chapter 2. The National Anti-vaccination Societies and the Schools

1. Benjamin Waterhouse, *Kine Pock Inoculation: Rules to Be Attended to during the Vaccination* (Cambridge, MA, 1809), n.p., RBCWL. See José Esparza et al., "Early Smallpox Vaccine Manufacturing in the United States: Introduction of the 'Animal Vaccine' in 1870, Establishment of 'Vaccine Farms,' and the Beginnings of the Vaccine Industry," *Vaccine* 38 (May 2020): 4773–79.

2. John Bolton, *Spurious Vaccination in the Confederate Army: Read before the Richmond, Virginia, Academy of Medicine, November 15, 1866*, RBCWL; Joseph Jones, *Researches upon "Spurious Vaccination," or the Abnormal Phenomena Accompanying and Following Vaccination in the Confederate Army during the Recent American Civil War, 1861–1865* (Nashville, TN: University Medical Press, 1867), RBCWL. Also see Jeffrey S. Sartin, "Infectious Diseases during the Civil War: The Triumph of the "Third Army," *Clinical Infectious Diseases* 16, no. 4 (April 1993): 580–84.

3. Robert D. Johnston makes this argument in *The Radical Middle Class: Populist Democracy and the Question of Capitalism in Progressive Era Portland, Oregon* (Princeton, NJ: Princeton University Press, 2003), xii, 220. See also Nadja Durbach, *Bodily Matters: The Anti-vaccination Movement in England, 1853–1907* (Durham, NC: Duke University Press, 2005), 204; Elena Conis, *Vaccine Nation: America's Changing Relationship with Immunization* (Chicago: University of Chicago Press, 2015), 4; Bernice L. Hausman, *Anti-Vax: Reframing the Vaccination Controversy* (Ithaca, NY: Cornell University Press, 2019), 9.

4. Michael Stolberg, " 'You Have No Good Blood in Your Body': Oral Communication in Sixteenth-Century Physicians' Medical Practice," *Medical History* 59, no. 1 (Jan. 2015): 63–82.

5. David M. Morens, "Death of a President," *NEJM* 342 (Dec. 9, 1999): 1845–50.

6. Samuel Thomson, *New Guide to Health; or, Botanic Family Physician* (Boston: J. Howe, Printer, 1832), 145.

7. Wooster Beach, *The American Practice of Medicine* [. . .] *on Vegetable or Botanical Principles* [. . .] (New York: Kelley & La Tourrette, 1836). For eclectic medicine, see John S. Haller Jr., *Medical Protestants: The Eclectics in American Medicine, 1825–1939* (Carbondale: Southern Illinois University Press, 1994), 151. Also see Harvey Wickes Felter, "Wooster Beach," in *History of the Eclectic Medical Institute, Cincinnati, Ohio, 1845–1902* (Cincinnati, OH: Alumnal Association of the Eclectic Medical Institute, 1902), 81–83. For the history of medical schools in the United States, see William G. Rothstein, *American Medical Schools and the Practice of Medicine: A History* (New York: Oxford University Press, 1987).

8. See James C. Whorton, *Nature Cures: The History of Alternative Medicine in America* (New York: Oxford University Press, 2004), 49–76.

9. John S. Haller, *The History of American Homeopathy: From Rational Medicine to Holistic Health Care* (New Brunswick, NJ: Rutgers University Press, 2009), 17.

10. "Hahnemann's Correspondence to Dr. Schreter, in Lemberg," *British Journal of Homeopathy* 6, no. 25 (1848): 415.

11. Beach, *The American Practice of Medicine*, 466–68; the quote is on p. 466.

12. Lois N. Magner, *A History of Infectious Diseases in the Microbial World* (New York: Praeger, 2009), 19–48; Haller, *Medical Protestants*, 151.

13. Alexander Wilder, *An Address Delivered before the Eclectic Medical Society of the State of New York* [. . .] *June, 1869* (Albany, NY: Weed, Parsons and Co., 1869), 7. For the growing disputes and divisions between allopathic and alternative physicians after the Civil War, see Paul Starr, *The Social Transformation of American Medicine: The Rise of a Sovereign Profession and the Making of a Vast Industry* (New York: Basic Books, 1982), 93–106. For boundary-work in the context of disputes over scientific theories, see Thomas F. Gieryn, "Boundary Work and the Demarcation of Science from Non-science: Strains and Interests in Professional Ideologies of Scientists," *American Sociological Review* 48, no. 6 (Dec. 1983): 781–95.

14. Wilder was coeditor of the society's journal, *The Medical Eclectic*. See Howard A. Kelly and Walter L. Burrage, *American Medical Biographies* (Baltimore, MD: Norman, Remington Co., 1920), 1235. Robert A. Gunn, *Vaccination: Its Fallacies and Evils* (New York: Munroe & Metz, [1877?]), 6, NIH.

15. Michael A. Willrich, *Pox: An American History* (New York: Penguin, 2011), 182–83.

16. Haller, *Medical Protestants*.

17. William Tebb, "Anti-Vaccination in the United States and Canada: Notes of a Recent Tour," *Vaccination Inquirer and Health Review* 1, no. 2 (1879): 155.

18. "Opposed to Vaccination: Doctors Who Condemn It—An Englishman's Views on the Subject," *New York Times*, October 11, 1879, 5. Wilder was coeditor of the society's journal, *Medical Eclectic*. He also served on the board of trustees of

the New York Homeopathic Medical College. See Kelly, *A Cyclopedia of American Medical Biography* [...] *1610 to 1910*, 1235.

19. "Opposed to Vaccination." For anti-vaccination activism in England, see Durback, *Bodily Matters*; Dorothy Porter and Roy Porter, "The Politics of Prevention: Anti-vaccinationism and Public Health in Nineteenth-Century England," *Medical History* 32 (July 1988): 231–52. For anti-vaccination movements in Europe from the eighteenth to the twenty-first centuries, see Françoise Salvadori and Laurent-Henri Vignaud, *Antivax: La résistance aux vaccins du XVIIIe siècle à nos jours* (Paris: Vendémiaire, 2019).

20. "Synopsis of Meetings of First Anti-Vaccination League of America" (handwritten entry in a bound notebook of the league), Anti-Vaccination Society of America, Minutes, Correspondence, etc., 1895–1898, Historical Medical Library of the College of Physicians of Philadelphia (hereafter AVSA, HMLCPP). The two laymen on the leadership team were Secretary J. R. Nickels and William Tebb, a member of the executive committee. The five doctors were President Alexander Wilder, Treasurer M. L. Holbrook, and executive committee members J. E. Briggs, Thomas A. Granger, and Robert A. Gunn. The books of the league are lost, and only a brief synopsis of meetings remains.

21. William Tebb, "Anti-Vaccination in the United States and Canada," 154, 155.

22. "The First Anti-Vaccination League," *Gloucester County (NJ) Democrat*, Oct. 16, 1879, 4. This news item was reprinted in other newspapers. Similar reports appeared in "An Anti-Vaccination League Organized in New York: *New York Sun*, Oct. 11," *Chicago Tribune*, Oct. 14, 1879, 7; and "Vaccination: Is Vaccine Virus Poison?," *Reno (NV) Gazette-Journal*, Oct. 20, 1879, 1.

23. "Anti-vaccination," *Detroit Free Press*, Oct. 14, 1879, 4.

24. "Anti-vaccination Folly," *Brown County World* (Hiawatha, KS), Nov. 20, 1879, 1. This is a reprint of an article appearing in *Scientific American*, Nov. 15, 1879.

25. Alexander Wilder, "A Crime against Nature," *Evening Gazette* (Port Jervis, NY), Dec. 6, 1879), 1.

26. Gunn, *Vaccination*, 3.

27. Gunn, *Vaccination*, 1. Alexander Ross is quoted in *Vaccination in Canada: A Reply to Pamphlet Published by the Provincial Board of Health, Ontario* (Toronto: Anti-Vaccination League of Canada, 1907), 43–44.

28. For contemporary information about the need to revaccinate every five years, see Austin Flint, *A Treatise on the Principles and Practice of Medicine* (Philadelphia: Henry C. Lea, 1873), 971. Today the CDC states that the smallpox vaccine confers immunity for only three to five years. See "Smallpox: Vaccine Basics," https://www.cdc.gov/smallpox/vaccine-basics/index.html.

29. See Robert N. Proctor, "Agnotology: A Missing Term to Describe the Cultural Production of Ignorance (and Its Study)," in *Agnotology: The Making and Unmaking of Ignorance*, ed. Robert N. Proctor and Londa Schiebinger

(Stanford, CA: Stanford University Press, 2008), 1–36. Also see A. J. Angulo, ed., *Misinformation: A History of Ignorance-Making in America and Abroad* (Baltimore, MD: Johns Hopkins University Press, 2016), 1–12.

30. Alfred Russel Wallace, *On Miracles and Modern Science: Three Essays* (London: James Burns, 1875). Alexander Wilder cites Wallace, Herbert Spencer, and other scientists opposed to vaccination in *The Fallacy of Vaccination* (New York: Metaphysical Publishing Co., 1899). Alfred Russel Wallace, *The Wonderful Century: Its Successes and Failures* (New York: Dodd, Mead & Co., 1898), 213–316. Also see Martin Fichman and Jennifer Keelan, "Resister's Logic: The Anti-vaccination Arguments of Alfred Russel Wallace and Their Role in the Debates over Compulsory Vaccination in England, 1870–1907," *Studies in History and Philosophy of Biological and Biomedical Sciences* 38, no. 3 (Sept. 2007): 585–607.

31. See Thomas P. Weber, "Alfred Russel Wallace and the Antivaccination Movement in Victorian England," *Emerging Infectious Diseases* 16 (April 2010): 664–68. For the particulars of the Leicester Method, see Stuart M. Fraser, "Leicester and Smallpox: The Leiester Method," *Medical History* 24 (July 1980): 315–32.

32. Magner, *A History of Infectious Diseases in the Microbial World*, 19–48; Sylvia Noble Tesh, *Hidden Arguments: Political Ideology and Disease Prevention Policy* (New Brunswick, NJ: Rutgers University Press, 1988), 7–32.

33. Historians of science generally identify the period from 1890 to 1900 as the time when germ theory gained broad acceptance. See John Waller, *The Discovery of the Germ: Twenty Years That Transformed the Way We Think about Disease* (New York: Columbia University Press, 2002).

34. Alexander Wilder, "Micro-organisms in Disease: The Microbian Craze," *Metaphysical Magazine* 1, no. 6 (June 1895): 502.

35. "Opposed to Vaccination," *New York Times*, Feb. 17, 1882, 2.

36. Alexander M. Ross, ed., *The Anti-Vaccinator, and Advocate of Cleanliness* (Montreal), Oct. 1885, 1, NLM.

37. Alexander Wilder, *Vaccination: A Medical Fallacy* (n.d., 1875?), 7, NLM.

38. Wilder, "A Crime against Nature," 1.

39. James Martin Peebles, *Vaccination a Curse and a Menace to Personal Liberty: With Statistics Showing Its Dangers and Criminality* (Battle Creek, MI: Peebles Publishing Co., 1913), 221.

40. For example, see Charles Michael Higgins, *Horrors of Vaccination Exposed and Illustrated* (Brooklyn, NY: Chas. M. Higgins, 1920), 9.

41. "Editorial Notes," *Oregon Sentinel* (Jacksonville), Dec. 23, 1882, 2.

42. "Comment and Opinion," *Indianapolis Journal*, Oct. 30, 1885, 5.

43. "Anti-Vaccination League of America," *San Jose Herald*, Feb. 25, 1882, 2. For plaintiffs' use of anti-vaccination arguments in court cases reaching state supreme courts, see chapter 3.

44. The league maintained about one hundred members from 1882 to 1885. Although scholars have commonly conflated these two groups, a handwritten account indicates the AVLA and AVSA were separate organizations and states that the books of the league were lost. See "Synopsis of Meetings of First Anti-Vaccination League of America" (handwritten entry in a bound notebook of the league), Anti-Vaccination Society of America, Minutes, Correspondence, etc., 1895–1898, AVSA, HMLCPP.

45. "The Anti-Vaccination Society of America: Special Announcements," *Vaccination* 1, no. 7 (Aug.–Sept. 1898): 14; Frank D. Blue, "Editorial," *Vaccination* 2, no. 3 (April 1899): 4.

46. Montague Leverson, "To All Who Care for Human Rights," speech at the AVSA New York meeting, June 5, 1895, AVSA, HMLCPP.

47. The treasurer and four members of the Executive Committee were all doctors. "Certificate of Incorporation of the Anti-Vaccination Society of America, December 2, 1885: Incorporated in the City and County of New York," AVSA, HMLCPP.

48. A list of officers and affiliates is printed on the back of all 1895 stationary of the Anti-Vaccination Society of America. In AVSA, HMLCPP.

49. Seven of the society's nine Executive Committee members possessed medical degrees. Of the 136 vice presidents who represented affiliated societies, 9 were women, and of these, 7 possessed medical degrees, a reflection of women's slow but gradual entry into medicine. The AVSA had 149 members in 1895, according to a list of officers and affiliates printed on the back of all 1895 stationary in AVSA, HMLCPP. For women in medicine during this period, see Ruth J. Abram, ed., *Send Us a Lady Physician: Women Doctors in America, 1835–1920* (New York: W. W. Norton, 1986); Thomas Neville Bonner, *To the Ends of the Earth: Women's Search for Education in Medicine* (Cambridge, MA: Harvard University Press, 1992).

50. "The Anti-Vaccination Society of America: Officers," *Vaccination* 3, no. 12 (January 1900): front matter. Of the eight officers listed in 1900, three were doctors.

51. For advances in medicine during this period, see Peter Conrad and Joseph W. Schneider, "Professionalization, Monopoly, and the Structure of Medical Practice," in *The Sociology of Health and Illness: Critical Perspectives*, ed. Peter Conrad (New York: Worth Publishers, 2009), 194–99.

52. "Tetanus from Anti-Diphtheria Serum," *JAMA* 37, no. 19 (Nov. 9, 1901): 1255. Julie B. Millen, "Regulation of Vaccines: Strengthening the Science Base," *Journal of Public Health Policy* 25, no. 2: 173–89. Esparza et al., "Early Smallpox Vaccine Manufacturing in the United States."

53. W. H. Hanchett, "Scarlet Fever," *North American Journal of Homeopathy* 42 (Jan. 1894): 673–84. The quote is on p. 674. Robert A. Baker, *The American Medical Ethics Revolution: How the AMA's Code of Ethics Has Transformed*

Physicians' Relationships to Patients, Professionals, and Society (Baltimore, MD: Johns Hopkins University Press, 1999), 70–90. The quote is on p. 84.

54. Baker, *The American Medical Ethics Revolution*, 84; Starr, *The Social Transformation of American Medicine*, 107.

55. "Frank D. Blue Early Identified with Pennsylvania," *Daily Tribune* (Terre Haute, IN), Feb. 7, 1903, 10. Emma Elizabeth Colket married Frank D. Blue in 1885. Genealogical information is in Henry Oscar Rockefeller, ed., *The Transactions of the Rockefeller Family Association for the Five Years, 1910–1914 with Genealogy* (New York: J. J. Little & Ives Co., 1915), 267.

56. *The Journal of Hygeio-Therapy and Anti-vaccination: A Monthly; Devoted to a Correct Method of Living, and a Scientific and Successful System of Treating the Sick without the Use of Drugs* 6 (March 1892): 9. Gifford and Blue are listed as members on the back of all 1895 AVSA stationary in AVSA, HMLCPP.

57. For Blue's case, see chapter 3. For Piehn, see D. D. Palmer and B. J. Palmer, *The Science of Chiropractic: Its Principles and Adjustments* (Davenport, IA: Palmer School of Chiropractic, 1906), 377–79.

58. "Frank D. Blue," *Anzeiger des Westens* (St. Louis, MO), Nov. 11, 1896, 8.

59. "Anti-virus Cranks after Judge Andy, *Atlanta Constitution*, Dec. 28, 1897, 7.

60. The quote is from Mary Baker Eddy, "Obey the Law," *Christian Science Journal* 18 (March 1901): 724. Also see Rennie B. Schoepflin, *Christian Science on Trial: Religious Healing in America* (Baltimore, MD: Johns Hopkins University Press, 2003).

61. M. R. Leverson, "To the President and Members of the Anti-Vaccination Society of America, New York, May 18, 1897," AVSA, HMLCPP.

62. "Vaccination Must Go!," *Kneipp Water Cure Monthly* 2 (Nov. 1901): 295; M. R. Leverson to "Respected Friend," May 18, 1898, AVSA, HMLCPP. Leverson notes that Blue "is hereby appointed Secretary to the Society." The 1902 membership card is in Anti-Vaccination Scrapbook, 1882–1903, AVSA, HMLCPP.

63. Details of Blue's life are from "Frank D. Blue's Death Sudden," *Tribune* (Terre Haute, IN), May 18, 1948, 13.

64. M. R. Leverson, "To the President and Members of the Anti-Vaccination Society of America, New York, May 18, 1897"; Leverson to "Respected Friend," May 18, 1898, AVSA, HMLCPP.

65. "The Anti-Vaccination Society of America: Special Announcements," 14.

66. "To the Members of the Anti-Vaccination Society of America," *Vaccination* 2, no. 9 (Oct. 1899): 8.

67. Frank D. Blue, "Quiet Talks to the Faithful," *Vaccination* 7, no. 6 (July 1904): 69; Blue, "How to Prevent Smallpox," *Vaccination* 9, no. 12 (Jan. 1906): 88. Blue's philosophy of healing was similar to that of other nineteenth-century naturopaths. For naturopathy, see Susan E. Cayleff, *Nature's Path: A History of*

Naturopathic Healing in America (Baltimore, MD: Johns Hopkins University Press, 2016), 144–77.

68. "Is Light Coming?" *Vaccination* 1, no. 1 (Feb. 1899): 8.

69. "Letters and Comment: Dr. Leverson's Work," *Health Culture* (ed. Elmer Lee) 23 (May 1917): 231. For a biography of Leverson, see Frederick Nolan, *The West of Billy the Kid* (Norman: University of Oklahoma Press, 1998), 116.

70. Blue, as cited in "Vaccination Harmful, Is Declaration," *Vancouver (BC) Sun*, Oct. 30, 1923, 1.

71. Frank D. Blue, "Quiet Talks to the Faithful," *Vaccination* 7, no. 7 (Aug. 1904): 1.

72. "The Anti-Vaccination Society of America: Special Announcements," 14; Blue, "Editorial," 4.

73. Frank D. Blue to M. R. Leverson, May 20, 1898, AVSA, HMLCPP.

74. Membership data is reported in the *Brooklyn Daily Eagle Almanac, 1901* (Brooklyn, NY: Brooklyn Daily Eagle), 308. Frank D. Blue to M. R. Leverson, May 12, 1898, AVSA, HMLCPP. Blue, "Executive Committee Notes," *Vaccination* 2, no. 11 (December 1899): 4. "Anti-Vaccination League," *New York Times*, Jan. 6, 1901.

75. Lawrence O. Gostin, "*Jacobson v. Massachusetts* at 100 Years: Police Power and Civil Liberties in Tension," *American Journal of Public Health* 95, no. 4 (Apr. 2005): 576–81; Willrich, *Pox*, 285–97; John Marshall Harlan, "Opinion," in *Jacobson v. Massachusetts*, Cornell Law School, Legal Information Institute, https://www.law .cornell.edu/supremecourt/text/197/11. Also see Karen L. Walloch, *The Antivaccine Heresy: Jacobson v. Massachusetts and the Troubled History of Vaccination in the United States* (Rochester, NY: University of Rochester Press, 2015).

76. Frank D. Blue, "Once Again," *Vaccination* 8, no. 7 (July 1905): 47. "Random Notes," *Homeopathic Recorder*, 21 (Oct. 1906): 478.

77. For Lora Little's activism, see Johnston, *The Radical Middle Class*, 192–213; Carley Roche, *Lora Little: The Vaccine Liberator* (blog), Feb. 10, 2017, The History of Vaccines, College of Physicians of Philadelphia, https://history ofvaccines.org/blog/lora-little-the-vaccine-liberator; Lora Little, *Crimes of the Cowpox Ring: Some Moving Pictures Thrown on the Dead Wall of Official Silence* (Minneapolis, MN: Liberator Publishing Co., 1906).

78. Arthur Allen, *Vaccine: The Controversial Story of Medicine's Greatest Lifesaver* (New York: W. W. Norton, 2007), 102–3.

79. For the emergence of *variola minor* in the nineteenth century, see Frank Fenner, "Smallpox: Emergence, Global Spread, and Eradication," *History and Philosophy of the Life Sciences* 15, no. 3 (Sept. 1993): 397–420. Also see Willrich, *Pox*, 41–74.

80. "Anti-vaccination Reports on Alleged Casualties from Compulsory Vaccination in the Philadelphia Area," HMLCPP. For the Philadelphia League, see Allen, *Vaccine*, 102–3; James Colgrove, *State of Immunity: The Politics of Vaccination in Twentieth-Century America* (Berkeley: University of California Press, 2006),

46–47; CDC, "Side Effects of Smallpox Vaccination," https://www.cdc.gov /smallpox/vaccine-basics/vaccination-effects.html. For statistics of deaths from the smallpox vaccine in the twentieth century, see J. Michael Lane et al., "Complications of Smallpox Vaccination, 1968," *NEJM* 281 (Nov. 27, 1969): 1201–8.

81. Data calculated from entries in the "Anti-Vaccination League of Pennsylvania Receipts," HMLCPP.

82. Receipts show that from 1906 to 1911, doctors represented 16 percent of paid members on average. Women's paid memberships averaged 20 percent. Membership data is calculated from entries in "Anti-Vaccination League of Pennsylvania Receipts, October 4, 1906–June 11, 1913," HMLCPP. Porter F. Cope, "Compulsory Vaccination," *Columbus Medical Journal* 32 (Jan. 1908): 360–62. In this article, Cope describes the league's success in procuring passage of the Watson Anti-vaccination Bill, which was vetoed by Governor Edwin S. Stuart.

83. "Start War on Vaccination," *Leavenworth (KS) Post*, Oct. 21, 1908, 1; "Oppose Vaccination," *Los Angeles Times*, Oct. 19, 1908, 1.

84. Allen, *Vaccine*, 102–3.

85. John Pitcairn, *Vaccination* (Philadelphia: Anti-Vaccination League of Pennsylvania, 1907), 1.

86. *First Report of the National League for Medical Freedom* (New York: National League for Medical Freedom, 1910), 6.

87. *First Report of the National League*, 6. See James C. Whorton, *Crusaders for Fitness: The History of American Health Reformers* (Princeton, NJ: Princeton University Press, 2014), 147.

88. United States, 61st Congress, 1909–11, House, *Hearings before the Committee on Interstate and Foreign Commerce of the House of Representatives on Bills Relating to Health Activities of the General Government, Part 1* (Washington, DC: GPO, 1910) 607. Also see Manfred Waserman, "The Quest for a National Health Department in the Progressive Era," *Bulletin of the History of Medicine* 49, no. 3 (Fall 1975): 353–80; Stephen Petrina, "Medical Liberty: Drugless Healers Confront Allopathic Doctors, 1910–1931," *Journal of Medical Humanities* 29, no. 4 (Dec. 2008): 205–30.

89. Karen Walloch, *"A Hot Bed of the Anti-vaccine Heresey": Opposition to Compulsory Vaccination in Boston and Cambridge, 1890–1905* (Boston: Proquest, 2007), 7.

90. Lora Little to John Pitcairn, quoted in Robert D. Johnston, "The Myth of the Harmonious City," *Oregon Historical Quarterly* (Fall 1998): 273.

91. Lora C. Little, "Nature-Cure Applied by an Expert," *Morning Oregonian* (Portland, OR), July 17, 1909, 13; Little, "Be Your Own Doctor," *Morning Oregonian*, Oct. 14, 1913, 14; and "Lora C. Little, Health Expert," *Morning Oregonian*, July 3, 1916, 13.

92. Patrick B. Hinfey et al., "What Is the Mortality Rate for Tetanus (Lockjaw)?," Medscape, Jan. 18, 2019, https://www.medscape.com/answers/229594-5925

/what-is-the-mortality-rate-for-tetanos-lockjaw. For the rise and popularization of naturopathy, see Cayleff, *Nature's Path*, 13–72.

93. Lora C. Little, as cited in Johnston, *The Radical Middle Class*, 204.

94. "Lora Little Charged with Anti-war Work," *Bismarck (ND) Tribune*, Mar. 30, 1918, 1; "Woman Convicted Here to Have Hearing on Appeal Week from Wednesday," *Bismarck Tribune*, May 14, 1918, 2; "Mrs. Lora Little," *Los Angeles Times*, June 30, 1918, 117.

95. Blue is reported as president in "Resolutions Adopted at Banquet, Second Annual Meeting: American Medical Liberty League, Chicago, October 26, 1920," in George Starr White, *Think: Side Lights, What Others Say, Clinical Cases, Etc.* (Los Angeles: George Starr White, 1920), 417–19.

96. Irving Fisher, "National Health and Medical Freedom: Both Sides of a Question of Public Interest," *Century Illustrated Monthly Magazine* 85 (Feb. 1913): 513–14. Also see Ronald Hamowy, *Government and Public Health in America* (Cheltenham, UK: Edard Elgar Publishing, 2007), 343–44. Medical journals during this period frequently noted the involvement of patent medicine interests in the league. See J. Morgan Sims, "The Owen Bill," *Illinois Medical Journal* 21(Mar. 2012): 383–85.

97. B. O. Flower, "The National League for Medical Freedom: Its Aim and Its Contention," *National Magazine* 36 (Apr.–Sept. 1912): 113–19. The quote is on p. 115. The editor's note to this article states that the organization "now has over a quarter of a million members," but there is no way to verify this claim.

98. "The Propaganda for Reform," *JAMA* 79 (July 1922): 396. "The Ensign Remedies," *Suggestion* 13 (1904): n.p. (the Ensign advertisement appears with other pages at the back of this Chicago monthly spiritualist magazine), accessed Feb. 11, 2018, http://www.iapsop.com/archive/materials/suggestion/suggestion _v13_adverts_and_loose_pages.pdf. For contemporary discussion of the Ensign remedies, see "A Cure for Disappointed Love," *Twenty-First Annual Report of the Dairy and Food Commissioner of the Sate of Michigan for the Year Ending June 30, 1914* (Lansing, MI: Wynkoop Hallenbeck Crawford Co., 1915), 195–96.

99. Blue announced his forthcoming role as superintendent of the Kokomo Invalids' Home Sanitarium in "Important Notice," *Vaccination* 7, no. 8 (Sept. 1904): 64. In March, vol. 8 of the journal was published in Kokomo, Indiana. For the AMA's campaign against fraud, see Eric W. Boyle, *Quack Medicine: A History of Combating Health Fraud in Twentieth Century America* (Santa Barbara, CA: Praeger, 2013), 61–90. For a history of the AMA, see James G. Burrow, *AMA: Voice of American Medicine* (Baltimore, MD: Johns Hopkins University Press, 1963).

100. See "Table 1.2: Flexner's Impact on U.S. and Canadian Schools," in William F. Rayburn and Jay Schulkin, eds., *Changing Landscape of Academic Women's*

Health Care in the United States (Berlin: Springer, 2011), 7. For the impact of the report on homeopathy, see Paolo Bellavite et al., "Immunology and Homeopathy: Historical Background," *Evidence-Based Complementary and Alternative Medicine* 2 (Dec. 2005): 441–52.

101. "Peebles, James Martin," *National Cyclopaedia of American Biography* (Clifton, NJ: James T. White & Co., 1901), 11:423–24; "Dr. Peebles Institute of Health: A Fraudulent and Dangerous 'Cure' for Epilepsy," *JAMA* 64 (Jan. 1915): 455–56.

102. R. Swinburne Clymer, *Vaccination Brought Home to You* (Terre Haute, IN: Frank D. Blue, 1904), 27.

103. "The Propaganda for Reform," 395; "Antis Soundly Flay Progress of Surgery," *Eugene (OR) Guard*, Oct. 31, 1923, 6.

104. Gretchen A. Condran, "The Elusive Role of Scientific Medicine in Mortality Decline: Diphtheria in Nineteenth- and Early Twentieth-Century Philadelphia," *Journal of the History of Medicine and Allied Sciences* 63, no. 4 (Oct. 2008): 484–522.

105. Rhea ex rel., *Rhea v. Board of Education*, 41 N.D., 171 N.W. 103 (1919).

106. "School Officials Have Right to Enforce Vaccination, Says Judge Buttz," *Grand Forks (ND) Herald*, May 8, 1918, 4.

107. "Medical Freedom Column," *Ottawa Citizen* (Canada), June 21, 1919, 2.

108. Michael Willrich and others have argued the anti-vaccinationists were libertarian. Willrich, *Pox*, 269–72; Johnston, *The Radical Middle Class*, 203–4.

109. For the role of collective identity in social movements, see Francesca Polleta and James M. Jasper, "Collective Identity and Social Movements," *Annual Review of Sociology* 27 (2001): 283–305.

110. According Harry B. Anderson, a former secretary of the National League, the organization was active until 1916, and in 1919 its records were turned over to a new medical liberty organization called the Citizens Medical Reference Bureau. "Statement of H. B. Anderson, Secretary, Citizens Medical Reference Bureau, Inc.," in US Congress, Senate, National Health Program, *Hearings before the Committee on Education and Labor [. . .] Seventy-Ninth Congress, Second Session on S. 1606* (Washington DC: GPO, 1946), 2448.

111. James Colgrove, " 'Science in a Democracy': The Contested Status of Vaccination in the Progressive Era and the 1920s," *Isis* 96, no. 2 (June 2005): 175, 190.

112. A search of online booksellers conducted in 2022 revealed many offering these texts.

113. *City Health: Monthly Bulletin, Detroit Department of Health* 2, no. 15 (Dec. 1919), 5. For Americans' widespread resistance to vaccination in the early twentieth century, see Willrich, *Pox*, 1–14, 246–84.

114. Linsly R. Williams, deputy commissioner of health, New York State, "The Smallpox Epidemic at Niagara Falls," paper presented at the American Public Health Association, Jacksonville, FL, Dec. 1, 1914, 426.

115. Dr. W. M. Dickie, secretary of the California State Department of Health, quoted in "Children Pay the Penalty," *Boston Medical and Surgical Journal* 187, no. 131 (Sept. 28, 1922): 491.

Chapter 3. Taking Schools to Court

1. "The Vaccination Law: A Test Case Advanced on the Supreme Court Calendar," *Daily Alta California* (San Francisco), Oct. 12, 1889, 1; "A Pioneer Editor Passes to Reward," *Sonoma West Times and News* (Sebastopol, CA), Jan. 21, 1921, 1.

2. G. G. Tyrrell, "Report of the Permanent Secretary," *Eleventh Biennial Report of the State Board of Health of California* (Sacramento, CA: J. D. Young, 1890), 40; "The Vaccination Law."

3. *D. K. Abeel et al. v. D. C. Clark*, 84 Cal. 226, no. 13511, May 31, 1890, Caselaw Access Project, Harvard Law School, https://cite.case.law/cal/84/226.

4. G. W. Miles, "Compulsory Vaccination," *ASBJ* 2, no. 11 (Nov. 1900): 2, 15. "Higher Court Decisions: Important Ruling on Question of Vaccination," *Indianapolis Journal*, Feb. 2, 1900, 2.

5. Michael Willrich, *Pox: An American History* (New York: Penguin, 2011), 11–12; Robert Johnston, *The Radical Middle Class: Populist Democracy and the Question of Capitalism in Progressive Era Portland, Oregon* (Princeton, NJ: Princeton University Press, 2003), 190.

6. Jeffrey K. Taubenberger and David M. Morens, "1918 Influenza: The Mother of All Pandemics," *Emerging Infectious Diseases* 12, no. 1 (Jan. 2006): 15–22.

7. *Henning Jacobson v. Commonwealth of Massachusetts*, 197 U.S. 11, 49. L. Ed. 643, 25S Ct 358 (Feb. 20, 1905).

8. "Indiana State News," *Hope (IN) Republican*, Nov. 30, 1893, 3; "Opposed to Vaccination," *Crawfordsville (IN) Review*, Nov. 18, 1893, 7; "General State News," *Indianapolis News*, Nov. 24, 1893, 6; "Terre Haute Vaccination Row," *Evening Messenger* (Marsha, TX), Nov. 24, 1893, 1; "Unvaccinated Children Shut Out," *Daily Inter Ocean* (Chicago), Nov. 22, 1893, 6; "Telegraphic Topics," *Akron (OH) Beacon Journal*, Nov. 23, 1893, 1. For Blue's views on contagion, see chapter 2.

9. By Nov. 11, 1893, of 147 smallpox cases in Muncie, 21 people died. See "Another Smallpox Death," *Indianapolis Journal*, Nov. 11, 1893, 2; "Indiana Anti-Vaccination League," *Indianapolis News*, Dec. 13, 1893, 6. William G. Eidson, "Confusion, Controversy, and Quarantine: The Muncie Smallpox Epidemic of 1893," *Indiana Magazine of History* 86 (Dec. 1990): 374–98; Kelly Hacker Jones, "Rebelling against Lawful Authority? The Vaccination Controversy during the Smallpox Epidemic at Muncie, Indiana, 1893," *Journal of the Indiana Academy of the Social Sciences* 14, no. 1 (2010): 74–87.

10. "Dr. Andrew R. Mock," *A Portrait and Biographical Record of Delaware and Randolph Counties, Ind.* (Chicago: A. W. Bowen & Co., 1894), 387–88;

"Dr. Lewis Payton," Frank D. Haimbaugh, ed., *History of Delaware County Indiana, Vol. 2* (Indianapolis, IN: Historical Publishing Co., 1924), 156. Clark is described as a member of the Homeopathic Medical Society in "Vaccination No Safeguard against Smallpox," *Indianapolis News*, Feb. 7, 1894, 8. Gifford published the *Journal of Hygeio-Therapy and Anti-Vaccination*. See "The Late Dr. T. V. Gifford," *Phrenological Journal and Science of Health* (Nov. 1903): 164.

11. "Against Vaccination," *Indianapolis News*, Dec. 12, 1893, 1. The executive committee included "Mr. Ensign, of Union City; Dr. Clarke; Dr. Allen, of Logansport; Dr. Payton, Dr. Gifford, and Frank D. Blue."

12. "Think It Is a Crime," *Indianapolis Journal*, Dec. 13, 1893; "Vaccination Not Compulsory: Important Decision of Judge Taylor of Terre Haute," *Indianapolis Journal*, Dec. 23, 1893, 2.

13. "An Important Case," *Indianapolis Journal*, Mar. 25, 1894, 4.

14. Connecticut State Board of Health, *Seventeenth Annual Report of the State Board of Health of the State of Connecticut* (New Haven, CT: Tuttle, Morehouse & Taylor, 1895), 13.

15. "New Britain," *Hartford (CT) Daily Courant*, Jan. 4, 1893, 6.

16. J. N. Bartlett to William H. Brewer, May 15, 1894, *Seventeenth Annual Report of the State Board of Health of the State of Connecticut*, 14; W. H. Brewer to J. N. Bartlett, May 16, 1894, in *Seventeenth Annual Report of the State Board of Health of the State of Connecticut*, 15. For homeopathic vaccination, see Edmund Fisher, *A Hand-Book on the Diseases of Children and Their Homeopathic Treatment* (Chicago: Medical Century Co., 1985), 263–64.

17. "Unique Court Case Relating to School Children Not Vaccinated," *Morning Record* (Meriden, CT), April 28, 1894, 1. Confirmation of Bissell's membership in the Universalist Church is in "Connecticut Universalists's Annual Meeting," *Meriden (CT) Daily Republican*, Apr. 11, 1894, 7.

18. *Bissell v. Davidson*, 65 Conn. 183 (Dec. 1, 1894), 185.

19. The discussion in this paragraph is based on my analysis of sixty-seven school health textbooks housed in Cubberley Education Library, Stanford University. See Kim Tolley, "Textbook Health: What Children Learned about Vaccination in the Progressive Era," paper presented at the History of Education Society Annual Meeting Virtual Conference, 2020, https://www.researchgate.net /publication/361241891_Textbook_Health_What_Children_Learned_about _Vaccination_in_the_Progressive_Era.

20. Tolley, "Textbook Health." For the temperance movement, see Jonathan Zimmerman, *Distilling Democracy: Alcohol Education in America's Public Schools, 1880–1925* (Lawrence: University Press of Kansas, 1999).

21. See Mary Waring and Brian Bainbridge, "The Roots of Curriculum Inertia," *Journal of Biological Education* 17, no. 4 (1983): 273–75; Denis Lawton, *Theory*

and Practice of Curriculum Studies (New York: Routledge, 2012), 273; Ruth Elson, *Guardians of Tradition: American Schoolbooks of the Nineteenth Century* (Lincoln: University of Nebraska Press, 1964).

22. See Tolley, "Textbook Health."
23. "Report of the Committee on the Teaching of Hygiene in Public Schools," *Bulletin of the American Academy of Medicine* 7, no. 1 (June 1905): 1–72. The quote is on p. 24.
24. "Supreme Court Decision," *Williamsport (PA) Sun-Gazette,* July 12, 1894, 5.
25. Addendum to Benjamin Lee, "The Necessity for the More Careful Instruction of Medical Students in the Diagnosis of Preventable Diseases," *Pennsylvania Medical Journal* 7, no. 2 (Nov. 1903): 68–69.
26. "Can Enforce Vaccination," *Inquirer* (Lancaster, PA), Feb. 24, 1894, 8; "Compulsory Vaccination," *Wilkes-Barre (PA) Times Leader, Evening News,* Mar. 17, 1894, 4; "Vaccination Denounced," *Times* (Philadelphia, PA), July 18, 1894, 3.
27. "Opposed to Vaccination," *Green Bay (WI) Weekly Gazette,* Feb. 21, 1894, 2. For discussion of alternative physicians in Milwaukee, see Judith W. Leavitt, *The Healthiest City: Milwaukee and the Politics of Health Reform* (Madison: University of Wisconsin Press, 1996), 42–43, 80. For the introduction of homeopathy in the United States by German immigrant physicians, see Naomi Rogers, *An Alternative Path: The Making and Remaking of Hahnemann Medical College and Hospital of Philadelphia* (New Brunswick, NJ: Rutgers University Press, 1998), 3–7.
28. "A Decision on Vaccination," *ASBJ* 6, no. 6 (June 1894): 4.
29. "Vaccination Test," *Wisconsin State Journal* (Madison), Mar. 21, 1896, 3.
30. "Judge Bennett Wipes Out the Vaccination Ruling," *Mineral Point (WI) Weekly Tribune,* Mar. 26, 1896, 3; *State ex rel. Adams v. Burdge,* 95 Wis. 390; M. R. Leverson, "To the President and Members of the Anti-Vaccination Society of America, New York, May 18, 1897," AVSA, HMLCPP.
31. "Schools and Vaccination," *ASBJ* 6, no. 1 (Jan. 1894): 5.
32. "The Vaccination Question," *ASBJ* 6, no. 3 (Mar. 1894): 1.
33. "Vaccination and School Boards," *ASBJ* 6, no. 9 (Sept. 1894): 14.
34. "Think It Is a Crime," 6.
35. *D. K. Abeel et al. v. D. C. Clark,* 84 Cal. 226, no. 13511 (May 31, 1890), 230–31.
36. *Frank D. Blue v. Fannie Beach and Orville E. Connor,* 155 Ind. 121 (Feb. 1, 1900), 136–37; *Henning Jacobson v. Commonwealth of Massachusetts,* 197 US 11 (Feb. 20, 1905).
37. The case was argued Dec. 19, 1889 and decided Feb. 25, 1890. *George W. Lawton et al. v. William N. Steele,* 23 NE 878 (N.Y. 1890).
38. *Abeel v. Clark,* 230.
39. "Law of Wisconsin Establishing a State Board of Health," in *First Annual Report of the State Board of Health of Wisconsin for the Year Ending Dec. 31, 1876* (Madison, WI: E. B. Bolens, 1876), vi.

40. *State ex rel. Adams v. Burdge*, 95 Wis. 390 (Feb. 23, 1897), 400.

41. *Potts vs. Breen*, 167 Ill. (May 10, 1897), 67.

42. *Henry Bissell v. Edward H. Davison*, 65 Conn. 183 (Dec. 1, 1894), 192.

43. *Andrew J. Duffield v. Williamsport School District*, 162 Pa. 476 (July 11, 1894), 137–38.

44. *Re Rebenack*, 62 Mo. App. 8 (Apr. 2, 1895).

45. *Blue v. Beach*. Rehearing denied June 20, 1900, in *Reports of Cases Argued and Determined in the Supreme Court of Judicature of the State of Indiana, Vol. 155* (Indianapolis, IN: Levey Bros., 1901), 124–25.

46. *Blue v. Beach*, 127.

47. *Blue v. Beach*, 121–42. The quotes are on pp. 127 and 128, respectively.

48. *Morris v. City of Columbus*, 102 Ga. 792 (1898), 797–98. Georgia's highest court was quoting from an earlier case, *People ex rel. Nechamcus v. Warden of the City Prison*, 144 N.Y. 529 (1895), 535.

49. *Blue v. Beach*, 131.

50. *Blue v. Beach*. Quotes are on pp. 135 and 136, respectively.

51. *Blue v. Beach*, 141.

52. *Blue v. Beach*, 135.

53. John L. Pyle to E. E. Collins, Jan. 13, 1900, in John L. Pyle, *Report of the Attorney General of the State of South Dakota for the Years 1899–1900* (Huron, SD: Huronite Printing House, 1900). The quotes are on pp. 152 and 154, respectively.

54. "Fourteenth Amendment," Constitution Annotated, constitution.congress.gov. For information about the case, see Lawrence O. Gostin, "*Jacobson v. Massachusetts* at 100 Years: Police Power and Civil Liberties in Tension," *American Journal of Public Health* 95, no. 4 (Apr. 2005): 576–81.

55. Gostin, "*Jacobson v. Massachusetts* at 100 Years." Willrich, *Pox*, 285–97. *Henning Jacobson v. Commonwealth of Massachusetts*. In Jacobson's case, Harlan ruled that the medical exemption did not apply.

56. *Jacobson v. Massachusetts*, 7.

57. Gostin, "Jacobson v. Massachusetts at 100 Years"; Willrich, *Pox*, 285–97.

58. O. S. Haines, "Monthly Retrospect of Homeopathic Materia Medica and Therapeutics," *Hahnemannian Monthly* 39 (Jan., 1904): 74. "Question of Vaccination," *Baltimore Sun*, May 30, 1904, 7; "Dr. Long's Reply to Dr. Fowler," *Bakersfield (CA) Morning Echo*, Nov. 15, 1908, 2, 3.

59. John B. Garrison, "Vaccination by the Internal Method," in *Transactions of the Homeopathic Medical Society of the State of New York for the Year 1910*, vol. 54, ed. Bert B. Clark (New York: n.p.), 251–57.

60. John B. Garrison, "Vaccination by the Internal Method—The Use of Variolinum as a Prophylactic in Smallpox," *North American Journal of Homeopathy* 58, no. 12 (1910): 775–81. "Judge Macy Decides in Favor of Homeopaths," *Gazette* (Cedar Rapids, IA), Nov. 8, 1905, 8.

61. "Lee vs. Borger," *Pittsburgh Legal Journal* 57 (August 1910): 459–64. W. R. Stephens is mentioned as a member of the Wilkinsburg health board in "Notes of the Courts," *Pittsburgh Daily Post*, Mar. 23, 1907, 14.

62. "Court News," *Pittsburgh Daily Post*, Dec. 4, 1909, 5.

63. "Lee v. Marsh," *Second Decennial Edition of the American Digest, Volume 5* (St. Paul, MN: West Publishing Co., 1919), 742.

64. "Denies Ottofy's Statement," *St. Louis (MO) Globe-Democrat*, Nov. 1, 1910, 2; "To Test Board's Right to Vaccinate," *Pine Bluff (AR) Daily Graphic*, Feb. 16, 1912, 3.

65. "St. Louis, Sept. 5," *St. Joseph (MO) Gazette*, Sept. 6, 1913, 5.

66. "Court Gives Opinion: Judge Shafer Holds That Law Is That Old-Style Method Is Required in Schools," *Pittsburgh Daily Post*, Dec. 24, 1909, 2.

67. *People ex rel. Jenkins v. Board of Education*, 234 Ill. 422 (1908), Caselaw Access Project, Harvard Law School, https://cite.case.law/ill/234/422.

68. *Rhea ex rel. Rhea v. Board of Education*, 41 N.D., 171 N. W. 103 (1919), Caselaw Access Project, Harvard Law School, https://cite.case.law/nd/41/449.

69. *Reynolds v. United States*, 98 US 145 (1879).

70. *City of New Braunfels et al. v. Fritz Waldschmidt et al.*, Texas Supreme Court Reports 109 (Dec. 1918): 302–11. The quote is on p. 308.

71. "Plans for Convention of School Directors," *York (PA) Dispatch*, Dec. 5, 1905, 6.

72. "Judge Rowe Holds Vaccination Law Is Valid," *People's Register* (Chambersburg, PA), Dec. 15, 1905, 1.

73. *Stull v. Reber*, 64 A. 419 (PA 1906), 157; 161.

74. "School Laws," *ASBJ* 33, no.1 (July 1906): 2.

75. "Objects to Vaccination; Fined," *Pitts Burgh (PA) Daily Post*, Feb. 1, 1916, 2; "Anti-Vaccination Society Decides to Appeal Case," *Pittsburgh Post-Gazette*, Mar. 31, 1916, 1; *Commonwealth v. Aiken*, Pa. Super. 96, 1916.

76. "Asks $30,000 for Requiring Vaccination," *San Antonio (TX) Evening News*, Mar. 25, 1919, 1.

77. "Vaccination Case at San Antonio Is in Supreme Court," *St. Louis (MO) Star and Times*, May 17, 1921, 2.

78. "Another San Antonio Antivaccination Lawsuit," *Texas Medicine* 15, no.1 (May 1919): 25.

79. *Zucht v. King*, 260 U.S. 174, 67 L. Ed. 194, 43 S. Ct. 24 (1922), 260; "Supreme Court Hold Vaccination Laws Legal: Decision Removes Doubt of Validity of State and City Legislation Affecting School Students," *Missouri Herald* (Hayti, MO), Nov. 17, 1922, 2.

Chapter 4. Schools against Vaccination Mandates

1. "To Check the Fever, Board of Health May Order All Schools Closed," *Seattle Post-Intelligencer*, May 12, 1895, 8; "No Power to Close: School Board Will Contest Health Board's Order," *Seattle Post Intelligencer*, May 15, 1985, 5.

2. Stephen Woolworth, "'The Warring Boards': Sanitary Regulation and the Control of Infectious Disease in the Seattle Public Schools, 1892–1900," *Pacific Northwest Quarterly* 96, no. 1 (Winter 2004/2005): 14–23.

3. See *First Annual Report of the State Board of Health, State of Kansas, from Its Organization April 10, 1885 and Ending December 31, 1885* (Topeka, KS: T. D. Thacher, State Printer, 1885), 58, 132, 134, 146, 151–52.

4. Quoted in James Colgrove, *State of Immunity: The Politics of Vaccination in Twentieth-Century America* (Berkeley: University of California Press, 2006), 73.

5. See Woolworth, "'The Warring Boards.'" Also see Colgrove, *State of Immunity*, 45–80, 200.

6. National Board of Health, "State and Municipal Boards of Health in the United States," *National Board of Health Bulletin* 1, no. 47 (May 22, 1880): 366–78.

7. G. G. Tyrrell, "Report of the Permanent Secretary," *Eleventh Biennial Report of the State Board of Health of California* (Sacramento, CA: J. D. Young, 1890), 40; "Test Case Advanced on the Supreme Court Calendar," *Daily Alta California* (San Francisco), Oct. 12, 1889, 1; *Abeel v. Clark*, 84 Cal. 226, no. 13511 (May 31, 1890).

8. Tyrrell, "Report of the Permanent Secretary," 41.

9. California Legislature, *Appendix to the Journals of the Senate and Assembly of the Twenty-Eighth Session of the Legislature of the State of California, Volume 6* (Sacramento CA: J. D. Young, 1889), 40.

10. "Must Be Heard: Alameda," *San Francisco Call*, Sept. 20, 1894, 9.

11. These five Californians are identified as AVSA members on the list of officers and affiliates printed on the back of all 1895 stationary of the Anti-Vaccination Society of America in AVSA, HMLCPP. The physicians included G. M. Pease, a homeopathic physician from San Francisco, and J. Fearn, a practitioner of eclectic medicine from Oakland who served as president of the Eclectic Medical Society of the State of California in 1910. For Pease, see "Homeopathic Physicians," in J. Pettet, *The North American Homeopathic Directory for 1877–78* (Cleveland, OH: Robison, Savage & Co., 1878), 9. For Fearn, see "Dr. Fearn" in *California Eclectic Medical Journal* 3 (January 1910): 192, 211–15. A third affiliate was Malinda Elliott Cramer, coeditor of the journal *Harmony*, which carried articles on theosophy, metaphysics, and the "Christ Method of Healing." The two lay affiliates were F. H. Brooks, an officer of the Oakland chapter of the Knights Templar, and Wilbur Walker. Information about Walker is in *San Francisco Call*, Jan. 25, 1904, 4. For Brooks, see Alameda County, California, *History of Alameda County, California* (Oakland, CA: M. W. Wood, 1883), 752.

12. "[Berkeley] Directors Object to Having Pupils Vaccinated—They Say It Is Useless," *San Francisco Call*, Aug. 24, 1896, 9; "Medical Men Oppose the Action of the Board of Trustees," *San Francisco Call*, Jan. 22, 1897, 11.

13. "The School Directors' President Davis' Comprehensive Address: His Practical Suggestions after a Conference with the Board of Health; Vaccination among Pupils Is Decided Upon," *Los Angeles Herald*, Jan. 10, 1899, 8.

14. "Don't Like Virus: Anti-Compulsory Vaccination Meeting Held at Music Hall," *Los Angeles Times*, Jan. 19, 1899, 10; "Vaccination Reprieve," *Los Angeles Herald*, Jan. 24, 1899, 5.

15. "Opposing Vaccination: Petition Being Sent to the Legislature Asking Repeal of the Law," *Morning Press* (Santa Barbara), Feb. 24, 1899, 3.

16. "To Abolish Vaccination Law," *Santa Cruz Sentinel*, Jan. 21, 1903, 1.

17. Woolworth, "'The Warring Boards.'" For California law, see art. 9, sec. 3, "Constitution of the State of California Adopted in Convention, at Sacramento, March Third, Eighteen Hundred and Seventy-Nine," in *Statutes of California Passed at the Twenty-Third Session of the Legislature, 1880* (Sacramento, CA: J. D. Young, 1880), xxxiii, https://archives.cdn.sos.ca.gov/collections/1879/archive/1879-constitution.pdf.

18. Jackie M. Blount, *Destined to Rule the Schools: Women and the Superintendency, 1873–1995* (Albany: State University of New York Press, 1998).

19. Although the proceedings of these early county superintendents' meetings apparently no longer exist, newspapers reprinted excerpts. This excerpt is from "Convention Adjourns: School Superintendents Conclude Their Business. Proceedings of Yesterday," *Santa Barbara Weekly Press*, May 19, 1904, 2.

20. "Bitter Fight against Law," *San Francisco Call*, Aug. 12, 1904, 4; "Will Raise Money to Fight Vaccination Law," *Oakland Tribune*, Sept. 9, 1904, 7. For Wilson, see Charles Wollenberg, *Berkeley: A City in History* (Berkeley: University of California Press, 2008), 71. Wilbur Walker's participation in the Berkeley organization is mentioned in "Anti-vaccine Organization," *Morning Press* (Santa Barbara), Sept. 7, 1904, 2.

21. "Child's Death Suggests Suit: Persons Who Oppose Compulsory Vaccination Want Some One to Pay Damages," *San Francisco Call*, Sept. 8, 1904, 6.

22. "Anti-vaccine Organization," *Morning Press* (Santa Barbara), Sept. 7, 1904, 2.

23. California State Library, "George Pardee," Governors of California, http://www.californiagovernors.ca.gov/h/biography/governor_21.html.

24. The quotes are from "Vaccination Bill Vetoed," *San Francisco Call*, Mar. 9, 1905, 4. For the full text of Pardee's message, see *The Journal of the Senate during the Thirty-Sixth Session of the Legislature of the State of California* (Sacramento, CA: W. W. Shannon, 1905), 1445.

25. Michael A. Willrich, *Pox: An American History* (New York: Penguin, 2011), 280; "First California Presents the Tattered Flag of Many Battles to the State's Keeping," *Morning Tribune* (San Luis Obispo), Feb. 24, 1905, 4. The quote is from "Vaccination Bill Vetoed," *San Francisco Call*, Mar. 9, 1905, 4.

26. Mrs. N. E. Davidson, Kings County's superintendent of schools, forwarded a copy of the proceedings to a newspaper in Hanford. The quote is from "Compulsory Vaccination of School Children as Viewed by School Superintendents," *Hanford (CA) Sentinel*, Nov. 26, 1906, 8. Information about Baker is from the Charlotte Baker Diary Collection, MS 173, San Diego History Center Document Collection, San Diego, CA.

27. "Education Law Cause of Row," *San Bernardino Sun*, Jan. 15, 1907, 1. The superintendents reiterated their motion at the 1908 state superintendents' convention at Lake Tahoe, as reported in "Proposed Legislation Outlined," *Amador (CA) Ledger-Dispatch*, Oct. 2, 1908, 8.

28. N. K. Foster, "Report of the State Board of Health," *Twentieth Biennial Report of the State Board of Health of California* (Sacramento, CA: W. W. Shannon, 1908), 19.

29. "Berkeley School Board Has Puzzle to Solve," *San Francisco Call*, Apr. 25, 1907, 6.

30. "Vaccination Law Still in Force," *Los Angeles Herald*, Feb. 9, 1907, 2.

31. "Vaccination Not in Favor," *Santa Cruz Evening News* Aug. 28, 1909, 5. In February 1910, superintendents in Watsonville and Los Gatos also refused to comply with the law, as described in "County Superintendent Opposed to Vaccination: Watsonville Trustees Stand Pat and Await the Outcome of Legal Proceedings," *Santa Cruz Sentinel*, Feb. 9, 1910, 1.

32. These percentages are calculated from "Summary of Statistics: Primary and Grammar Schools," in *Appendix to the Journals of the Senate and Assembly of the Thirty-Seventh Session of the Legislature of the State of California, Vol. 1* (Sacramento, CA: W. W. Shannon, 1907), 259; "Summary of Statistics. Primary and Grammar Schools," in *Appendix to the Journals of the Senate and Assembly of the Thirty-Ninth Session of the Legislature of the State of California, Vol. 1* (Sacramento, CA: Friend Wm. Richardson, 1912), 52.

33. Tae Hynog Kim, Jennie Johnstone, and Mark Loeb, "Vaccine Herd Effect," *Scandinavian Journal of Infectious Diseases* 43, no. 9 (Sept. 2011): 683–89.

34. *State Board of Health of State of California v. Board of Trustees of Watsonville School District of Santa Cruz County* 13 Cal. App. 514 (Cal. Ct. App. 1910).

35. C. P. Pomeroy, *Reports of Cases Determined in District Courts of Appeal of the State of California, Vol. 13* (San Francisco: Bancroft-Whitney, 1911), 514–15. The quote is on p. 515.

36. "Anti-vaccination Societies Forming throughout State," *Morning Press* (Santa Barbara), Sept. 16, 1910, 3.

37. For the libertarianism among anti-vaccinationists, see Michael Willrich, "'The Least Vaccinated of Any Civilized Country': Personal Liberty and Public Health in the Progressive Era," *Journal of Policy History* 20, no. 1 (2008): 76–93. For homeopathy and alternative medicine, see Natalie Robins, *Copeland's Cure:*

Homeopathy and the War between Conventional and Alternative Medicine (New York: Knopf Doubleday, 2009); Nadav Davidovitch, "Negotiating Dissent: Homeopathy and Anti-vaccinationism at the Turn of the Twentieth Century," in *The Politics of Healing: Histories of Alternative Medicine in Twentieth-Century North America*, ed. Robert D. Johnston (New York: Routledge, 2004), 11–28.

38. "Compulsory Vaccination Law Sustained by the Court," *Los Angeles Herald*, Feb. 18, 1910, 2; "Supreme Court Upholds the Vaccination Law," *Press Democrat* (Santa Rosa), Aug. 14, 1910, 6.

39. William F. Snow, "Smallpox and the State Board of Health," *California State Board of Health Monthly Bulletin* 6, no. 2 (Aug. 1910): 71–86.

40. "State Health Board Milder on Vaccination: Demurely Asks Opinions of Citizens Opposed to Method," *Morning Press* (Santa Barbara), Sept. 3, 1910, 8.

41. Santon Pope, "The Antivaccinationists' Standpoint," *California State Board of Health Monthly Bulletin* 6, no. 2 (Aug. 1910): 52–55.

42. Snow, "Smallpox and the State Board of Health," 72.

43. "Anti-vaccination Societies Forming throughout the State," 3.

44. "Anti-vaccination Societies Forming throughout the State," 3.

45. "School Enrollment Threatened by Sudden Vaccination Edict," *Morning Press* (Santa Barbara), Aug. 26, 1910, 8.

46. "Vaccination Law in Doctors' Hands," *San Francisco Call*, Dec. 2, 1910, 2; "To Urge Stricter Vaccination Law: State Board of Health Fathers Compulsory Bill," *Sacramento Union*, Jan. 8, 1911, 30.

47. "Vaccination Fight Will Be Reopened," *Sacramento Union*, Feb. 2, 1909, 2.

48. "Baldwin Predicts Good School Legislation," *San Diego Union and Daily Bee*, Feb. 2, 1911, 8.

49. For repeal of California's 1889 vaccination law, see "Introduction and First Reading of Bills," *Journal of the Senate during the Thirty-Eighth (Extra) Session of the Legislature of California* (Sacramento, CA: W. W. Shannon, 1911), 443; "Act 3690—An Act to Encourage and Provide for a General Vaccination for All Public and Private Schools of California [. . .] Approved February 20, 1889," W. F. Henning, ed., *General Laws of California* (San Francisco: Bender-Moss Co., 1914), 1493. Also see "Complete List of School Bills Passed by Last Legislature," *Sacramento Union*, Apr. 12, 1911), 6; "Educational Bills That the Governor Has Signed," *Press Democrat* (Santa Rosa), Apr. 22, 1911, 9.

50. "The Schools and the New Vaccination Law," *California State Board of Health Monthly Bulletin* 7, no. 1 (July 1911): 7.

51. "The Schools and the New Vaccination Law," 6.

52. *Twenty-Sixth Biennial Report of the State Board of Health of California for the Fiscal Years from July 1, 1918, to June 30, 1920* (Sacramento, CA: State Printing Office [hereafter SPO], 1921), 14.

53. *Twenty-Ninth Biennial Report of the State Board of Health of California for the Fiscal Years from July 1, 1924, to June 30, 1926* (Sacramento, CA: SPO, 1926), 23; "Less Vaccination, More Smallpox," *San Bernardino Sun*, May 3, 1926, 12.

54. "High Lights from Biennial Report," *California State Board of Health Weekly Bulletin*, Nov. 20, 1926, 1. For the emergence of *variola minor*, see Willrich, *Pox*, 337–38.

55. John N. Force, "Symposium on Smallpox: Epidemiological Study of Smallpox in California," *American Journal of PublicHealth* 11, no. 1 (Jan. 1921): 119–25. The quotes are on p. 121.

56. "Education Board Defies Health Rule, *Sacramento Union*, Mar. 5, 1912, 1.

57. "Vaccination Law Is Responsible for Some Schools Losing Money," *San Diego Union and Daily Bee*, Mar. 4, 1913, 2.

58. "Vaccination Law Is Responsible for Some Schools Losing Money."

59. "School Doors May Not Open," *Sacramento Union*, Aug. 3, 1919, 3.

60. "Southern California News Tersely Told," *Coronado (CA) Eagle and Journal*, Nov. 10, 1917, 4.

61. For information about Crutcher, see "Vaccination in Public Schools Commented On," *Morning Press* (Santa Barbara), Sept. 26, 1919, 10.

62. Crutcher is quoted in Thos. G. McConkey, "Psora, Sycosis and Syphilis as Causative Factors in the Chronic Diseases," *Journal of the American Institute of Homeopathy*, ed. Willis A. Dewey and J. Richey Horner (New York: Medical Century Publishing, 1910), 1:113–14.

63. "Charges against Dr. Lewis P. Crutcher Contained in Dr. Brem's Article Refuted," *Los Angeles Herald*, Dec. 14, 1920, 6.

64. *Report of the Commissioner of Education for the Year Ended June 30, 1918* (Washington, DC: GPO, 1918), 59.

65. See William Reese, *Power and Promise of School Reform: Grassroots Movements during the Progressive Era* (New York: Teachers College Press, 2002), 186–212; John Duffy, "School Vaccination: The Precursor to School Medical Inspection," *Journal of the History of Medicine and Allied Sciences* 33, no. 3 (July 1978): 344–55. For contemporary accounts of medical inspection in schools, see Luther Halsey Gulick and Leonard P. Ayres, *Medical Inspection of Schools* (New York: Russell Sage Foundation, 1913), 7–20. Also see Leonard P. Ayres, "What American Cities Are Doing for the Health of School Children," *Annals of the American Academy* 37 (Mar. 1911): 250–60.

66. Sally Lucas Jean, "First Out of Town Speech, Association House, 5150 West North Avenue, Chicago," ca. 1917, Sally Lucas Jean Papers, series 1, box 7, fol. 48, SHC.

67. For the rise of school medical inspections as a factor in Progressive Era anti-vaccination protest, see Robert D. Johnston, *The Radical Middle Class: Populist Democracy and the Question of Capitalism in Progressive Era Portland,*

Oregon (Princeton, NJ: Princeton University Press, 2003), 177–220; James Colgrove, "'Science in a Democracy': The Contested Status of Vaccination in the Progressive Era and the 1920s," *Isis* 96, no. 2 (June 2005): 167–91; Reese, *Power and Promise of School Reform*, 200–208; Willrich, *Pox*, 246–84.

68. "Constitution Change Is League's Object: School Protective Society Plans Initiative at Annual Meeting," *Los Angeles Times*, Oct. 28, 1919, part II, 3.

69. "Prohibiting Compulsory Vaccination" [California Proposition 6], in "Amendments to Constitution and Proposed Statutes with Arguments Respecting the Same, To Be Submitted to the Electors of the State of California at the General Election on Tuesday, November 2, 1920," 21, in Ballot Pamphlets, 1912–1932, CSA.

70. "Statement of the Public School Protective League," *Coronado (CA) Eagle and Journal*, Sept. 13, 1919, 6; "A Law That Needs to Be Changed," *Mill Valley (CA) Record*, Apr. 2, 1921, 4; Gerrie Schipske, "Parents and School Board Fight against Vaccinations—1907," *Beachcomber*, Sept. 14, 2017, https://beachcomber .news/content/parents-and-school-board-fight-against-vaccinations---1907.

71. Crutcher claimed that the California State Board of Health had announced this statistic, but a search of the published health reports for 1919 reveal this was not the case. His remark was reported in "Constitution Change Is League's Object." For the outcome of the vote, see "Prohibiting Compulsory Vaccination: California Proposition 6 (1920)," Hastings Law Scholarship Repository, http://repository .uchastings.edu/ca_ballot_props/135U.C.

72. "Senate Committee Opposed to Compulsory Vaccination," *Sacramento Union*, Mar. 24, 1921, 1.

73. James Colgrove, *State of Immunity: The Politics of Vaccination in Twentieth-Century America* (Berkeley: University of California Press, 2006).

74. C.-E. A. Winslow, "The Untilled Fields of Public Health," *Science* 60, no. 1306 (Jan. 9, 1920): 30. Also see Willrich, *Pox*, 337–38.

75. "Senate Committee Opposed to Compulsory Vaccination."

76. S.B. 408's language was amended in the Senate to give the California State Board of Health control over smallpox. "Amended in Senate, March 28, 1921," Original Bill File: S.B. 408, Bill Files, CSA. Also see William Fowler, *Smallpox Vaccination Laws, Regulations, and Court Decisions* (Washington DC: GPO, 1927), 17; William Fowler, "Principal Provisions of Smallpox Vaccination Laws and Regulations in the United States," *PHR (1896–1970)* 56, no. 5 (Jan. 31, 1941): 167–89.

77. For advances in medicine during this period, see Peter Conrad and Joseph W. Schneider, "Professionalization, Monopoly, and the Structure of Medical Practice," in *The Sociology of Health and Illness: Critical Perspectives*, ed. Peter Conrad (New York: Worth Publishers, 2009), 194–99; Julie B. Millen, "Regulation of Vaccines: Strengthening the Science Base," *JPHP* 25, no. 2: 173–89. For declining anti-vaccinationist sentiment during the 1930s, see

Colgrove, "'Science in a Democracy.'" For the rise of persuasive policies among public health professionals, see Willrich, *Pox*, 337–38.

78. John W. Ritchie and Joseph S. Caldwell, *Primer of Hygiene, California State Series: Revised by the State Text-Book Committee and Approved by the State Board of Education* (Sacramento, CA: W. W. Shannon, Superintendent of State Printing, 1911), 138–39. This wording appears only in this version of their text.

79. John Woodside Ritchie, *Primer of Sanitation* (Yonkers-on-Hudson, NY: World Book Co., 1913), 126–27.

80. CDPH, "San Luis Obispo Guards against Smallpox," *State Board of Health Weekly Bulletin for March 8, 1924*, 15.

81. For example, "Dr. Telfer to Urge Vaccination of Pupils," *Madera (CA) Mercury*, Oct. 30, 1924, 1; "Chamber of Commerce Favors Vaccination," *Healdsburg (CA) Enterprise*, Jan. 20, 1927, 8; "Intensive Vaccination in Schools Starts Tuesday," *San Bernardino Sun*, May 7, 1934, 3.

82. "School Doctor Directs Appeal on Vaccination," *Press Democrat* (Santa Rosa), Sept. 8, 1920, 8.

83. "Public Health Nurses Meet with Teachers," *Morning Tribune* (San Luis Obispo), Dec. 5, 1925, 1; "Red Cross Nurse Reports on Work in Homes and Schools," *Santa Cruz Evening News*, Dec. 9, 1929, 7. For public health nurses in the schools, see Diane Allensworth et al., eds., *Schools and Health: Our Nation's Investment* (Washington, DC: National Academies Press, 1997), 34–35; Richard A. Meckel, *Classrooms and Clinics: Urban Schools and the Protection and Promotion of Child Health, 1870–1930* (New Brunswick, NJ: Rutgers University Press, 2013), 62–63.

84. "School Children to Be Immunized from Diphtheria," *Colusa (CA) Herald*, Oct. 28, 1926, 1.

85. "Report of the Secretary," *Twenty-Ninth Biennial Report of the State Board of Health of California* (Sacramento, CA: John E. King, State Printer, 1926), 23. A search for "Public School Protective League" in the California Digital Newspaper Collection reveals no mention of this organization after 1926.

86. Giles S. Porter, "Report of the Director," *Thirty-Second Biennial Report of the Department of Public Health of California* (Sacramento, CA: Superintendent of State Printing, 1931), 23.

87. Lyman A. Best, "Proper Sanitation of the Schoolroom," in *Proceedings of the Fifth Congress of the American School Hygiene Association, Vol. 3* (Springfield, MA: American Physical Education Review, 1911), 130–31.

88. *California State Board of Health Monthly Bulletin* 17, no. 4 (Oct. 1921): 171.

89. Walter M. Dickie, "Report of the Director," *Thirtieth Biennial Report of the California Department of Public Health of California* (Sacramento, CA: SPO, 1929), 12.

90. Thomas D. Wood, Committee on the School Child, "Section III—Education and Training," White House Conference on Child Health and Protection, *The Administration of the School Health Program* (New York: New Century Co., 1932), 29n15.

91. Walter M. Dickie, "Report of the Director," 12.

Chapter 5. Schools and the Campaign against Polio

1. Richard Daggett, *Not Just Polio: My Life Story* (Bloomington, IN: iUniverse, 2010), 28, 31; Daniel J. Wilson, *Living with Polio: The Epidemic and Its Survivors* (Chicago: University of Chicago Press, 2005).

2. "Global Immunization: What Is Polio?," CDC, https://www.cdc.gov/polio/what-is-polio/index.htm.

3. CDC, "Surveillance of Poliomyelitis in the United States, 1958–61," *PHR* 77, no. 12 (Dec. 1962): 1011–20; Philip J. Smith, David Wood, and Paul M. Darden, "Highlights of Historical Events Leading to National Surveillance of Vaccination Coverage in the United States," *PHR* 126, suppl. 2 (July 2011): 3–12.

4. Oral history interview with Mary Duncan [unedited], conducted by Tom Gatewood, July 19, 1982, RHCOHP, https://www.kyhistory.com/digital/collection/Ohist/id/2055/rec/7.

5. CDPH, *California Public Health Report, July 1, 1951 to June 30, 1952* (CDPH, 1952), 4, 71.

6. M.-J. Freyche, A.M.-M. Payne, and C. Lederrey, "Table 1. Notified Cases of, and Deaths from Poliomyelitis: Various Countries, 1949–53," in "Poliomyelitis in 1953," *Bulletin of the World Health Organization* 12 (1955): 600.

7. Ronald Moser, "Better Organization Needed for Vaccine," *San Jose (CA) Mercury News Group*, Jan. 19, 2021, A6.

8. See Bernard Seytre and Mary Shaffer, *The Death of a Disease: A History of the Eradication of Poliomyelitis* (New Brunswick, NJ: Rutgers University Press, 2005); David W. Rose, *March of Dimes* (Mount Pleasant, SC: Arcadia Publishing, 2003); Stephanie True Peters, *Epidemic! The Battle against Polio* (New York: Marshall Cavendish, 2005); David M. Oshinsky, *Polio: An American Story* (New York: Oxford University Press, 2005).

9. Oshinsky, *Polio*, 216–42, documents the American government's lack of involvement and preparation during the early 1950s, which led to vaccine shortages and contamination of the supply. Naomi Rogers and other scholars have highlighted racial discrimination in access to polio prevention and treatment. See Rogers, "Race and the Politics of Polio: Warm Springs, Tuskegee, and the March of Dimes," *Public Health Then and Now* 97, no. 5 (May 2007): 784–95; Stephen E. Mawdsley, "'Dancing on Eggs': Charles H. Bynum, Racial Politics, and the National Foundation for Infantile Paralysis, 1938–1954," *Bulletin of the History of Medicine* 84, no. 2 (Summer 2010): 217–47; Heather

Green Wooten, *The Polio Years in Texas: Battling a Terrifying Unknown* (College Station: Texas A&M University Press, 2009), 46–48, 51–53, 82–83, 142, 146; Linda Logan, *A Summer without Children: An Oral History Wythe County, Virginia's 1950 Polio Epidemic* (Wytheville, VA: Town of Wytheville Department of Museums, 2005), 39.

10. Amy L. Fairchild, "The Polio Narratives: Dialogues with FDR," *Bulletin of the History of Medicine* 75, no. 3 (Fall 2001): 488–534. Also see David W. Rose, *March of Dimes* (Mount Pleasant, SC: Arcadia Publishing, 2003).

11. March of Dimes, "Origin of Our Name," https://www.marchofdimes.org /mission/eddie-cantor-and-the-origin-of-the-march-of-dimes.aspx.

12. Franklin Delano Roosevelt, *The Public Papers and Addresses of Franklin D. Roosevelt: The Continuing Struggle for Liberalism, 1938* (New York: Random House, 1938), 73.

13. Sally Lucas Jean to Basil O'Connor, "Progress Report—Education, June 1944–January 1945," 1, in Sally Lucas Jean Papers (hereafter SLJ Papers), series 1, box 9, folder 59, SHC.

14. Kim Tolley, "Textbook Health: What Children Learned about Vaccination in the Progressive Era," paper presented at the History of Education Society Annual Meeting Virtual Conference, 2020, doi: 10.13140/RG.2.2.25617.71520.

15. Oshinsky, *Polio*, 68.

16. Franklin Delanor Roosevelt, "Annual Appeal for the National Foundation for Infantile Paralysis: Radio Broadcast, January 29, 1944," *Public Papers of the Presidents of the United States: Franklin D. Roosevelt, 1944–45*, vol. 13 (New York: Random House, 1949), 61–62.

17. Charles C. Wilson, John L. Bracken, and John C. Almack, *Life and Health* (Indianapolis, IN: Bobbs-Merrill, 1945), 252–53.

18. R. Will Burnett, *To Live in Health* (New York: Silver Burdett Co., 1944), 64.

19. SLJ Papers collection overview, SHC; Marguerite Vollmer, *Sally Lucas Jean, 1878–1971: Health Education Pioneer* (Geneva: International Journal of Health Education, 1973), 74–79.

20. Sally Lucas Jean, "The National Foundation for Infantile Paralysis: Proposed Health Education Program Feb. 1, 1944)," SLJ Papers, series 1, box 3, folder 24, SHC.

21. Sally Lucas Jean, "The National Foundation for Infantile Paralysis Abstract of Progress Report, Sept. 1, 1944, The Education Service," 1, in SLJ Papers, series 1, box 3, folder 24, SHC. This is also discussed in "National Foundation for Infantile Paralysis Health Education Advisory Committee Meeting, Nov. 30, 1949," 9, in SLJ Papers, series 1, box 9, folder 59, SHC.

22. "Conquering Germ Diseases," Jessie Williams Clemensen, Thomas Gordon Lawrence, Howard S. Hoyman, William Ralph La Porte, *Your Health and Safety* (New York: Harcourt, Brace and Co., 1957), 411–55. For a similar insert, also

see Harold S. Diehl and Anita D. Laton, *Health and Safety for You* (New York: McGraw-Hill Book Co., 1954), chap. 24.

23. Sally Lucas Jean, "If Polio Comes: Thru Instruction and Observation, the Teacher Can Help Protect the Child," *National Education Association Journal* 39, no. 4 (April 1950): 268–69; Sally Lucas Jean to Health Education Advisory Committee, National Foundation for Infantile Paralysis Education Service Report, Dec. 1949–June 1950, in SLJ Papers, series 1, box 9, folder 59, SHC.

24. Elsa Schneider and Simon A. McNeely, *Teachers Contribute to Child Health*, Bulletin No. 8 (Washington DC: GPO, HEW, 1951), foreword, 4–5. One journal referred to this bulletin as "widely used." See "Simon A. McNeely," *Journal of Health, Physical Education, and Recreation* 34, no. 6 (June 1963): 56.

25. "Students Help March of Dimes," *Whittier (CA) News*, Feb. 3, 1955, 27.

26. "Routt Students Conducting Own March of Dimes," *Jacksonville (IL) Daily Journal*, Jan. 27, 1954, 12. Such class drives often made front-page news. For example, see "Student Council Starts March of Dimes Drive, *Comstock (NE) News*, Jan, 28, 1954, 1.

27. "Plans Completed for March of Dimes in Rayne," *Weekly Acadian* (Rayne, LA), Jan. 31, 1952, 2.

28. "Schoolchildren Give $286.96 to March of Dimes," *Alexandria (IN) Times-Tribune*, Feb. 1, 1954, 1.

29. "Student Council Starts March of Dimes Drive," *Comstock (NE) News*, Jan, 28, 1954, 1; "March of Dimes Hits $1,300 Total," *Houston Home Journal* (Perry, Houston County, GA), Feb. 11, 1954, 1.

30. "School Children Will Participate in Study of New Polio Vaccine," *El Sereno (CA) Star*, Jan. 21, 1954, 8.

31. Melvin Glasser, "M-Day for Polio," *Adult Leadership* 3, no. 3 (Sept. 1954): 5–7. The quote is on p. 6.

32. Hart E. Van Riper, *SL* 36, no. 5 (Feb. 1954): 69–70. The quote is on p. 70.

33. "Turn on Your Porch Light for Mothers' March on Polio," *Healdsburg (CA) Tribune, Enterprise and Scimitar*, Jan. 28, 1954, 1; "La Habra Mothers March on Polio Tuesday Night," *La Habra (CA) Star*, Jan. 28, 1954, 1.

34. In 1955, Sally Lucas Jean worked as consultant to the School Health Bureau and authored some of its reports. Jean, "The 1955 Report of the School Health Bureau to the Members of the Advisory Educational Group"; "School Health Bureau Staff Meeting on Correspondence, November 1955," 5, 6, in SLJ Papers, series 1, box 8, folder 54, SHC.

35. Marian V. Miller of the National Foundation describes some classroom practices in "Pupils Pioneer against Polio," *SL* 37, no. 5 (Oct. 1954): 4–5. For school segregation during the program, see Rogers, "Race and the Politics of Polio," 10.

36. See William Schupmann, "Public Schools as Loci for Human Experimentation: Implications of Using Public Schools to House the Polio Vaccine Field Trial of

1954," *Penn History Review* 23, no. 2 (Fall 2016): 61–86; Jeffrey P. Baker, "History Lesson: Vaccine Trials in the Classroom," *American Journal of Public Health* 108, no. 8 (Aug. 2018): 976–77.

37. For an overview of medical ethics in the Salk and other trials, see Sydney A. Halpern, *Lesser Harms: The Morality of Medical Research* (Chicago: University of Chicago Press, 2004), 91–116.

38. "March of Dimes: Protestant, Catholic and Jewish Leaders Back Drive," *Whittier (CA) News*, Jan. 9, 1954, 7; "Leaders of All Faiths Appeal for Support of Polio Campaign," *News-Messenger* (Fremont, OH), Jan. 7, 1954; "Church Leaders Support March against Polio," *Florence (SC) Morning News*, Jan. 22, 1955, 2.

39. "Calendar of Vaccine Standards and Distribution," *PHR* 70, no. 8 (Aug. 1955): 747–51, quote on 749; CDC, "50th Anniversary of the First Effective Polio Vaccine—April 12, 2005," *MMWR* 54, no. 13 (April 8, 2005): 335–36, quote on 335.

40. Dwight D. Eisenhower, "Statement by the President on the Polio Vaccine Situation, May 31, 1955," *Public Papers of the Presidents of the United States Containing the Public Messages, Speeches, and Statements of the President, January 1 to December 31, 1955* (Washington DC: GPO, 1959), 559–63.

41. Public Law 377, chap. 863, August 12, 1955 [S. 2501], Poliomyelitis Vaccination Assistance Act of 1955, https://www.govinfo.gov/content/pkg/STATUTE-69 /pdf/STATUTE-69-Pg704.pdf.

42. See Simon A. McNeely, "Planning for 1955 Polio Vaccine Program," *SL* 37, no. 5 (Feb. 1955): 67.

43. Wooten, *The Polio Years in Texas*, 146–47. Coordination in California involving PTA members and school officials is described in City of Mill Valley, "Vaccine Dreams: Looking Back to Marin's "K.O. Polio" Campaign," https://www .cityofmillvalley.org/news/displaynews.htm?NewsID=2954&TargetID=57; "Polio Shots Start Here Saturday," *Coronado (CA) Eagle and Journal*, Apr. 14, 1955, 1.

44. "Growing Number of States Opposed to Vaccinations," *Pittston (PA) Gazette*, June 3, 1955, 1; Smith, Wood, and Darden, "Highlights of Historical Events Leading to National Surveillance of Vaccination Coverage in the United States"; Paul Offit, "The Cutter Incident, 50 Years Later," *NEJM* 352, no. 10 (Mar. 10, 2005): 1411–12; Oshinsky, *Polio*, 216–21.

45. Eleanor McBean, *The Poisoned Needle: Suppressed Facts about Vaccination* (Mokelumne Hill, CA: Health Research, 1956). The quote is from chap. 10, n.p., Internet Archive, https://archive.org/details/the_poisoned_needle _mcbean/page/196/mode/2up.

46. "Dr. Benjamin P. Sandler, Nutritionist, 77, Is Dead," *New York Times*, May 23, 1979, 22.

47. Benjamin P. Sandler, *Diet Prevents Polio* (Milwaukee, WI: Lee Foundation for Nutritional Research, 1951), 7.

48. Information about Miller is in "Two New Polio Cases Reported at Key West," *News Tribune* (Fort Pierce, FL), Oct. 1, 1953, 6.

49. Miller's comments are included in an anti-vaccine advertisement in "If the Salk Vaccine Is So Good Now Is the Time to Accept the Challenge," *Telegraph-Bulletin* (North Platte, NE), Apr. 7, 1955, 5. For his idea about soft drinks, see "Indict Critic of Polio Scientist," *Daily Times* (New Philadelphia, OH), Apr. 5, 1954, 9.

50. "If the Salk Vaccine Is So Good Now Is the Time to Accept the Challenge," 5.

51. "Polio Libel Case Gets Underway," *Courier News* (Blytheville, AR), Apr. 26, 1954, 10; "Indict Critic of Polio Scientist," 9.

52. "Fighting Polio," *Times Record* (Troy, NY), Apr. 27, 1954, 14.

53. Robert C. Davis, *The Public Impact of Science in the Mass Media* (Ann Arbor: University of Michigan Survey Research Center, 1958), 179.

54. Selwyn D. Collins, "Frequency and Volume of Doctors' Calls among Males and Females in 9,000 Families, Based on Nation-Wide Periodic Canvasses, 1928–31," *PHR* 55 (Nov. 1, 1940): 1987–88. For the rise of allopathic medicine in the United States, see Paul Starr, *The Social Transformation of American Medicine* (New York: Basic Books, 1982).

55. Paul Offit, "The Cutter Incident, 50 Years Later," *NEJM* 352, no. 10 (Mar. 10, 2005): 1411–12; Smith, Wood, and Darden, "Highlights of Historical Events Leading to National Surveillance of Vaccination Coverage in the United States"; Oshinsky, *Polio*, 216–21.

56. William C. Bruce, ed., "A School Opportunity," *ASBJ* 130, no.6 (June 1955): 50.

57. California State Legislature, S.B. No. 1988, "An Act to Add Section 16444 to the Education Code, Relating to the Administering of Poliomyelitis Vaccine to Pupils of the Public School [. . .]," *Senate Bills, Original and Amended* (Sacramento, CA: State Printing Office, 1955).

58. "Polio Vaccine to Be Distributed," *Dade County (GA) Times*, Oct. 20, 1955, 6.

59. For resistance to integration, see Derrick A. Bell Jr., "*Brown v. Board of Education* and the Interest-Convergence Dilemma," *Harvard Law Review* 93, no. 3 (Jan. 1980): 518–33.

60. "Polio Vaccination Program Begun for Houston Children," *Houston Home Journal* (Perry, GA), Apr. 21, 1955, 1.

61. "White Students in First–Second Grades to Get Salk Polio Shots Thursdays," *Jackson (GA) Progress-Argus*, Apr. 21, 1955, 1.

62. "Salk Polio Shots to Be Delayed until Government Checks Safety of Vaccine," *Jackson (GA) Progress-Argus*, May 12, 1955, 1.

63. Leila Calhoun Deasy, "Socio-economic Status and Participation in the Poliomyelitis Vaccine Trial," *American Sociological Review* 21, no. 2 (Apr. 1956): 185–91. Also see Leo Morris, "Further Analysis of National Participation in the Inactivated Poliomyelitis Vaccination Program, 1955–61," *PHR* 79 no. 6

(June 1964): 469–80. A large survey in California drew similar conclusions—
see CDPH, *California Health Survey 1956, Vol. 1* (Berkeley: CDPH, 1958).

64. This event is briefly described in multiple sources, e.g., Oshinsky, *Polio*, 198;
Jane S. Smith, *Patenting the Sun: Polio and the Salk Vaccine* (New York: W.
Morrow, 1990), 273; Rogers, "Race and the Politics of Polio," 793.

65. Black children in Butler received their shots at the Choctaw County Training
School at Lisman. The other centers included the American Legion Hall in
Butler and the Reserve Armory at Gilberton, where both whites and Blacks
received their shots. The article makes no mention of segregation imposed at
the legion hall and armory, though it may have occurred. "854 County Pupils
Receive Salk Polio Vaccine Shots," *Choctaw Advocate* (Butler, AL), Apr. 28,
1955, 1.

66. John C. Belcher, "Acceptance of the Salk Polio Vaccine," *Rural Sociology* 23,
no. 2 (June 1958): 158–70.

67. Belcher, "Acceptance of the Salk Polio Vaccine," 164–65.

68. Belcher, "Acceptance of the Salk Polio Vaccine," 170. Chart 5.3 includes the four
most important sources of information for Blacks identified in Belcher's table.
The only category of response not included is "never heard of it."

69. Belcher, "Acceptance of the Salk Polio Vaccine," 163.

70. Belcher, "Acceptance of the Salk Polio Vaccine," 163.

71. CDPH, *California Health Survey 1956, Vol. 1*, chap. 1, 8.

72. *California Health Survey, Vol. 1*, chap. 3, 2–3.

73. *California Health Survey, Vol. 1*, chap. 3, 5, 11.

74. Tables 401 and 411, *California Health Survey, Vol. 1*, chap. 4 appendix, n.p.

75. *California Health Survey 1956*, chap. 1, 3. "US Health Authorities Still Confident
of Salk Vaccine," *Santa Cruz (CA) Sentinel*, Apr. 28, 1955, 1; "Vaccine Held Up;
Napa Supply Ready," *Napa Valley (CA) Register*, May 19, 1955, 1.

76. *California Health Survey, Vol. 1*, chap. 4, 3.

77. *California Health Survey, Vol. 1*, chap. 4, 12.

78. Monroe G. Sirkin, "National Participation Trends, 1955–61 in the Poliomyelitis
Vaccination Program," *PHR* 77, no. 8 (Aug. 1962): 667. For the decline in cases,
see "Table 2. Poliomyelitis Cases Reported in 1956 and 1957 by State and
Paralytic Status," in Lauri D. Thrupp, Helen E. Forester, and Jacob A. Brody,
"Poliomyelitis in the United States, 1957," *PHR* 74, no. 6 (June 1959): 540.

79. HEW, *Annual Report, 1958* (Washington DC: GPO, 1958), 58.

80. Smith, Wood, and Darden, "Highlights of Historical Events Leading to National
Surveillance of Vaccination Coverage in the United States." For statistics on race
and vaccination from 1955–61, see Morris, "Further Analysis of National
Participation in the Inactivated Poliomyelitis Vaccination Program, 1955–61."

81. Reimert T. Ravenholt, "Poliomyelitis in an Immunized Community," *PHR* 76,
no. 2 (Feb. 1961): 166–78. The quote is on p. 166.

82. Morris, "Further Analysis of National Participation in the Inactivated Poliomy-elitis Vaccination Program, 1955–61."

83. *SL* 39 (Mar. 1957): 4.

84. Irwin Rosenstock, Mayhew Derryberry, and Barbara Carriger, "Why People Fail to Seek Poliommyelitis Vaccination," *PHR* 74, no. 2 (Feb. 1959): 98–103.

85. Joseph G. Molner and George H. Agate, "Final Report of Poliomyelitis Epidemic in Detroit and Wayne County, 1958," *PHR* 75, no.11 (Nov. 1960): 1031–43.

86. "Des Moines Has Polio Epidemic," *Desert Sun* (Palm Springs, CA), July 10, 1959, 1.

87. Tom D. Y. Chin and William M. Marine, "The Changing Pattern of Poliomy-elitis Observed in Two Urban Epidemics," *PHR* 76, no. 7 (July 1961): 553–63.

88. "Polio Still Powerful," *Calexico (CA) Chronicle*, Nov. 15, 1958, 2; "Polio Epidemic May Still Strike State Unless More Take Vaccine," *Calexico Chronicle*, Dec. 27, 1958, 2. In some areas of the country, a lack of funding made problems worse, because by 1959, March of Dimes coffers were running low.

89. In 1941, only eighteen states required vaccination against smallpox or other diseases for school attendance regardless of the threat of disease, and fourteen allowed for the exclusion of unvaccinated students only when smallpox threatened. See William Fowler, "Principal Provisions of Smallpox Vaccination Laws and Regulations in the United States," *PHR* 56, no. 5 (Jan. 31, 1941): 173.

90. HEW, "Georgia," *State School Legislation, 1957* (Washington DC: GPO, 1958), 44–45. The quote is on p. 44. Charles L. Jackson, "State Laws on Compulsory Immunization in the United States," *PHR* 84, no. 9 (Sept. 1969): 787–95.

91. Oshinsky, *Polio*, 255–68. Marc A. Shampo, Robert A. Kyle, and David P. Steensma, "Albert Sabin—Conqueror of Poliomyelitis," *Mayo Clinic Proceedings* 86, no. 7 (July 2011): 44.

92. Oral history interview with Mary Duncan, RHCOHP.

93. "Should Polio Shots Be Made Compulsory?," *Evening Times* (Sayre, PA), June 7, 1961, 4.

94. Elena Conis and Jonathan Kuo, "Historical Origins of the Personal Belief Exemption to Polio Vaccination Mandates: The View from California," *Journal of the History of Medicine and Allied Sciences* 76, no. 2 (Feb. 24, 2021): 173–75.

95. "A.B. 1940, chap. 837, [1961], Governor's Chapter Bill files, Governor's Papers, CSA; California State Department of Education, "Health and Safety: Legal Provisions for Polio Immunization Changed in California Administrative Code," *California Schools* 33, no. 1 (1962): 30. Also see discussion in chapter 7.

96. US Congress, *Hearings before the Committee on Interstate and Foreign Commerce: Eighty-Seventh Congress, Second Session on H.R. 10541, May 15 and 16, 1962* (Washington DC: GPO, 1962), 14; CDC, *Measles Surveillance: Report, No. 10, 1973–1976* (Atlanta, GA: CDC, 1977), 20; US Congress, *A Review of Selected Federal Vaccine and Immunization Policies Based on Case Studies of*

Pneumococcal Vaccine (Washington, DC: GPO, 1979), 86. As of 1969, twenty-six states and the District of Columbia had passed new school vaccination laws requiring inoculation against polio. All state laws allowed exemptions for medical reasons. California's law also allowed religious or philosophical exemptions. "New Law Now in Effect in State: Polio Shots Needed by All School Kids," *Mill Valley (CA) Record*, Jan. 17, 1962, 5; California Legislature, "Assembly Bill no. 1940," *Assembly Bills, Original and Amended, Number 1901–2050* (Sacramento, CA: State Printing Office, 1961); CDC, "Polio Elimination in the United States," https://www.cdc.gov/polio/what-is-polio/polio-us.html.

97. HEW, "Table 1–9. Death Rates for 60 Selected Causes, by 10-Year Age Groups, Color, and Sex, United States, 1962," *VSUS, 1962, Volume II—Mortality, Part A* (Washington DC: GPO, 1964), sec. 1–10.

98. "Kennedy Calls for 'Mass Immunization' against Diseases," *Wall Street Journal*, Jan. 12, 1962), 2; US Senate Committee on Labor and Public Welfare, *Vaccination Assistance Act of 1962: Report to Accompany H.R. 10541* (Washington DC: GPO, 1962); CDC, "Polio Elimination in the United States."

99. By 1962, seven states had passed laws requiring vaccination against polio: California, Kansas, Kentucky, Michigan, Missouri, North Carolina, and Ohio, and by 1969, twenty-six states plus the District of Columbia had passed laws requiring vaccination against polio and other childhood diseases for school admission. US Congress, *Hearings before the Committee on Interstate and Foreign Commerce: Eighty-Seventh Congress, Second Session on H.R. 10541, May 15 and 16, 1962*, 14; CDC, *Measles Surveillance: Report, No. 10, 1973–1976*, 20; U.S. Congress, *A Review of Selected Federal Vaccine and Immunization Policies Based on Case Studies of Pneumococcal Vaccine*, 86.

100. CDC, "Polio Elimination in the United States."

Chapter 6. Schools in the Age of Eradication

1. "President Kennedy Calls for 'Quest for Peace': Brief Address Follows Oath Taking Rite," *Daily News-Post* (Monrovia, CA), Jan. 20, 1961, 1–2. The quote is on p. 2.

2. "President Seeks Mass Immunization," *Times Record* (Troy, NY), Jan. 11, 1962, 12.

3. For the shift toward eradication, see F. Fenner, A. J. Hall, and W. R. Dowdle, "What Is Eradication?," in *The Eradication of Infectious Diseases*, ed. W. R. Dowdle and D. R. Hopkins (New York: John Wiley & Sons, 1998), 9; James Colgrove, *State of Immunity: The Politics of Vaccination in Twentieth-Century America* (Berkeley: University of California Press, 2006), 149–85. Also see Frank M. Snowden, *Epidemics and Society: From the Black Death to the Present* (New Haven, CT: Yale University Press, 2019), 385–87.

4. Michael Dwyer, *Strangling Angel: Diphtheria and Childhood Immunization in Ireland* (Liverpool, UK: Liverpool University Press, 2018), 1–12; John R.

Murphy, "Corynebacterium Diphtheriae," in *Medical Microbiology*, ed. Samuel Baron, 4th ed. (Galveston: University of Texas Medical Branch at Galveston, 1996), chap. 32, https://www.ncbi.nlm.nih.gov/books/NBK7971.

5. Murphy, "Corynebacterium Diphtheriae"; Dwyer, *Strangling Angel*, 1–12.

6. "A Patent for Diphtheria Antitoxin Recently Granted in the United States," *Lancet* 2 (Aug. 20, 1898): 502; Colgrove, *State of Immunity*, 81–84.

7. Edward S. Godfrey, "Division of Communicable Diseases," in *Forty-Fifth Annual Report of the State Department of Health for the Year Ending December 31, 1924* (Albany, NY: J. B. Lyon Co., 1925), 1:137.

8. Anna M. Acosta et al., "Diphtheria," in *Epidemiology and Prevention of Vaccine-Preventable Diseases*, ed. Elisha Hall, A. Patricia Wodi, Jennifer Hamborsky, et al., 14th ed. (Washington, DC: Public Health Foundation, 2021), https://www.cdc.gov/vaccines/pubs/pinkbook/downloads/dip.pdf; United States, *Mortality Statistics 1933: Thirty-Fourth Annual Report* (Washington DC: GPO, 1936), 37.

9. S. P. Tejpratap et al., "Tetanus," in *Epidemiology and Prevention of Vaccine-Preventable Diseases*, https://www.cdc.gov/vaccines/pubs/pinkbook/tetanus.html.

10. E. Kuchar, M. Karlikowska-Skwarnik, S. Han, and A. Nitsch-Osuch, "Pertussis: History of the Disease and Current Prevention Failure," in *Pulmonary Dysfunction and Disease*, ed. Mieczyslaw Pokorski (Cham, Switzerland: Springer, 2016), 77–82.

11. Abraham Ribicoff to John W. McCormack, Speaker of the House of Representatives, Feb. 27, 1962, in US Congress, House Committee on Interstate and Foreign Commerce, *Intensive Immunization Programs* (Washington, DC: GPO, 1962), 1–2.

12. "Kennedy Calls for 'Mass Immunization' against Diseases," *Wall Street Journal*, Jan. 12, 1962, 2; US Senate Committee on Labor and Public Welfare, *Vaccination Assistance Act of 1962: Report to Accompany H.R. 10541* (Washington, DC: GPO, 1962).

13. William Kelsay, a colleague of Teague's in Kentucky, provides a brief overview of Teague's career in "Oral History Interview with William Kelsay," RHCOHP.

14. "Statement of Dr. Russell E. Teague, Commissioner of Health, Frankfort, KY., on Behalf of the American Public Health Association," US Congress, House, *Hearings before the Committee on Interstate and Foreign Commerce: Eighty-Seventh Congress, Second Session on H.R. 10541, May 15 and 16, 1962* (Washington, DC: GPO, 1962), 8–9.

15. "Statement of Dr. Russell E. Teague," 13.

16. Fenner, Hall, and Dowdle, "What Is Eradication?" 9; Colgrove, *State of Immunity*, 154–56.

17. "Statement of Dr. Russell E. Teague," 13–14. According to the list Teague provided Congress, the states with compulsory vaccination laws requiring

immunization against smallpox were Arkansas, California, District of Columbia, Hawaii, Kansas, Kentucky, Maryland, Massachusetts, Michigan, Missouri, New Hampshire, New Mexico, New York, North Carolina, Ohio, Pennsylvania, Rhode Island, South Carolina, Virginia, and West Virginia. Of these, California, North Carolina, and Ohio had added polio, and West Virginia had added diphtheria. Hawaii required immunization against smallpox, diphtheria, and typhoid. Kansas, Kentucky, Michigan, Missouri, North Carolina, and Ohio were already requiring vaccination against the four diseases recommended in the proposed act.

18. "Statement of Dr. Russell E. Teague," 13.
19. Thomas D. Wood, Committee on the School Child, "Section III—Education and Training," White House Conference on Child Health and Protection, *The Administration of the School Health Program* (New York: New Century Co., 1932), 29n15.
20. Oral history interview with William Kelsay, conducted by Tom Gatewood, July 14, 1982, RHCOHP.
21. "Statement of Miss Frances Adelhardt, McLean, VA," in US Congress, House, *Hearings before the Committee* [. . .] *H.R. 10541*, 40–41. The quote is on p. 41. "Statement of Mrs. Iva Perdue," in US Congress, House, *Hearings before the Committee* [. . .] *H.R. 10541*, 128–29.
22. "Statement of Dr. J. Buroughs Stokes," in US Congress, House, *Hearings before the Committee* [. . .] *H.R. 10541*, 24–40. The quotes are on p. 25.
23. "Statement of Clinton R. Miller, Assistant to the President, National Health Federation, Washington D.C.," US Congress, House, *Hearings before the Committee* [. . .] *H.R. 10541*, 80–86.
24. US Congress, House, H.R. 10541—Public Law 87-868, approved Oct. 23, 1962, 1156, https://www.govinfo.gov/content/pkg/STATUTE-76/pdf/STATUTE-76-Pg1155.pdf.
25. James Colgrove and Abigail Lowin, "A Tale of Two States: Mississippi, West Virginia, and Exemptions to Compulsory School Vaccination Laws," *Health Affairs* 35, no. 2 (Feb. 2016): https://doi.org/10.1377/hlthaff.2015.1172; "Not Immunized: Schools Could Reject 1,500," *Buckley (WV) Post-Herald*, May 5, 1957, 1.
26. Colgrove and Lowin, "A Tale of Two States." For religious exemptions, see CDC, *Measles Surveillance Report No. 11, 1977–1981* (Atlanta, GA: CDC, 1982), 29. For the rise in personal belief exemptions, see chapter 8.
27. US Congress, House, *Hearings before the Committee* [. . .] *H.R. 10541*, 60–62.
28. Michigan State Board of Health, "Table 2. Exhibiting, Relative to 96 Outbreaks, 927 Cases of Measles, in Michigan, in 1887," in *Sixteenth Annual Report of the Secretary of the State Board of Health of the State of Michigan* [. . .] *June 30, 1888* (Lansing MI: Darius D. Thorp, 1889), 270. Also see Brooklyn Department of Health, "Table of Measles, 1893," in *Annual Report of the Commissioner*

of the Department of Health of the City of Brooklyn [. . .] *for the Year 1893* (Brooklyn, NY, 1894), 23.

29. CDC, "Measles (Rubeola)," https://www.cdc.gov/measles/about/index.html, accessed Oct. 1, 2021.

30. US Congress, Senate, *Labor—Health, Education and Welfare Appropriations for Fiscal Year 1967: Hearings before the Subcommittee of the Committee on Appropriations, United States Senate, Eighty-Ninth Congress, Second Session on H.R. 14745* (Washington, DC: GPO, 1966), 642.

31. John F. Kennedy Library, "John F. Kennedy and People with Intellectual Disabilities, https://www.jfklibrary.org/learn/about-jfk/jfk-in-history/john-f -kennedy-and-people-with-intellectual-disabilities.

32. "Discuss Elimination of Child Diseases," *Waukesha (WI) Daily Freeman*, Apr. 22, 1966, 5.

33. "Many Children Suffer Needlessly: U.S. Has Power to Stop Measles," *Greenville (OH) Advocate*, Sept. 26, 1967, 2.

34. "Measles Shots Will Be Given 6,700 Children," *Idaho State Journal* (Pocatello), Dec. 31, 1967, 2.

35. The Lions Club in Liberty, Texas, helped publicize the effort there. See "Remember Those Measles 'Shots,'" *Liberty Vindicator* (Liberty, TX), May 25, 1967, 4.

36. Senator Gordon Cologne to Governor Ronald Reagan, July 31, 1967; Vernon L. Sturgeon and Jack B. Lindsey, "Bill Memorandum" to Governor Reagan, Aug. 7, 1967; "Senate Bill No. 288," S.B. 288 Reg. Sess., chap. 1021, Governor's Chapter Bill Files, Governor's Papers, CSA.

37. Kay Rogers to Ronald Reagan, August 6, 1967, S.B. 288 Reg. Sess., chap. 1021, Governor's Chapter Bill Files, Governor's Papers, CSA.

38. Charles L. Jackson, "State Laws on Compulsory Immunization in the United States," *PHR* 84 (1969): 787–95. The seventeen states that passed laws requiring measles vaccination for school were Arkansas, California, Georgia, Hawaii, Illinois, Kansas, Kentucky, Louisiana, Massachusetts, Michigan, Minnesota, Mississippi, New Jersey, New York, Rhode Island, Tennessee, and West Virginia. "Common Measles—Once Nearly Wiped Out—Sweep U.S.," *Amarillo (TX) Globe-Times*, Mar. 11, 1970, 6.

39. CDC, *MMWR* 20, no. 5 (Feb. 6, 1971): 33; CDC, "Table 1: Reported Cases of Measles [. . .]," *Measles Surveillance Report No. 9, 1972 Summary* (Atlanta, GA: CDC, 1973), 2.

40. "Apathy Blamed for Rise in Children's Diseases," *Idaho Free Press* (Nampa), Sept. 26, 1975, 3.

41. *Statement by Dr. Foege in Departments of Labor and Health, Education, and Welfare Appropriations for 1978: Hearings before a Subcommittee of the Committee on Appropriations, House of Representative,. Ninety-Fifth Congress, First Session, Wed. March 2, 1977* (Washington, DC: GPO, 1977), 38.

42. "Doctor Sees Red in Measles Fight," *Grand Prairie (TX) Daily News*, June 8, 1971; "Measles on Rise in Nation," *Waxahachie (TX) Daily Light*, July 29, 1971, 9; "Measles Epidemic Predicted 1972–73," *Waco (TX) Citizen*, Oct. 28, 1971. The quote is on p. 12.

43. "Accent on Health," *Fredericksburg (TX) Standard*, June 4, 1975, 10. Lon Gee and R. F. Sowell Jr., "A School Immunization Law Is Successful in Texas," *PHR* 90, no. 1 (Jan.–Feb. 1975): 21–24.

44. CDC, "Surveillance Summary: Measles—United States, First 40 Weeks, 1972," *MMWR* 21, no. 47 (Nov. 25, 1972): 403.

45. A search of "student immunization" in Wisconsin newspapers on www.newspapers .com reveals this was a common practice across the state. "Immunization Clinics Set Up in Manitowoc," *Manitowoc (WI) Herald-Times*, Oct. 5, 1974, 2.

46. See "Childhood Diseases Reported on the Rise," *Waukesha (WI) Daily Freeman*, Dec. 16, 1974, 1. "Immunization Remains Important," *Waukesha Daily Freeman*, Mar. 1, 1975. The quote is on p. 6.

47. "State Immunization Law Now Being Implemented," *Reporter* (Fond du Lac, WI), Sept. 25, 1975, 2.

48. CDC, *Immunization against Disease 1980* (Atlanta, GA: 1980).

49. US Department of Health and Human Services, "Prevention Highlights," *Prevention '80* (Washington, DC: GPO, 1980), 3.

50. J. P. Middaugh and L. D. Zyla, "Enforcement of School Immunization Law in Alaska," *JAMA* 239, no. 20 (May 19, 1978): 2128–30.

51. US Congress, House of Representatives, *National Child Immunization Programs: Hearing before the Subcommittee on Oversight and Investigations* [...] *Ninety-Fifth Congress, First Session, August 31, 1977* (Washington, DC: GPO, 1977), 17.

52. US Congress, House of Representatives, *National Child Immunization Programs*, 51.

53. "Senate Bill no. 942," S.B. 942, Reg. Sess., chap. 1176, Chapter Bill Files, Governor's Papers, CSA (hereafter S.B. 942, Chapter Bill Files, CSA), 3–5. The quote is on p. 5.

54. Senator Omer L. Rains, Senate Democratic Caucus, May 25, 1977, Senate Democratic Caucus, Chapter Bill Files, CSA.

55. The Bill file includes a letter from Ronald R. McKinley, chief deputy superintendent of education to Gov. Edmund G. Brown and telegrams from school nurses and other individuals asking the governor to veto the bill because it no longer included the funding necessary to do the work. S.B. 942, Chapter Bill Files, CSA.

56. US Congress, *National Child Immunization Programs*, 60.

57. "Measles Prober: School Lax on Vaccination Law," *Daily Herald* (Chicago), May 26, 1971, 37.

58. Charles L. Jackson, "Effect of a State Law Intended to Require Immunization of Elementary School Children," Communicable Disease Control Conference, Houston Texas, March 13–16, 1972, 96–99.

59. Turrell quoted in US Congress, *National Child Immunization Programs*, 60.

60. Barry Ensminger, "Political Commitment to Immunization Programs at the Local Level," *15th Immunization Conference Proceedings, March 10–13, 1980, Denver, Colorado* (Atlanta, GA: CDC, 1980), 26–28. Also see Colgrove, *State of Immunity*, 202–3.

61. The quotes are from a later interview conducted with Gelati, in Gilda Williams, "Laws Shoot for Healthy Pupils, Society," *Southtown Star* (Tinley Park, IL), Mar. 31, 1991, 9.

62. US Congress, *National Child Immunization Programs*, 9.

63. Philip P. Landrigan, "Epidemic Measles in a Divided City," *JAMA* 221, no. 6 (1972): 567–70.

64. CDC, "Measles and School Immunization Requirements—United States," *MMWR* 27 (1978): 303–4; K. B. Robbins, A. D. Brandling-Bennett, and A. R. Hinman, "Low Measles Incidence: Association with Enforcement of School Immunization Laws," *American Journal of Public Health* 71 (1981): 270–74; "Percentage of Immunized Youths Tops," *Fairbanks (AK) Daily News*, Oct. 13, 1977, 2.

65. "Big Measles Outbreak on Coast Threatens Serious Complications," *New York Times*, Jan. 27, 1977, 14; Jon Nordheimer, "Measles Outbreaks Fuel Vaccine Debate, *New York Times*, May 16, 1977, 1.

66. Department of Health, Education, and Welfare, "Surgeon General Calls Immunization Levels 'A Dramatic Success,'" *Programs for the Handicapped* (Nov./Dec. 1979): 6.

67. See "Table 1–25. Deaths from 282 Selected Causes, by 5-Year Age Groups, Race, and Sex [...] 1980," in *VSUS 1980*, vol. 2, *Mortality*, part A (Washington, DC: GPO, 1985), 244.

68. Marie M. Ready, *Physical Education in American Colleges and Universities*, Bulletin No. 14, Department of the Interior, Bureau of Education (Washington, DC: GPO, 1927), 3, 47.

69. CDC, "Measles—United States, First 26 Weeks, 1984," *MMWR* 33, no. 35 (Sept. 7, 1984); "Measles Cases Point to Urgency of Shots," *Southtown Star* (Tinley Park, IL), Oct. 25, 1984, 21; CDC, "Current Trends: Immunization Practices in Colleges," *MMWR* 36, no. 14 (April 17, 1987): 209–12.

Chapter 7. Vaccine Hesitancy and the Rise of Personal Belief Exemptions

1. *Reyes v. Wyeth* 498 F.2d 1264 (5th Cir., 1974), *cert. denied*, 419 U.S. 1096, 95 S. Ct. 687, 42 L. Ed. 2d 688 (1974). An earlier precedent for this case is *Davis v. Wyeth*, 399 F.2d. 121 (1968).

2. In 1984, scientists working for the CDC's Immunization Program estimated that out of 3.2 million doses of Sabin vaccine, one person had been infected with

paralytic polio, a finding that made the news. See Walter A. Orenstein et al., "Risks from Polio Vaccination—Reply," *JAMA* 251, no. 6 (Feb. 10, 1984): 728–29; Philip Boffey, "Vaccine Liability Threatens Supplies," *New York Times*, June 26, 1984, C1.

3. "Better living through chemistry" is a popular shortening of a former DuPont Corporation tagline. Anna McCarthy, *The Citizen Machine: Governing by Television in 1950s America* (New York: New York University Press, 2013), 44.

4. Rachel Carson, *Silent Spring* (Cambridge, MA: Houghton Mifflin, 1962). "Pesticide Controversy," *Holland (MI) Evening Sentinel*, Aug. 9, 1965, 9; US Congress, Senate, *Interagency Environmental Hazards Coordination: Pesticides and Public Policy, 89th Congress, 2d Session* [. . .] *July 21, 1966* (Washington, DC: GPO, 1966). Elena Conis, *Vaccine Nation: America's Changing Relationship with Immunization* (Chicago: University of Chicago Press, 2015), 131–60.

5. For the Progressive Era back-to-nature movement and its twentieth-century revival, see Peter Schmitt, *Back to Nature: The Arcadian Myth in Urban America* (New York: Oxford University Press, 1969).

6. Wendy Kline, *Bodies of Knowledge: Sexuality, Reproduction, and Women's Health in the Second Wave* (Chicago: University of Chicago Press, 2010), 1–4, 73–74, 116–18.

7. Georgine M. Pion and Mark W. Lipsey, "What Have the Surveys Told Us?," *Public Opinion Quarterly* 45, no. 3 (Autumn 1981): 303–16; National Science Board, *Science at the Bicentennial: A Report from the Research Community* (Washington, DC: GPO, 1976), 71–91.

8. Pion and Lipsey, "What Have the Surveys Told Us?" 304.

9. CDC, "Public Health Service Recommendation on Smallpox Vaccination," *MMRW* 20, no. 38 (Sept. 25, 1971): 339. Michael A. Willrich, *Pox: An American History* (New York: Penguin, 2011), 339–40. For contemporary statistics of deaths from the smallpox vaccine, see J. Michael Lane et al., "Complications of Smallpox Vaccination, 1968," *NEJM* 281 (Nov. 27, 1969): 1201–8.

10. "Lawrence Lamb, 1926–2015," *San Antonio (TX) Express-News*, July 12, 2015; "The Doctor Says," *Salem (OH) News*, Aug. 23, 1972, 16.

11. "Board Will Discuss Vaccination Policy," *Bridgeport (CT) Post*, Jan. 3, 1972, 2. Information about Haberlin is in Connecticut newspapers, e.g., "Schools 'Catching Up' on Polio Vaccine Shots," *Bridgeport Telegram*, Apr. 17, 1963, 27. Dr. Harris's quote is in "School Board Will Consider End of Smallpox Vaccinations," *Bridgeport Post*, Jan. 12, 1972, 8.

12. "Smallpox Vaccination No Longer Health Requirement," *Zenia (OH) Daily Gazette*, Jan. 22, 1972, 7.

13. James Wisecup, "Teacher Bargaining Completed," *Piqua (OH) Daily Call*, Mar. 4, 1972, 4; "Madison Won't Require Smallpox Vaccinations," *News-Journal* (Mansfield, OH), Apr. 15, 1972, 11.

14. Mary Jane Griffin and her husband sued the US government under the Federal Tort Claims Act, 28 U.S.C. 1346(b), 2761 et seq.; *Griffin v. United States*, 351 F. Supp. 10 (Nov. 7, 1972).

15. Colgrove, *State of Immunity: The Politics of Vaccination in Twentieth-Century America* (Berkeley: University of California Press, 2006), 201–2.

16. US Congress, Senate, *Polio Immunization Program: Hearing before the Subcommittee on Health of the Committee on Labor and Public Welfare,* [. . .] *Ninety-Fourth Congress* (Washington, DC: GPO, 1976), 144; National Research Council (US) Division of Health Promotion and Disease Prevention, "Appendix E, Vaccine-Injury Compensation in Other Countries," in *Vaccine Supply and Innovation* (Washington, DC: National Academies Press, 1985).

17. National Academies of Sciences et al., *Reproducibility and Replicability in Science* (Washington, DC: National Academies Press, 2019), 1–5.

18. CDC, "DTP Vaccination and Sudden Infant Deaths—Tennessee," *MMWR* 28, no. 11 (Mar. 23, 1979): 131–32; Associated Press, "Baby Vaccine Recall Ordered," *San Bernardino County (CA) Sun*, Mar. 22, 1979, 1.

19. David L. Miller et al., "Pertussis Immunisation and Serious Acute Neurological Illness in Children," *British Medical Journal* 282 (May 16, 1981): 1595–99; Paul A. Offit, *Deadly Choices: How the Anti-vaccine Movement Threatens Us All* (New York: Basic Books, 2011), 17–18.

20. Canadian National Advisory Committee on Immunization, Minister of National Health and Welfare, National Advisory Committee on Immunization, *Canadian Immunization Guide*, 3rd ed. (Ottawa, Canada: Minister of National Health and Welfare, 1989), 78–83; Institute of Medicine, *Adverse Effects of Pertussis and Rubella Vaccines: A Report of the Committee to Review the Adverse Consequences of Pertussis and Rubella Vaccines* (Washington, DC: National Academies Press, 1991); James L. Gale et al., "Risk of Serious Acute Neurological Illness after Immunization with Diphtheria-Tetanus-Pertussis Vaccine: A Population-Based Case-Control Study," *JAMA* 271, no. 1 (Jan. 5, 1994): 37–41; Offit, *Deadly Choices*, 28–32.

21. *DPT: Vaccine Roulette*, WRC-TV (Washington, DC), Apr. 19, 1982; Offit, *Deadly Choices*, 2–6. The quote is on p. 2.

22. Schwartz quoted in "Parents Fight to Make Vaccines Safer," *Salina (KS) Journal*, Dec. 30, 1984, 23. Also see Arthur Allen, "Questions for Barbara Loe Fisher on the Costs of Vaccination," *New York Times*, May 6, 2001, https://www.nytimes.com/2001/05/06/magazine/questions-for-barbara-loe-fisher-on-the-costs-of-vaccination.html.

23. A search of digital newspaper collections reveals that papers across the country published the report, e.g., Chris Collins and John Hanchette, Gannett News Service, "Controversy Grows over Value, Safety of Vaccines," *San Bernardino County (CA) Sun*, Dec. 16, 1984, 1, 4.

24. US Congress, Senate, *Hearing before the Committee on Labor and Human Resources* [...] *Ninety-Ninth Congress* [...] *on S. 827* (Washington, DC: GPO, 1985).

25. "100 Stat. 3743, Public Law 99–660, Nov. 14, 1986, 99th Congress," https://www.govinfo.gov/content/pkg/STATUTE-100/pdf/STATUTE-100-Pg3743 .pdf#page=57; Health Resources and Services Administration, "National Vaccine Injury Compensation Program," in *Public Health Service Act (1986), Sect. 2111*, 1311–14, https://www.hrsa.gov/sites/default/files/hrsa/vaccine -compensation/about/title-xxi-phs-vaccines-1517.pdf. For an overview, see Institute of Medicine (US) Committee on Review of Priorities in the National Vaccine Plan, *Priorities for the National Vaccine Plan* (Washington, DC: National Academies Press, 2010); Violane S. Mitchell, Nalini M. Philipose, and Jay P. Sanford, eds., *The Children's Vaccine Initiative: Achieving the Vision* (Washington, DC: National Academies Press, 1993).

26. CDC, *Epidemiology and Prevention of Vaccine-Preventable Diseases*, ed. Elisha Hall et al., 14th ed. (Washington, DC: Public Health Foundation, 2021); Stanley A. Plotkin, Walter A. Orenstein, and Paul A. Offit, eds., *Vaccines* (Edinburgh, UK: Elsevier Health Sciences, 2012), 95.

27. See, e.g., Philip I. Markowitz, "Autism in a Child with Congenital Cytomegalo-virus Infection," *Journal of Autism and Developmental Disorders* 13 (Sept. 1983): 249–53; Marie M. Bristol et al., "State of the Science in Autism: Report to the National Institutes of Health," *Journal of Autism and Developmental Disorders* 26 (Apr. 1996): 121–54.

28. CDC, "Autism Spectrum Disorder (ASD)," https://www.cdc.gov/ncbddd /autism/facts.html; Andrew J. Wakefield et al., "Ileal-Lymphoid-Nodular Hyperplasia, Non-specific Colitis, and Pervasive Developmental Disorder in Children," *Lancet* 351, no. 9103 (Feb. 28, 1998): 637–41.

29. See Colgrove, *State of Immunity*, 229.

30. Richard Horton, "A Statement by the Editors of *The Lancet*," *Lancet* 363, no. 9411 (Mar. 6, 2004): https://doi.org/10.1016/S0140-6736(04)15699-7; Fiona Godlee, Jane Smith, and Harvey Marcovitch, "Wakefield's Article Linking MMR Vaccine and Autism Was Fraudulent," *BMJ* 342 (Mar. 15, 2011): https://doi.org/10.1136/bmj.d1678; Laura Eggertson, "*Lancet* Retracts 12-Year-Old Article Linking Autism to MMR Vaccines," *Canadian Medical Association Journal* 182, no. 4 (Mar. 9, 2010): 199–200; Reuters, "Update 1-Autism-Vaccine Researcher a 'Fraud'-Medical Journal," Jan. 5, 2011, https://www.reuters.com/article/autism-vaccines/update-1-autism-vaccine-researcher-a -fraud-medical-journal-idUSN053966320110106.

31. Institute of Medicine, *Vaccine Safety Research, Data Access, and Public Trust* (Washington, DC: National Academies Press, 2004).

32. Department of Developmental Services, *Autistic Spectrum Disorders: Changes in the California Caseload; An Update; 1999 through 2002* (Sacramento: California

Health and Human Services Agency, 2003); "Best Practices for Designing and Delivering Effective Programs for Individuals with Autistic Spectrum Disorders: Recommendations of the Collaborative Work Group on Autistic Spectrum Disorders" (Sacramento: California Department of Education, 1997); "State Study Finds Sharp Rise in Autism Rate," *Los Angeles Times*, Apr. 16, 1999, https://www.latimes.com/archives/la-xpm-1999-apr-16-mn-28029-story.html.

33. Lisa A. Croen et al., "The Changing Prevalence of Autism in California," *Journal of Autism and Developmental Disorders* 32, no. 3 (June 2002): 207–15; Paul T. Shattuck, "The Contribution of Diagnostic Substitution to the Growing Administrative Prevalence of Autism in US Special Education," *Pediatrics* 117, no. 4 (2006): 1028–37; Marissa King and Peter Bearman, "Diagnostic Change and the Increased Prevalence of Autism," *International Journal of Epidemiology* 38, no. 5 (Oct. 2009): 1224–34; Ginny Russell et al., "Time Trends in Autism Diagnosis over 20 Years: A UK Population-Based Cohort Study," *Journal of Child Psychology and Psychiatry* (2021), doi: 10.1111 /jcpp.13505; Kristen Lyall et al., "The Association between Parental Age and Autism-Related Outcomes in Children at High Familial Risk for Autism," *Autism Research* 13, no. 6 (June 2020): 998–1010; Anita Thapar and Michael Rutter, "Genetic Advances in Autism," *Journal of Autism and Developmental Disorders* 51 (2021): 4321–32, https://doi.org/10.1007/s10803-020-04685-z.

34. Conis, *Vaccine Nation*, 213–15.

35. "Notice to Readers: Thimerosal in Vaccines; A Joint Statement of the American Academy of Pediatrics and the Public Health Service," *MMWR* 48, no. 26 (July 9, 1999): 563–65, https://www.cdc.gov/mmwr/preview/mmwrhtml/mm4826a3 .htm; Jeffrey P. Baker, "Mercury, Vaccines, and Autism: One Controversy, Three Histories," *American Journal of Public Health* 98, no. 2 (Feb. 2008): 244–53.

36. JAMA and Archives Journals, "Autism: Removing Thimerosal from Vaccines Did Not Reduce Autism Cases in California, Report Finds," *Science Daily* 8 (Jan. 2008), www.sciencedaily.com/releases/2008/01/080107181551.htm.

37. Salamone quoted in Jonathan Bor, "Polio Shots Safer Than Oral Vaccine," reprinted in *South Florida Sun-Sentinel* (Fort Lauderdale), Apr. 17, 1999, https://www.sun-sentinel.com/news/fl-xpm-1999-04-18-9904180354-story.html.

38. Offit, *Deadly Choices*, 77–80. Salamone is quoted on p. 80.

39. Melinda E. Wharton, "Measles Elimination in the United States," *Journal of Infectious Diseases* 189, suppl. 1 (May 2004): S1–S3; CDC, "Elimination of Rubella and Congenital Rubella Syndrome—United States, 1969–2004."

40. Arthur Allen, "Questions for Barbara Loe Fisher on the Costs of Vaccination," *New York Times*, May 6, 2001.

41. Norma J. Allred et al., "Parental Vaccine Safety Concerns: Results from the National Immunization Survey, 2001–2002," *American Journal of Preventative Medicine* 2 (Feb. 28, 2005): 221–24.

42. Quotes from Fisher, Kennedy, and Offit are in John Stossel, Kristina Kendall, and Patrick McMenamin, "Should Parents Worry about Vaccinating Their Children?," ABC News, Feb. 22, 2007, https://abcnews.go.com/2020/Health/story?id=2892683&page=1. For celebrities in the anti-vaccination movement, see Offit, *Deadly Choices*, 149–70.
43. Anna Kata, "A Postmodern Pandora's Box: Anti-vaccination Misinformation on the Internet," *Vaccine* 28 (2010): 1709–16.
44. Kim Tolley, "School Vaccination Wars: The Rise of Anti-science in the American Anti-vaccination Societies, 1879–1929," *History of Education Quarterly* 59, no. 2 (May 2019): 162, 193.
45. Associated Press, "1 in 4 Parents Buys Unproven Vaccine-Autism Link," KAIT8, Mar. 3, 2010, https://www.kait8.com/story/12075542/1-in-4-parents-buys-unproven-vaccine-autism-link; Gary L. Freed et al., "Parental Vaccine Safety Concerns in 2009," *Pediatrics* 125, no. 4 (April 2010): 654–59. Also see Kata, "A Postmodern Pandora's Box"; Paul Scullard, Clare Peacock, and Patrick Davies, "Googling Children's Health: Reliability of Medical Advice on the Internet," *Archives of Disease in Childhood* 95, no. 8 (Aug. 2010): 580–82.
46. Paul A. Offit et al., "Addressing Parents' Concerns: Do Multiple Vaccines Overwhelm or Weaken the Infant's Immune System?," *Pediatrics* 109, no. 1 (Jan. 2002): https://doi.org/10.1542/peds.109.1.124; CDC, *Epidemiology and Prevention of Vaccine-Preventable Diseases*; Plotkin, Orenstein, and Offit, *Vaccines*, 95.
47. Sarah Geoghegan, Kevin P. O'Callaghan, and Paul A. Offit, "Vaccine Safety: Myths and Misinformation," *Frontiers in Microbiology* 11, no. 372 (2020): doi: 10.3389/fmicb.2020.00372.
48. Robert Sears, *The Vaccine Book: Making the Right Decision for Your Child* (New York: Little, Brown & Co., 2007).
49. Philip J. Smith et al., "Parental Delay or Refusal of Vaccine Doses, Childhood Vaccination Coverage at 24 Months of Age, and the Health Belief Model," *PHR* 126, suppl. 2 (July–Aug. 2011): 135–46, doi: 10.1177/00333549111260S215.
50. Saad B. Omer et al., "Vaccine Refusal, Mandatory Immunization, and the Risks of Vaccine-Preventable Diseases," *NEJM* 360 (May 7, 2009): 1981–88.
51. "New Compulsory Immunization Law for Ohio Children Outlined," *Lancaster (OH) Eagle-Gazette*, July 18, 1959, 5. Also see "Act of July 7, 1959," Am H.B. no. 323, 1959 Ohio Laws, 707.
52. Adelaide M. Hunter, Robert Ortiz, and Joe Martinez, "Compulsory and Voluntary School Immunization Programs in the United States," *Journal of School Health* 33, no. 3 (Mar. 1963): 98–102.
53. Wallace F. Janssen, assistant to the commissioner of the Food and Drug Administration, HEW, "The Teacher vs. Quackery in Medicine," *Journal of the American Association for Health, Physical Education, and Recreation* (June 1954): 15–16. The quote is on p. 15.

54. For Hart's role in establishing the NHF, see Lewis A. Grossman, *Choose Your Medicine: Freedom of Therapeutic Choice in America* (New York: Oxford University Press, 2021), 128; National Health Federation, "About NHF," https://web.archive.org/web/20220306023532/https:/thenhf.com/about-nhf, accessed Oct. 13, 2022.

55. Fred J. Hart to Assemblyman Bert DeLotto [Umbert J. DeLotto], Mar. 20, 1961, Public Health Committee Files, Bill Files, Governor's Papers, CSA.

56. Don C. Matchan to Chairman William Bryon Rumford and members of the Assembly Public Health Committee, Mar. 29, 1961. Other letters referencing Sandler's book were Drusilla D. Lane to Bryon Rumford, Mar. 8, 1961; Walter L. and Jeanette M. Cooks to Bryon Rumford, Mar. 9, 1961, Public Health Committee files, CSA.

57. "Pupil Polio Shots Law Has Loophole," *Oakland (CA) Tribune*, Aug. 29, 1961, 2.

58. Fred J. Hart to Bryon Rumford, Apr. 7, 1961, Public Health Committee files, CSA.

59. Quoted in Elena Conis and Jonathan Kuo, "Historical Origins of the Personal Belief Exemption to Vaccination Mandates: The View from California," *Journal of the History of Medicine and Allied Sciences* 76, no. 2 (Feb. 24, 2021): 176.

60. *McCartney v. Austin*, 293 N.Y. S. 2d 188 (N.Y., Aug. 16, 1968).

61. *Sherr v. Northport-East Northport Union Free School Dist.*, 672 F. Supp. 81 (E.D.N.Y. 1987). Also see the earlier case, *Dalli vs. Board of Education et al.*, 358 Mass. 753, decided on Mar. 2, 1971.

62. James Colgrove and Abigail Lowin, "A Tale of Two Sates: Mississippi, West Virginia, and Exemptions to Compulsory School Vaccination Laws," *Health Affairs* 35, no. 2 (2016): 348–55; *Brown v. Stone*, 378 So.2d 218 (Miss. 1979).

63. *Boone v. Boozman*, 217 F. Supp. 2d 938 (E.D. Ark. 2002), 942. James Colgrove, *State of Immunity*, 249–50.

64. See Daniel P. Maher, "Vaccines, Abortion, and Moral Coherence," *National Catholic Bioethics Quarterly* 2, no. 1 (Spring 2002): 51–67; Edward J. Furton, "Vaccines and the Right of Conscience," *National Catholics Bioethics Quarterly* 4, no. 1 (Spring 2004): 53–62; Angel Rodríguez Luño, "Ethical Reflections on Vaccines Using Cells from Aborted Fetuses," *National Catholic Bioethics Quarterly* 6, no. 3 (Autumn 2006): 453–59.

65. CDC, "Elimination of Rubella and Congenital Rubella Syndrome—United States, 1969–2004"; Meredith Wadman, *The Vaccine Race: Science, Politics, and the Human Costs of Defeating Disease* (New York: Penguin, 2018), 107–32.

66. Elio Sgreccia to Debra L Vinnedge, June 9, 2005, Statement from the Pontifical Academy for Life, "Moral Reflections on Vaccines Prepared from Cells Derived from Aborted Human Foetuses," *National Catholic Bioethics Quarterly* 6, no. 3 (Autumn 2006): 549.

67. Tony Reichardt, David Cryanoski, and Quirin Schiermeier, "Religion and Science: Studies of Faith," *Nature* 432, no. 7018 (Dec. 9, 2004): 666–69;

Richard Kent Zimmerman, "Ethical Analysis of Vaccines Grown in Human Cell Strains Derived from Abortion: Arguments and Internet Search," *Vaccine* 22, nos. 31–32 (Oct. 22, 2004): 4238–44.

68. Saad B. Omer et al., "Nonmedical Exemptions to School Immunization Requirements: Secular Trends and Association of State Policies with Pertussis Incidence," *JAMA* 296, no. 14 (2006): 1757–63; Daniel A. Salmon et al., "Compulsory Vaccination and Conscientious or Philosophical Exemptions: Past, Present, and Future," *Lancet* (Feb. 2006): 436–42.

69. CDC, "Human Papillomavirus (HPV)," https://www.cdc.gov/hpv/index.html.

70. Becky Bright, "Majority of Americans Back HPV Vaccine, Poll Shows," *Wall Street Journal*, Aug. 8, 2006, https://www.wsj.com/articles/SB115464198706026167.

71. Editorial, "Flogging Gardasil: In Its Rush to Market Its Human Papillomavirus Vaccine, Merck Forgot to Make a Strong and Compelling Case for Compulsory Immunization," *Nature Biotechnology* 25, no. 3 (Mar. 2007): 3.

72. "Merck's Gardasil Vaccine Not Proven Safe for Little Girls: National Vaccine Information Center Criticizes FDA for Fast-Tracking Licensure," *PR Newswire*, June 27, 2006.

73. Lauri E. Markowitz et al., "Quadrivalent Human Papillomavirus Vaccine: Recommendations of the Advisory Committee on Immunization Practices (ACIP)," *MMWR* 56 (Mar. 23, 2007): 12–14. Barbara Loe Fisher, "Vaccine Freedom of Choice: Presented at the Rally for Conscientious Exemption to Vaccination October 16, 2008—Trenton, NJ," National Vaccine Information Center, https://www.nvic.org/informed-consent/freedomofchoice.aspx.

74. Diane Eicher, "Hepatitis B Vaccine Carries a Quandary: Debate Rages over Necessity of Wide Usage," *Denver Post*, June 27, 1994, F1. For debates over the hepatitis B vaccine, see Conis, *Vaccine Nation*, 194–202. For safety concerns regarding the vaccine, see Offit, *Deadly Choices*, 64–68, 87–88.

75. Laurie Udesky, "Push to Mandate HPV Vaccine Triggers Backlash in USA," *Lancet* 369, no. 9566 (Mar. 24, 2007). The mother's quote is on p. 979. "HPV," *Naples (FL) Daily News*, Feb. 23, 2007, 9.

76. Raphael P. Viscidi and Keerti V. Shah, "Should Human Papillomavirus Vaccination Be Mandatory?," *JAMA Journal of Ethics* 9, no. 12 (Dec. 2007): 823–26. The quote is on p. 824.

77. Quoted in Udesky, "Push to Mandate HPV Vaccine," 979. Also see Miriam J. Laugesen et al., "Early Policy Responses to the Human Papillomavirus Vaccine in the United States, 2006–2010," *Journal of Adolescent Health* 55, no. 5 (Nov. 2014): 659–64; "Bill Distracts from Real Cause of CPV Cancer," *Index-Journal* (Greenwood, SC), Feb. 6, 2007, 9.

78. Quoted in Udesky, "Push to Mandate HPV Vaccine," 979.

79. Virginia, Rhode Island, and Washington passed laws mandating that adolescents receive the HPV vaccine as a requirement for school admission. See Jessica

Keim-Malpass et al., "Legislative Activity Related to the Human Papillomavirus (HPV) Vaccine in the United States (2006–2015): A Need for Evidence-Based Policy," *Risk Management and Healthcare Policy* 10 (Mar. 13, 2017): https://doi.org/10.2147/RMHP.S128247.

80. Robert Griffin, Kathleen Stratton, and Rosemary Chalk, "Childhood Vaccine Finance Safety Issues," *Health Affairs* 23, no. 5 (2004): 106.

81. Andrew J. Pollard, "Childhood Immunisation: What Is the Future?," *Archives of Disease in Childhood* 92, no. 5 (May 2007): 426–33. The quote, from Paul Offit, is on p. 427.

Chapter 8. The Twenty-First-Century Effort to Preserve Immunity in Schools

1. Shots against hepatitis B and chicken pox, which the state had added to the list of required vaccines the previous year, were the inoculations children generally lacked. "Maryland School System Gets Tough, Threatens Parents with Jail for Not Vaccinating Their Kids," *Titusville (PA) Herald*, Nov. 17, 2007. The quote is on p. 11. Also see Matthew Baraakat, "Md. County Gets Tough on Vaccination," *Daily Intelligencer* (Doylestown, PA), Nov. 18, 2007, 11; "School Gets Tough on Shots," *Indiana (PA) Gazette*, Nov. 18, 2007, 12.

2. "Maryland School System Gets Tough," 11.

3. ABC News, "Md. Officials: Vaccinate Your Kids or Face Jail," Nov. 17, 2007, https://abcnews.go.com/GMA/WaterCooler/story?id=3880578&page=1.

4. All quoted in "Maryland School System Gets Tough," 11.

5. Jacqueline Gindler et al., "Acute Measles Mortality in the United States, 1987–2002, *Journal of Infectious Diseases* 189, suppl. 1 (May 2004): S69–S77. Pertussis cases increased from 4,570 in 1990 to 25,616 in 2005. CDC, "Pertussis Cases by Year (1922–2019)," https://www.cdc.gov/pertussis/surv-reporting/cases-by-year.html.

6. Saad B. Omer et al., "Vaccination Policies and Rates of Exemption from Immunization, 2005–2011," *NEJM* 367, no. 12 (Sept. 2012): 1170–71; National Vaccine Advisory Committee, "Assessing the State of Vaccine Confidence in the United States: Recommendations from the National Vaccine Advisory Committee, June 10, 2015," *PHR* 130 (Nov.–Dec. 2015): 582.

7. CDC, "Vaccination Coverage among Children in Kindergarten—United States, 2013–14 School Year," *MMWR* 63, no. 41 (Oct. 17, 2014): 913–20.

8. Daniel E. Salmon et al., "Health Consequences of Religious and Philosophical Exemptions from Immunization Laws: Individual and Societal Risk of Measles," *JAMA* 282, no. 1 (July 7, 1999): 47–53. Also see Thomas Novotny et al., "Measles Outbreaks in Religious Groups Exempt from Immunization Laws," *PHR* 103, no. 1 (Jan.–Feb. 1988): 49–54.

9. V. K. Phadke, R. A. Bednarczyk, and D. A. Salmon, "Association between Vaccine Refusal and Vaccine-Preventable Diseases in the United States: A Review of Measles and Pertussis," *JAMA* 315, no. 11 (2016): 1149–58. Also see D. R. Feikin, D. C. Lezotte, R. F. Hamman, et al., "Individual and Community Risks of Measles and Pertussis Associated with Personal Exemptions to Immunization," *JAMA* 284 (2000): 3145–50.

10. Douglas S. Diekema, "Personal Belief Exemptions from School Vaccination Requirements," *Annual Review of Public Health* 35 (2014): 280.

11. Douglas J. Opel and Douglas S. Diekema, "Finding the Proper Balance between Freedom and Justice: Why We Should Not Eliminate Vaccine Mandates," *Journal of Health Politics, Policy and Law* 37, no. 1 (Feb. 2012): 141–47; John D. Lantos, Mary Anne Jackson, and Christopher J. Harrison, "Why We Should Eliminate Personal Belief Exemptions to Vaccine Mandates," *Journal of Health, Politics, Policy and Law* 37, no. 1 (Feb. 2012): 131–40. For herd immunity, see Daniel A. Salmon et al., "Compulsory Vaccination and Conscientious or Philosophical Exemptions: Past, Present, and Future," *Lancet* 367, no. 9508 (May 4, 2006): 436–42.

12. *In re LePage*, Wyo. Stat. Ann. § 21-4-09(a) (2007). Also see *Turner v. Liverpool Central School*, 186 F. Supp. 2d 187, N.D.N.Y. (2002).

13. Anthony Ciolli, "Religious and Philosophical Exemptions to Mandatory School Vaccinations: Who Should Bear the Costs to Society?," *Missouri Law Review* 74, no. 2 (Spring 2009): 12.

14. Jennifer S. Rota et al., "Processes for Obtaining Nonmedical Exemptions to State Immunization Laws," *American Journal of Public Health* 91, no. 4 (April 2001): 645–48.

15. See Ellen De Lara, "Bullying and Violence in American Schools," in *Handbook of Children, Culture, and Violence*, ed. Nancy E. Dowd, Dorothy G. Singer, and Robin Fretwell Wilson (Thousand Oaks, CA: Sage Publications, 2006), 333–54.

16. See chapter 7 in this book.

17. US Department of Health and Human Services, *Healthy People 2000: National Health Promotion and Disease Prevention Objectives* (Washington DC: GPO, Public Health Service, 1991); Department of Health and Human Services, *HECAT: Health Education Curriculum Analysis Tool* (Atlanta, GA: CDC, 2007), 2.

18. Kylie Hall et al., "Immunization and Exemption Policies and Practices in North Dakota," North Dakota State University Center for Immunization Research and Education, June 13, 2016, https://www.health.nd.gov/sites/www/files /documents/Files/MSS/Immunizations/School_Childcare/Immunizationand ExemptionPoliciesandPracticesinNorthDakota_20160615.pdf. The quote is on

p. 3; Kylie Hall et al., "Enforcement Associated with Higher School-Reported Immunization Rates," *American Journal of Preventive Medicine* 53, no. 6 (Dec. 2017): 892–97; Warren Abrahamson, "North Dakota's Kindergarten Vaccination Rates Increase," NewsDakota.com, Feb. 27, 2017, https://www .newsdakota.com/2017/02/27/north-dakotas-kindergarten-vaccination-rates -increase.

19. Jouchens in quoted in Jennifer Brown, "Colorado's Near-Lowest Vaccination Rates Have Schools Ready to Enforce State Law to Prevent an Outbreak," *Colorado Sun* (Denver), Nov. 4, 2019, https://coloradosun.com/2019/11/04 /vaccination-exemptions-in-colorado-schools; Anusha Roy, "School Districts in Colorado Update Vaccination Policies to Comply with Decades-Old Law," 9NEWS, Nov. 4, 2019, https://www.9news.com/article/news/local/next /school-districts-in-colorado-update-vaccination-policies-to-comply-with -decades-old-law/73-1351be7b-c260-424a-bf6c-4343874acbec.

20. Ranee Seither et al., "Vaccination Coverage with Selected Vaccines and Exemption Rates among Children in Kindergarten—United States, 2019–20 School Year," *MMWR* 70, no. 3 (Jan. 22, 2021): 75–82.

21. Saad B. Omer et al., "Nonmedical Exemptions to School Immunization Requirements: Secular Trends and Association of State Policies with Pertussis Incidence," *JAMA* 296, no. 14 (Oct. 11, 2006): 1157–63; Eileen Wang et al., "Nonmedical Exemptions from School Immunization Requirements: A Systematic Review," *American Journal of Public Health* 104, no. 11 (Nov. 2014): e62–e84.

22. Denise F. Lillvis, Anna Kirkland, and Anna Frick, "Power and Persuasion in the Vaccine Debates: An Analysis of Political Outcomes in the United States, 1998–2012," *Milbank Quarterly* 92, no. 3 (Sept. 2014): 475–508.

23. Sarah Breitenback, "To Combat Disease, States Make It Harder to Skip Vaccines, PEW Charitable Trusts, May 25, 2016, https://www.pewtrusts.org/en /research-and-analysis/blogs/stateline/2016/05/25/to-combat-disease-states -make-it-harder-to-skip-vaccines; Wendy Underhill, Dan Diorio, and Kae Warnock, "State Vote: 2015 State Elections," National Conference of State Legislatures, Nov. 4, 2015, https://www.ncsl.org/research/elections-and -campaigns/statevote-2015-elections.aspx.

24. Lori Higgins, "More Michigan Parents Willing to Vaccinate Kids," *Detroit Free Press*, Jan. 28, 2016, https://www.freep.com/story/news/education/2016/01/28 /immunization-waivers-plummet-40-michigan/79427752.

25. James Colgrove and Abigail Lowin, "A Tale of Two States: Mississippi, West Virginia, and Exemptions to Compulsory School Vaccination Laws," *Health Affairs* 35, no. 2 (Feb. 2016): 348–55. Arkansas joined West Virginia and Mississippi in not allowing exemptions after a US district court ruled in 2002 that the state's religious exemption was unconstitutional. However, Arkansas legislators revised the law in 2003 to allow personal exemptions. See Daniel A.

Salmon et al., "Public Health and the Politics of School Immunization Requirements," *American Journal of Public Health* 95, no. 5 (May 2005): 778–83; *McCarthy v. Boozman*, 212 F. Supp. 2d 945 (W.D. Ark, 2002), 948.

26. Tony Yang, "Why Mississippi Hasn't Had Measles in over Two Decades," Conversation, Feb. 5, 2015, https://theconversation.com/why-mississippi-hasnt-had-measles-in-over-two-decades-37075.

27. Ciolli, "Religious and Philosophical Exemptions to Mandatory School Vaccinations," 287–99.

28. US Supreme Court, *Prince v. Commonwealth of Massachusetts*, 321 U.S. 158, Jan. 31, 1944, https://www.law.cornell.edu/supremecourt/text/321/158.

29. US Supreme Court, *Prince v. Commonwealth of* Massachusetts.

30. CDC, "Year in Review: Measles Linked to Disneyland," *Public Health Matters* (blog), https://blogs.cdc.gov/publichealthmatters/2015/12/year-in-review-measles-linked-to-disneyland; Assembly Committee on Health, "Analysis of SB 277," June 9, 2015, 10, California Legislative Information, https://leginfo.legislature.ca.gov/faces/billAnalysisClient.xhtml?bill_id=201520160SB277.

31. In 2014, California required immunization against diphtheria, haemophilus influenzae type b, measles, mumps, pertussis, poliomyelitis, rubella, tetanus, hepatitis b, and varicella. Senate Committee on Education, California Legislature, "Analysis of SB 277," April 22, 2015, 2–3, 5, California Legislative Information, https://leginfo.legislature.ca.gov/faces/billAnalysisClient.xhtml?bill_id=201520160SB277.

32. Senate Committee on Education, "Analysis of SB 277," April 22, 2015, 5.

33. Jessica E. Atwell et al., "Nonmedical Vaccine Exemptions and Pertussis in California, 2010," *Pediatrics* 132, no. 4 (Oct. 2013); 624–30; California Legislature, "Assembly Bill No. 2109 Chapter 821," Sept. 30, 2012, http://www.leginfo.ca.gov/pub/11-12/bill/asm/ab_2101-2150/ab_2109_bill_20120930_chaptered.pdf. The quote is on p. 94. Kathleen Winter et al., "California Pertussis Epidemic, 2010," *Journal of Pediatrics* 161, no. 6 (Dec. 1, 2012): 1091–96; Kathleen Winter, et al., "Pertussis Epidemic—California, 2014," *MMWR* 63, no. 48 (Dec. 5, 2014): 1129–32.

34. Robin Abcarian, "California Journal: From Young Cancer Patient's Parents, a Special Plea to Vaccinate," *Los Angeles Times*, Feb. 5, 2015, https://www.latimes.com/local/abcarian/la-me-abcarian-vaccinations-20150206-column.html.

35. Hannah Henry, interview on NAPABroadcasting.com, "The Immunization Debate Is in Sacramento, but It Hits Very Close to Home: One Napa School Is Seriously Under Immunized," n.d., http://napabroadcasting.com/one-napa-school-is-51-under-immunized-why-this-creates-risks-for-the-whole-community. Source: Vaccinatecalifornia.org, Mar. 2015.

36. Renee DiResta, "The Facebook Dilemma," interview with James Jacoby, *Frontline* (PBS), May 17, 2018, https://www.pbs.org/wgbh/frontline/interview/renee-diresta.

37. Leah Russin, cofounder and executive director of Vaccinate California, interview with author, Mar. 21, 2022; VaccinateCalifornia.org.

38. Leah Russin, interview with author, Mar. 21, 2022. Also see VaccinateCalifornia .org. For Pan's earlier bill, see California State Senate, "Dr. Richard Pan's 2013 Legislation Leads to More Vaccinated Children in Schools: Announces Bill to Further Empower Parents with Immunization Facts," Jan. 27, 2015, https://sd06 .senate.ca.gov/news/2015-01-27-dr-richard-pan's-2013-legislation-leads-more -vaccinated-children-schools-announces.

39. Senate Committee on Education, "Analysis of SB 277," Apr. 22, 2015, 6.

40. Leah Russin, interview with author, Mar. 21, 2022.

41. Russin, interview with author, Mar. 21, 2022.

42. DiResta, "The Facebook Dilemma."

43. California Legislature, "California Senate Floor Analyses, SB 277," June 26, 2015, 8–10, California Legislative Information, https://leginfo.legislature.ca.gov /faces/billAnalysisClient.xhtml?bill_id=201520160SB277.

44. Assembly Committee on Health, "Analysis of SB 277," June 19, 2015, 10, 15–16.

45. Association of American Physicians and Surgeons, "About AAPS," https:// aapsonline.org/about-aaps/; Stephanie Innes, "Tucson Group Fueling National Vaccine Fears," Tucson.com, Feb. 8, 2015, https://tucson.com/news/science /health-med-fit/tucson-group-fueling-national-vaccine-fears/article_8bee1d28 -75c0-59dd-b40f-15058df6cdf5.html.

46. "SB 277 Testimony: Barbara Loe Fisher, Co-founder & President, National Vaccine Information Center (NVIC), Assembly Committee on Health," June 9, 2015, https://www.nvic.org/cmstemplates/nvic/pdf/blf-ca-sb-277-testimony -2015.pdf.

47. California Legislature, "Senate Floor Analyses, SB 277," June 26, 2015, 10, California Legislative Information, https://leginfo.legislature.ca.gov/faces /billAnalysisClient.xhtml?bill_id=201520160SB277; California Right to Life, "About," https://www.calrighttolife.org/about, accessed Oct. 18, 2022.

48. Daniel K. Williams, *Defenders of the Unborn: The Pro-Life Movement before Roe v. Wade* (New York: Oxford University Press, 2015), 243–44. Also see March for Life, "Women of the Pro-life Movement: Nellie Gray," https://marchforlife .org/women-of-the-pro-life-movement-nellie-gray.

49. Ed Silverman, "Pro-life Groups Say Merck Is Partly to Blame for Measles Outbreaks," *Wall Street Journal*, Jan. 30, 2015, https://www.wsj.com/articles/BL -270B-1401.

50. Barbara Loe Fisher, "Over 1,000 Californians Show Up to Testify; Vermont Politicians Cut Parents out of the Democratic Process; Texas Pushes Back on Teacher Vaccine Mandates," NVIC.org, April 29, 2015, NVIC.org archives.

51. Barbara Loe Fisher, "Blackmail and the Medical Vaccine Exemption," NVIC .org, May 18, 2015, NVIC.org archives.

52. California Legislature, "Senate Judiciary Bill Analysis, SB 277, April 22, 2015,"
14; *Serrano v. Priest*, 5 Cal. 3d. 584 (1971); *Serrano v. Priest*, 18 Cal. 3d 728
(1976); *Serrano v. Priest*, 20 Cal. 3d 25 (1977).

53. Dorit Rubinstein Reiss, "A Few Hail Mary Passes: Immunization Mandate
Law, SB277, Brought to Court," Health Affairs, Feb. 28, 2018, doi: 10.1377
/forefront.20180226.699777.

54. California's School Safety Act passed in 1985. California Legislature, "SB 719
School Safety: Version 10/11/03," California Legislative Information, https://
leginfo.legislature.ca.gov/faces/billTextClient.xhtml?bill_id=200320040SB719.
For description of Allen's testimony, see Dorit Rubenstein Reiss, "Vaccines,
School Mandates, and California's Right to Education," *UCLA Law Review:
Discourse* 98 (2015): 114–15, https://repository.uchastings.edu/faculty
_scholarship/1483.

55. Reiss, "Vaccines, School Mandates." The quotes are on pp. 115 and 118.

56. California Legislature, "Senate Judiciary Bill Analysis, SB 277, April 22, 2015,"
15; Reiss, "A Few Hail Mary Passes."

57. California Legislature, "Senate Judiciary Bill Analysis, SB 277," 15; Reiss, "A Few
Hail Mary Passes."

58. California Legislature, "SB-277 Public Health: Vaccinations (2015–2016),"
California Legislative Information, https://leginfo.legislature.ca.gov/faces
/billNavClient.xhtml?bill_id=201520160SB277; Jacqueline K. Olive et al.,
"The State of the Antivaccine Movement in the United States: A Focused
Examination of Nonmedical Exemptions in States and Counties," *PLOSMed* 15,
no. 6 (June 2018): https://doi.org/10.1371/journal/pmed.1002578.

59. See cases in the appendix. Also see Dorit Rubinstein Reiss, "Litigating
Alternative Facts: School Vaccine Mandates in the Courts," *Journal of Constitutional Law* 21, no. 1 (Oct. 2018): 207–66.

60. *Whitlow et al. v. California Department of Education et al.*, 203 F. Supp.
3rd 1079 (S.D. Cal. 2016), 1089–90.

61. *Torrey-Love et al. v. State Dept. of Education et al.*, Super. Ct. No. SCV0039311,
Cal. (2018). The quotes are on pp. 14 and 3, respectively. See Reiss, "Litigating
Alternative Facts."

62. Donnelly is quoted in Jon Brooks, "Not over Yet: Tim Donnelly Files for
Referendum to Overturn California's New Vaccine Law," KQED, July 2, 2015,
https://www.kqed.org/stateofhealth/43117/california-vaccine-debate-not-quite
-over-tim-donnelly-files-referendum-to-overturn-new-law; Frances Kai-Hwa
Wang, "Anti-vaxers Fight to Unseat State Senator, Pediatrician Richard Pan,"
NBCnews, Aug. 6, 2015, https://www.nbcnews.com/news/asian-america/anti
-vaxxers-fight-unseat-state-senator-pediatrician-richard-pan-n405176.

63. LegiScan, "Roll Call: CA SB 277, 2015–2016 Regular Session," https://legiscan
.com/CA/rollcall/SB277/id/463827.

64. Assembly Committee on Health, "Analysis of SB 277," June 19, 2015, 15–16.

65. Leah Russin, interview with author.

66. Gustavo S. Mesch and Kent P. Schwirian, "Social and Political Determinants of Vaccine Hesitancy: Lessons Learned from the H1N1 Pandemic of 2009–2010," *American Journal of Infection Control* 43, no. 11 (Nov. 1, 2015): 1161–65.

67. Monica Anderson, "Young Adults More Likely to Say Vaccinating Kids Should Be a Parental Choice," Pew Research Center, Feb. 2, 2015, https://www .pewresearch.org/fact-tank/2015/02/02/young-adults-more-likely-to-say -vaccinating-kids-should-be-a-parental-choice.

68. For example, see NBC News, "By the Numbers: Republicans, Democrats and the Vaccination Debate," Feb. 2, 2015, https://www.nbcnews.com/politics/first -read/numbers-republicans-democrats-vaccination-debate-n298606.

69. Robert N. Lupton and Christopher Hare, "Conservatives Are More Likely to Believe Vaccines Cause Autism," *Washington Post*, March 1, 2015, https://www .washingtonpost.com/news/monkey-cage/wp/2015/03/01/conservatives-are -more-likely-to-believe-that-vaccines-cause-autism.

70. Pew Research Center, "*Roe v. Wade* at 40: Most Oppose Overturning Abortion Decision," Jan. 16, 2013, https://www.pewresearch.org/religion /2013/01/16/roe-v-wade-at-40; David Crary, "Evangelicals' Vaccine Skepticism Isn't Coming from the Pulpit," *Christianity Today*, Apr. 7, 2021, https://www.christianitytoday.com/news/2021/april/white-evangelicals -pastors-covid-vaccine-skepticism.html; Pew Research, "White Evangelical Protestants Less Likely to Have Been Vaccinated for COVID-19 Than Other Religious Groups," Sept. 17, 2021, https://www.pewresearch.org/ps_2021-09 -15_covid19-restrictions_a-01.

71. Seth Dowland, "Evangelical Homeschooling and the Development of 'Family Values,'" Georgetown University Berkley Center for Religion, Peace and World Affairs, Dec. 18, 2019, https://berkleycenter.georgetown.edu/responses /evangelical-homeschooling-and-the-development-of-family-values. Also see Seth Dowland, *Family Values and the Rise of the Christian Right* (Philadelphia: University of Pennsylvania Press, 2015); Adam Laats, *The Other School Reformers: Conservative Activism in American Education* (Cambridge, MA: Harvard University Press, 2015).

72. Daniel K. Williams, "Jerry Falwell's Sunbelt Politics: The Regional Origins of the Moral Majority," *Journal of Policy History* 22, no. 2 (Mar. 31, 2010): 125–47; Patrick Allitt, *Religion in America since 1945: A History* (New York: Columbia University Press, 2003), 148–85.

73. L. Whitehead and Samuel L. Perry, "How Culture Wars Delay Herd Immunity: Christian Nationalism and Anti-vaccine Attitudes," *Socius* 6 (Dec. 7, 2020): 1–12, https://doi.org/10.1177/2378023120977727; Jack Delehanty, Edgell Penny, and

Stewart Evan, 2019, "Christian America? Secularized Evangelical Discourse and Boundaries of National Belonging," *Social Forces* 97, no. 3 (Mar. 2019): 1283–1306. Also see Michelle Goldberg, *Kingdom Coming: The Rise of Christian Nationalism* (Washington, DC: National Geographic Books, 2007).

74. Nicholas Riccardi, AP, "Vaccine Skeptics Find Unexpected Allies in Conservative GOP," Feb. 6, 2015, https://www.pbs.org/newshour/health/vaccine -skeptics-find-unexpected-allies-conservative-gop.

75. Jeremy W. Peters and Richard Pérez-Peña, "Measles Outbreak Proves Delicate Issue to GOP Field," *New York Times*, Feb. 2, 2015, https://www.nytimes.com /2015/02/03/us/politics/measles-proves-delicate-issue-to-gop-field.html.

76. Richard Alan Rappeport, "Paul Calls Vaccination a Matter of Freedom," *New York Times*, Feb. 2, 2015, https://www.nytimes.com/politics/first-draft/2015/02 /02/paul-calls-vaccination-a-matter-of-freedom.

77. Louis S. Tavernise, "Vaccine Issue Arises at Republican Debate, to Doctors' Dismay," *New York Times*, Sept. 17, 2015, http://www.nytimes.com/2015/09/18 /health/republican-presidential-debate-vaccines.html. For Sears's recommendation, see Paul A. Offit and Charlotte A. Moser, "The Problem with Dr. Bob's Alternative Vaccine Schedule," *Pediatrics* 123, no. 1 (Jan. 2009): e164–69. Also see Sarah Geoghegan, Kevin P. O'Callaghan, and Paul A. Offit, "Vaccine Safety: Myths and Misinformation," *Frontiers in Microbiology* 11, no. 372 (2020): doi: 10.3389/fmicb.2020.00372.

78. See Matthew A. Baum, "Red State, Blue State, Flu State: Media Self-Selection and Partisan Gaps in Swine Flu Vaccinations," *Journal of Health Politics, Policy and Law* 36, no. 6 (Dec. 2011): 1021–59.

79. Dan M. Kahan, "Vaccine Risk Perceptions and Ad Hoc Risk Communication: An Empirical Assessment," Jan. 27, 2014, CCP Risk Perception Studies Report No. 17, Yale Law and Economics Research Paper #491, http://dx.doi.org/10 .2139/ssrn.2386034; Graham Dixon and Christopher Clarke, "The Effect of Falsely Balanced Reporting of the Autism-Vaccine Controversy on Vaccine Safety Perceptions and Behavioral Intentions," *Health Education Research* 28, no. 2 (Apr. 2013): 352–59.

80. Evan Simko-Bednarski, "Maine Bars Residents from Opting Out of Immunizations for Religious or Philosophical Reasons," CNN Health, May 27, 2019, https://www.cnn.com/2019/05/27/health/maine-immunization-exemption -repealed-trnd/index.html.

81. Sanderson is quoted in Riccardi, "Vaccine Skeptics Find Unexpected Allies in Conservative GOP"; Scott Thistle, "Maine Senate Reverses Course, Ends Religious Exemption for Vaccines," *Portland (ME) Press Herald*, May 14, 2019, https://www.pressherald.com/2019/05/14/maine-senate-reverses-course-ends -religious-exemption-for-vaccines.

82. National Conference of State Legislatures, "States with Religious and Philosophical Exemptions from School Immunization Requirements," Jan. 20, 2022, https://www.ncsl.org/research/health/school-immunization-exemption-state-laws.aspx; Bobby Allyn, "New York Ends Religious Exemptions for Required Vaccines, KQED (National Public Radio), June 13, 2019, https://www.npr.org/2019/06/13/732501865/new-york-advances-bill-ending-religious-exemptions-for-vaccines-amid-health-cris; Susan Haigh, "Connecticut Ends Its State Religious Vaccine Exemption," AP News, Apr. 28, 2021, https://apnews.com/article/connecticut-religion-health-education-government-and-politics-6d9ce9 16908bbdacce4e7a7840a57a87.

83. Amanda Vinicky, "Measles Vaccine Legislation Seeks Delicate Balance," NPR Illinois, Mar. 30, 2015, https://www.nprillinois.org/statehouse/2015-03-30/measles-vaccine-legislation-seeks-delicate-balance.

84. Illinois General Assembly, "Bill Status of SB0986, 99th General Assembly," Aug. 4, 2015, https://www.ilga.gov/legislation/BillStatus.asp?DocNum=986&GAID=13&DocTypeID=SB&SessionID=88&GA=99.

85. Montana Legislature, "Detailed Bill Information, 64th Regular Session [...] April 28, 2015: HB 158," accessed from Montana State Legislature Bill Lookup Information at https://leg.mt.gov/bill-info. For Republican control of the state's legislature that year, see Montana State Legislature, "Majority and Minority Party Numbers 1889–Present," https://leg.mt.gov/civic-education/facts/party-control.

86. Brissa Nuñez, Victoria Stuart-Cassel, and Deborah Temkin, "As COVID-19 Spreads, Most States Have Laws That Address How Schools Should Respond to Pandemics," Child Trends, Mar. 11, 2020, https://www.childtrends.org/blog/as-covid-19-spreads-most-states-have-laws-that-address-how-schools-should-respond-to-pandemics.

87. CDPH, "To School Leaders," Aug. 23, 2021, https://www.cdph.ca.gov/Programs/CID/DCDC/Pages/COVID-19/Requirement-for-Universal-Masking-Indoors-at-k-12-.

88. Jeanine Santucci, "Name-Calling, Canceled Meetings, Please from Students: A Week of School Mask Mandate Chaos," *USA Today*, Aug. 15, 2021, https://www.usatoday.com/story/news/nation/2021/08/15/school-mask-mandates-spark-protests-parents-covid-cases-rise/8124375002.

89. California, Connecticut, Delaware, Hawaii, Illinois, Louisiana, Nevada, New Jersey, Oregon, Washington, and the District of Columbia adopted the CDC's recommendations. At the time, control of Louisiana's legislature was divided between Democrats and Republicans. The eight Republican-controlled states that forbade masks in school were Arizona, Arkansas, Florida, Iowa, Oklahoma, South Carolina, Texas, and Utah. See Christine Vestal, "10 States Have School

Mask Mandates While 8 Forbid Them," PEW Research, Aug. 10, 2021, https://www.pewtrusts.org/en/research-and-analysis/blogs/stateline/2021/08 /10/10-states-have-school-mask-mandates-while-8-forbid-them. Information regarding legislative partisanship in 2021 is from National Conference of State Legislatures, "2021 State and Legislative Partisan Composition," Feb. 1, 2021, https://www.ncsl.org/documents/elections/Legis_Control_2-2021.pdf. For the use of masks during the influenza epidemic, see John M. Barry, *The Great Influenza: The Story of the Deadliest Pandemic in History* (New York: Penguin Books, 2004), 214, 215, 315–16, 343–44, 358–59.

90. Kevin McElrath, "Nearly 93% of Households with School-Age Children Report Some Form of Distance Learning during COVID-19," US Census, Aug. 26, 2020, https://www.census.gov/library/stories/2020/08/schooling-during-the -covid-19-pandemic.html.

91. Hemi Tewarson, Katie Greene, and Michael R. Fraser, "State Strategies for Addressing Barriers during the Early US COVID-19 Vaccination Campaign," *American Journal of Public Health* 111, no. 6 (June 2021): 1073–77, doi: 10.2105/AJPH.2021.306241.

92. Karen Weintraub, "Operation Warp Speed Is Living Up to Its Name, but COVID-19 Immunizations Are Going 'Slower' Than Expected, Officials Say," *USA Today*, Dec. 23, 2020, https://www.usatoday.com/story/news/health /2020/12/23/covid-19-vaccines-slower-operation-warp-speed/4032188001.

93. HHS, "Biden Administration Purchases Additional Doses of COVID-19 Vaccines from Pfizer and Moderna," Feb. 11, 2021, https://www.hhs.gov/about /news/2021/02/11/biden-administration-purchases-additional-doses-covid-19 -vaccines-from-pfizer-and-moderna.html.

94. "Monthly Trend in COVID-19 Vaccination by Party ID," in Lydia Saad, "More in U.S. Vaccinated after Delta Surge, FDA Decision," Gallup, Sept. 29, 2021, https://news.gallup.com/poll/355073/vaccinated-delta-surge-fda-decision.aspx.

95. Joseph R. Biden Jr., "Executive Order on Requiring Coronavirus Disease 2019 Vaccination for Federal Employees," Sept. 9, 2021, https://www.whitehouse.gov /briefing-room/presidential-actions/2021/09/09/executive-order-on-requiring -coronavirus-disease-2019-vaccination-for-federal-employees.

96. White House Briefing Room, "Fact Sheet: Biden Administration Announces Details of Two Major Vaccination Policies," Nov. 4, 2021, https://www .whitehouse.gov/briefing-room/statements-releases/2021/11/04/fact-sheet -biden-administration-announces-details-of-two-major-vaccination-policies. The quotes are on p. 1.

97. Reuters, "U.S. Congress Republicans Attack Biden's Vaccination Mandates," Sept. 9, 2021, https://www.reuters.com/world/us/us-congress-republicans -attack-bidens-vaccination-mandates-2021-09-09; Associated Press, "Lawsuits

over Workplace Vaccine Rule Focus on States' Rights," Nov. 5, 2021, https:// www.usnews.com/news/business/articles/2021-11-05/11-states-file-suit-against -bidens-business-vaccine-mandate.

98. *Joseph R. Biden, Jr. v. Missouri*, 595 U.S. Jan. 13, 2022.

99. Leo Morris, "Further Analysis of National Participation in the Inactivated Poliomyelitis Vaccination Program, 1955–61," *PHR* 79, no. 6 (June 1964): 469–80.

100. "Statement by Dr. Jane Wooten, Chairman, Polio Committee, Wake County Medical Society, Raleigh, NC," June 3, 1964, series 1.1, box 90, folder 1041, John William Harden Papers, SHC.

101. Lindsay M. Monte, "Household Pulse Survey Shows Many Don't Trust COVID Vaccine, Worry about Side Effects," US Census Bureau, Dec. 28, 2021, https://www.census.gov/library/stories/2021/12/who-are-the-adults-not -vaccinated-against-covid.html.

102. William Al Galston, "For COVID-19 Vaccinations, Party Affiliation Matters More Than Race and Ethnicity," Brookings Institution, Oct. 1, 2021, https:// www.brookings.edu/blog/fixgov/2021/10/01/for-covid-19-vaccinations-party -affiliation-matters-more-than-race-and-ethnicity.

103. WHO and UNICEF, "COVID-19 Pandemic Fuels Largest Continued Backslide in Vaccinations in Three Decades," July 15, 2022, https://www.who .int/news/item/15-07-2022-covid-19-pandemic-fuels-largest-continued -backslide-in-vaccinations-in-three-decades.

104. Stephanie A. Kujawski et al., "Impact of the COVID-19 Pandemic on Pediatric and Adolescent Vaccinations and Well Child Visits in the United States: A Database Analysis," *Vaccine* 40, no. 5 (Jan. 31, 2022): 706–13.

105. Melissa Suran, "Why Parents Still Hesitate to Vaccinate Their Children against COVID-19," *JAMA* 327, no. 1 (Dec. 15, 2021): doi: 10.1001/jama.2021.21625.

106. For common false claims about COVID-19 vaccines, see Gabor David Kelen and Lisa Maragakis, "COVID-19 Vaccines: Myth versus Fact," John Hopkins Medicine, Mar. 10, 2022, https://www.hopkinsmedicine.org/health/conditions -and-diseases/coronavirus/covid-19-vaccines-myth-versus-fact.

107. HealthGuard, "The Top COVID-19 Myths Spreading Online," Britannica, Feb. 1, 2021, https://www.britannica.com/list/the-top-covid-19-vaccine-myths -spreading-online.

108. Riccardo Gallotti et al., "Assessing the Risks of 'Infodemics' in Response to COVID-19 Epidemics," *Nature Human Behavior* 4 (Oct. 29, 2020): 1285–93, doi: 10.1038/s41562-020-00994-6. For common false claims about COVID-19 vaccines, see Kelen and Maragakis, "COVID-19 Vaccines"; Katie Schoolov, "Why It's Not Possible for the COVID Vaccines to Contain a Magnetic Tracking Chip That Connects to 5G," CNBC, Oct. 1, 2021, https://www.cnbc.com/2021/10/01 /why-the-covid-vaccines-dont-contain-a-magnetic-5g-tracking-chip.html.

109. Megan Messerly and Krista Mahr, "Covid Vaccine Concerns Are Starting to Spill Over into Routine Immunizations," Politico, Apr. 18, 2022, https://www.politico.com/news/2022/04/18/kids-are-behind-on-routine-immunizations-covid-vaccine-hesitancy-isnt-helping-00025503.

110. Apoorva Mandavilli and Euan Ward, "Britain Declares National Incident after Poliovirus Found in London," *New York Times*, June 22, 2022, https://www.nytimes.com/2022/06/22/health/uk-polio-london-poliovirus.html.

111. Nuzzo quoted in Mike Stobbe, "New York Reports 1st US Polio Case in Nearly a Decade," AP News, July 21, 2022, https://apnews.com/article/polio-case-new-york-4c1e2512145a1d897982f27507259d83. See also Will Sullivan, "First Polio Case in U.S. since 2013 Detected in New York State," *Smithsonian Magazine*, July 22, 2011, https://www.smithsonianmag.com/smart-news/first-polio-case-in-us-since-2013-detected-in-new-york-state-180980459.

112. "Frequently Asked Questions on Schooling at Home," in California Department of Education, "Schooling at Home," https://www.cde.ca.gov/sp/ps/homeschool.asp, accessed Oct. 24, 2022.

113. Donya Khalili and Arthur Caplan, "Off the Grid: Vaccinations among Homeschooled Children," *Journal of Law, Medicine & Ethics* 35, no. 3 (Fall 2007): 471–77.

114. Hannah Henry, interview on NAPABroadcasting.com.

Conclusion

1. Rebecca Klein and Caroline Preston, "How the Science of Vaccination Is Taught (or Not) in US Schools," *Hechinger Report*, May 23, 2020, https://hechingerreport.org/how-the-science-of-vaccination-is-taught-or-not-in-us-schools. Also see Arianna Prothero, "Many Schools Don't Teach about the Science of Vaccines: Here's Why They Should," *Education Week*, July 2, 2021, https://www.edweek.org/teaching-learning/many-schools-dont-teach-about-the-science-of-vaccines-heres-why-they-should/2021/07.

2. National Vaccine Advisory Committee, "Assessing the State of Vaccine Confidence in the United States: Recommendations from the National Vaccine Advisory Committee, June 10, 2015," *PHR* 130 (Nov.–Dec. 2015): 573–95.

3. Frank Bruni, "Russia, Where All the News Is Fake," *New York Times*, Mar. 10, 2022. For lingering misinformation in schoolbooks, see chapter 3.

4. This quote is ubiquitous, e.g., BrainyQuote, "Heraclitus Quotes," https://www.brainyquote.com/quotes/heraclitus_107157, accessed July 23, 2022. Translations from the Greek vary. Brooks Haxton translates Heraclitus's words as: "Just as the river where I step is not the same, and is, so I am as I am not." See *Heraclitus*, trans. Brooks Haxton (New York: Penguin Books, 2003), 81.

5. CDC, "Clinical Considerations: Mycarditis and Pericarditis after Receipt of mRNA COVID-19 Vaccines among Adolescents and Young Adults," https://www.cdc.gov/vaccines/covid-19/clinical-considerations/myocarditis.html, accessed July 23, 2022; "Topline Report on COVID-19 Vaccination in the United States: Survey Waves 6–8, January 10–February 27, 2001," Delphi Group at Carnegie Mellon University in Partnership with Facebook, Mar. 12, 2021), https://www.cmu.edu/delphi-web/surveys/CMU_Topline_Vaccine _Report_20210312.pdf.

6. Public Religion Research Institute (PRRI), "Survey: Only 1 in 10 Americans Say COVID-19 Vaccinations Conflict with Religious Beliefs," Dec. 9, 2021, https://www.prri.org/press-release/survey-only-1-in-10-americans-say-covid-19 -vaccinations-conflict-with-religious-beliefs/; PRRI, "Religious Identities and the Race against the Virus: American Attitudes on Vaccination Mandates and Religious Exemptions (Wave 3), Dec. 9, 2021, https://www.prri.org/research /religious-identities-and-the-race-against-the-virus-american-attitudes-on -vaccination-mandates-and-religious-exemptions. For surveys of vaccine resistance among chiropractors, see Iben Axén et al., "Misinformation, Chiropractic, and the COVID-19 Pandemic," *Chiropractic & Manual Therapies* 28, no. 65 (Nov. 18, 2020): doi: 10.1186/s12998-020-00353-2. Also see Anna Karina Mascarenhas et al., "Dental Students' Attitudes and Hesitancy toward COVID-19 Vaccine," *Journal of Dental Education* 85 (Sept. 2021): 1504–10; Filice E. Dubé et al., "Vaccination Discourses among Chiropractors, Naturo- paths and Homeopaths: A Qualitative Content Analysis of Academic Literature and Canadian Organizational Webpages," *PLOS One* 15, no. 8 (Aug. 12, 2020): https://doi.org/10.1371/journal.pone.0236691.

7. Riccardo Gallotti et al., "Assessing the Risks of 'Infodemics' in Response to COVID-19 Epidemics," *Nature Human Behavior* 4 (Oct. 29, 2020): 1285–93, doi: 10.1038/s41562-020-00994-6. For common false claims about COVID-19 vaccines, see Gabor David Kelen and Lisa Maragakis, "COVID-19 Vaccines: Myth versus Fact," John Hopkins Medicine, Mar. 10, 2022, https://www .hopkinsmedicine.org/health/conditions-and-diseases/coronavirus/covid-19 -vaccines-myth-versus-fact; Katie Schoolov, "Why It's Not Possible for the COVID Vaccines to Contain a Magnetic Tracking Chip That Connects to 5G," CNBC, Oct. 1, 2021, https://www.cnbc.com/2021/10/01/why-the-covid -vaccines-dont-contain-a-magnetic-5g-tracking-chip.html.

8. See Rebecca Randall, "Not Worth a Shot: Why Some Christians Oppose Vaccination on Moral Grounds," *Christianity Today*, Apr. 26, 2019, https://www .christianitytoday.com/ct/2019/april-web-only/why-christians-refuse-measles -vaccinations-moral-grounds.html; David Crary, AP, "Evangelicals' Vaccine Skepticism Isn't Coming from the Pulpit," *Christianity Today*, Apr. 7, 2021,

https://www.christianitytoday.com/news/2021/april/white-evangelicals
-pastors-covid-vaccine-skepticism.html; Katie E. Corcoran, Christopher P.
Scheitle, and Bernard D. DiGregorio, "Christian Nationalism and COVID-19
Vaccine Hesitancy and Uptake," *Vaccine* 39, no. 45 (Oct. 29, 2021): 6614–21.

9. Cynthia G. Whitney et al., "Benefits from Immunization during the Vaccines
for Children Program Era—United States, 1994–2013," *MMWR* 63, no. 16
(Apr. 25, 2014): 352–55.

10. Krawitt quoted in Kari Brenner, "Marin Teen Reprises Role as Vaccination
Advocate," *Marin (CA) Independent Journal*, Oct. 30, 2021, https://www
.marinij.com/2021/10/30/marin-teen-reprises-role-as-vaccination-advocate.

Archival and Digitized Sources

Archives

California

California State Archives
- Ballot Pamphlets
- Bill Files
- Governors' Chapter Bill Files

San Diego History Center
- Charlotte Baker Diary Collection

San Francisco Public Library Government Information Center
- California Department of Public Health Biennial Reports, 1929–42
- California Public Health Statistical Reports, 1954–60
- California State Department of Public Health Reports, 1947–52

Stanford University
- Cubberley Education Library
  - Historical Textbook Collection
  - Historical US State and City School Reports
- Green Library
  - Special Collections: Rare Books
- Lane Medical Library
  - California State Board of Health Monthly Bulletins, 1915–21
  - California State Board of Public Health Biennial Reports, 1882–1926

Kansas

Dwight D. Eisenhower Presidential Library and Museum, Abilene
Kansas Historical Society, Topeka
    Journal of John Hawkins Clark
    Letters of Julia Louisa Lovejoy

Kentucky

Kentucky Historical Society, Rural Health Care Oral History Project, Frankfort
    Oral history interview with Mary Duncan
    Oral history interview with William Kelsay

North Carolina

Wilson Library, University of North Carolina, Chapel Hill
    Rare Books Collection
    Southern Historical Collection
        John William Harden Papers, 1914–86
        Sally Lucas Jean Papers, 1914–66

Pennsylvania

Historical Medical Library of the College of Physicians of Philadelphia
    Anti-Vaccination League of Pennsylvania Records
    Anti-Vaccination Society of America Minutes, Correspondence, etc.

Digitized Historical Texts, Records, and Reports

American Presidency Project, University of California, Santa Barbara, http://www
    .presidency.uscb.edu
HathiTrust Digital Library, www.hathitrust.org
Internet Archive, www.archive.org
Library of Congress, www.loc.gov
Medical Heritage Library, https://www.medicalheritage.org
National Library of Medicine (United States), https://www.nlm.nih.gov
Wellcome Library (London), https://wellcomecollection.org

Historical Newspaper Collections

California Digital Newspaper Collection, https://cdnc.ucr.edu
Chronicling America, https://chroniclingamerica.loc.gov
Georgia Historic Newspapers, https://gahistoricnewspapers.galileo.usg.edu
Hoosier State Chronicles: Indiana's Digital Historic Newspaper Program, https://
    newspapers.library.in.gov
Newspapers.com, https://newspapers.com
Washington Digital Newspapers, https://washingtondigitalnewspapers.org

Index

Page numbers in *italics* refer to charts, figures, and tables.

demographics. *See* race; socioeconomic
status

Dickie, Walter M., 132, 138, 140

diphtheria, 3, 7, 9, 12, 20, 53, 56, 82;
alternative remedies, 69, 70–71;
antitoxin, 57, 71, 178; bacterium,
177–78; eradication, 196; fatality
rates, 138, 177; immunization, 178,
205, 218, 229, 260, *261*, 265; Lora
Little's son, 63, 71; Schick skin test,
178; tainted antitoxin, 57; voluntary
immunization programs, 136–38,
273. *See also* DPT vaccine

DiResta, Renee, 244, 245, 246

Dissatisfied Parents Together (DPT),
207–8

Donnelly, Tim, 253

DPT vaccine, 166, 178, 179, 187, 205–6,
214. See also *Vaccine Roulette*

Duffield v. Williamsport, 83–84, 88, 90,
95, *285*

Eclectic Medical Society of New York,
45–46

eclectic medicine, 44–46, 48, 50, 57, 112,
120

Eddy, Mary Baker, 59

education laws. *See* compulsory education
laws

educators. *See* school boards; school
principals; school superintendents;
schoolteachers

Eisenhower, Dwight D., 155

enforcement of school vaccination laws:
decline of disease outbreaks, 30–31,
193; efforts to strengthen, 236–40,
260, 261, 268; health board authority,
80, 86, 92, 95, 127; municipal
authority, 90–91; resistance from
school leaders, 4–5, 109–23, 177,
189–92, 196, 274; school board

authority, 84–86; state authority,
23, 63, 88–90. *See also* Childhood
Immunization Initiative; *Zucht v.
King*

England, 18, 24, 27, 206; anti-vaccination
in, *47*, 47–58; Leicester, 52–53.
See also Tebb, William

Ensign Remedies Company, 68–69

eradication of disease in the US: era of,
176–96; as policy, *7*; measles and polio,
173–74, 185, 213; smallpox, 40, 202.
See also Vaccination Assistance Act

Europe, 3, 20, 24, 31, 52

evangelical Christians, 8–9, 224, 255,
282

exemptions from vaccination: concerns
over, 234–36, 238; increase in states
allowing, 217, 224–25; medical, 96,
183; legislation from 2015 to 2016,
259; nonmedical (conscientious or
philosophical), 107, 113, 123–27, *225*;
public demand for, 230–31; public
health officials' support for, 217–18,
219–20, 235; religious, 102, 107,
219, 220–24, 235–36, 241; school
exemption forms, 126–27, 232–33,
239; school exemption rates, 259–60,
261. *See also* enforcement of school
vaccination laws

Female Boarding School, Salem, NC, 26

feminism, 200–201

fetal cell lines in vaccine development,
223–24; opposition to, 224

Fisher, Barbara Loe, 207, 214, 226, 233,
247, 248. *See also* National Vaccine
Information Center

Fisher, Irving, 68

Flexner, Abraham, 69–70; Flexner
Report, 70

Florida, 110, 157–58, 228, 259

in California, 247; opposition to vaccines, 226; and vaccine skepticism, 214

National Vaccine Program, 208–9

Native Americans, 3, 20–21

naturopathy, 44, 66–68

Nebraska, 110, 152, 258

New Britain Anti-Vaccination Society. See *Bissell v. Davidson*

New Hampshire, 34

New Mexico, 34, 35, 156, 259

news media: anti-vaccination reports in, 48–55, 73, 159; "back to nature" and "natural health" concerns, 200opposition to vaccination requirements in newspapers, *49, 98, 112, 159*; polio campaign and, 152, 159, 163, *164, 165*, 174; criticism of vaccine policy in, 208, 213; public confidence in, *201*. See also *Vaccine Roulette*

New York, 1, 34, 35; and Brooklyn anti-vaccination league, 62; conflicts between health and school boards, 191–92; concerns over liability for vaccine injury, 204; and health board composition, 109; legislation to eliminate nonmedical exemptions, 259–60; and religious exemption from vaccination, 220–21; schools' reluctance to enforce state vaccination law, 191–92; tightening requirements for exemptions, 240. See also *Viemeister v. White*

New York City: and alternative medicine, 44, 45; and Anti-Vaccination League of America (1879–1885), 46–48; and the Anti-Vaccination Society of America (1885–1906), 55–56; and conflicts between health and school officials, 109; and Cutter Labs

incident, 156; and diphtheria immunization, 137; polio case in 2021, 267; and public health nurses in, 135–36; school administrators and failure to enforce state vaccination law, 191–192

New York Medical Society, 35, 39

Nicolaier, Arthur, 53

North Carolina, 11, 26, 34, 172, 180, 259, 264; and 1821 vaccine controversy, 28

North Dakota, 71, 101; and schools' enforcement of vaccination law, 237–38. See also *Rhea ex rel. Rhea v. Board of Education*

North Dakota Freedom League, 68

nurses: and concerns about disease reemergence, 267; and enforcement of vaccination policies, 232, 239; protesting unfunded vaccination mandates, 190; in school immunization campaigns, 135–36, 137–38, 144–45, 153, 154, 164, 172, 197; School Nurses Association, 247. *See also* Jean, Sally Lucas

O'Connor, Basil, 152

Ohio, 34, 172, 180, 195, 203, 218

Oklahoma, 191, 240, 259

Operation Polio, 152–55

Oregon, 34, 54, 129, 156, 239–40, 259; Lora Little in, 67–68

Pan, Richard, 244; and anti-vaccination recall effort, 253

Pardee, George C., 116–17

parents, 5–6; advocacy for vaccination, 35, 242–46, 248–49; anti-vaccination activism, 120–21; decision to vaccinate, 169–170; preference for persuasion, 181; polio campaigns and, 152, 154–55, 159–162, 164–66,

school boards, 5–6, 35, 36, 55, 110;
    advocacy for vaccination, 35, 36,
    160–61, 247; compliance with
    vaccination laws, 86, 111–15, 274;
    127–28, 202–3; concerns over
    enrollment loss, 118–20, 125–26,
    127–28, 139, 190; fear of litigation,
    86, 204, 274; opposition to health
    mandates, 97, 108–9, 115; polio
    campaign and, 160–61. *See also*
    court cases
school curriculum: germ theory, *82*,
    133–34, *148*; outdated information,
    82–83; polio, 147–50; vaccination
    marginalized in, 236–37, 274–75
school principals: conflicts with health
    authorities, 108; enforcement of
    vaccination laws, 189, 191–92;
    exclusion of unvaccinated students,
    273; exemption certificates and,
    126–27; polio vaccination campaign,
    153–54; targets of anti-vaccination
    campaigns, 55, 62; targets of lawsuits,
    75, 79, 81, 91, 98, 103, 221–22
schools: communication with parents,
    165–66; contagion spread in, 3, 18,
    271–72; vaccination sites and
    154–55, 162–68. *See also* school
    boards; school curriculum; school
    principals; school superintendents;
    schoolteachers; school vaccination
    laws
school superintendents: acceptance of
    vaccination in California, 139–40;
    exclusion of unvaccinated students,
    191, 238; opposition to vaccination
    requirements in California, 107,
    109–10, 114–15, 117–19, 128;
    professional priorities, 139, 191–92;
    supporting the polio vaccination
    campaign, 162–63

schoolteachers: and compulsory
    vaccination in California, 122,
    124–25; and misinformation, 124;
    and National Foundation for
    Infantile Paralysis, 147; promoting
    polio vaccination, 150–51, 153–54,
    163–64; and public health nurses,
    135–36; as targets of anti-vaccination
    campaigns, 62. *See also* parent-teacher
    associations
school vaccination laws, 3–4, 33–34,
    34, *194*, 272–73, 282; compulsory
    education laws and, *38*, 102–7,
    278; disease eradication and, 180;
    disease outbreaks and, 193; financial
    concerns about, 190–91, 196;
    late-twentieth-century rise of, 168,
    171–73, *173*, 175, 185–88, 194–95;
    opposition reported in newspapers,
    49, *98*, *112*, *159*; polio vaccine and,
    173; types of laws, 11–12, *259*;
    twenty-first-century movement to
    strengthen, 232–33, 236–40,
    260–61. *See also* attitudes toward
    vaccination; court cases; enforcement
    of school vaccination laws; exemptions
    from vaccination; Vaccination
    Assistance Act
Seattle, 108–9
segregation: during polio campaign,
    151–52, 161–62; of unvaccinated
    students, 122
smallpox, 3; declining rates of, 64, 76–77;
    eradication in US, 202; fatality rates,
    3, 21–22, 37, 75, 77, 83–84, 137;
    infection and spread, 20–21; types
    of, 21–22; variola strains, 136; variola
    virus, 20, *22*. *See also* smallpox vaccine
smallpox vaccine: adverse effects, 30,
    32, 39–40, 64, 81, 95, 114, 116,
    120; development, *7*, 19–26;